"For more than forty years, I have enjoyed a special relationship with our local Cystic Fibrosis Foundation chapter, and shared a passion with its leaders, people living with CF and their families, for finding a cure. It was, perhaps, a chance—or maybe routine—request to help out a good friend and fellow athlete already involved with the CFF that led to my devotion to the foundation. Pee Wee Reese, a local Major League baseball legend, invited me to be part of the Celebrity Dinner Party (CDP) as a celebrity 'bartender' in the early days of this fundraiser, and a commitment was born.

"I enjoyed the annual event, but even more, I made cherished friendships with young people with CF, their families, and the organization working so hard to raise money to find a cure. I eventually took over as host, along with my wife, Susan Sweeney Crum, until we turned over those duties to then University of Louisville Head Coach Chris Mack; however, our commitment to the CFF will continue.

"Over those forty-plus years, I've developed treasured friendships through the CFF, and I've also shared the heartbreak of losing young people to CF. However, I've been able to see breakthroughs in research and tremendous advances in treatments. People are surviving, and thriving, well into adulthood, raising families and living lives—at one time thought impossible—and that is why I am so proud to support the CF Warrior Project, which is revealing many of these incredible stories.

"I am blessed and thankful to see so much hope in the cystic fibrosis community in my lifetime and continue to look forward to the day when the ultimate cure for CF is discovered."

—DENNY CRUM

Head Coach, University of Louisville Men's Basketball Team 1971–2001
Three-time National Coach of the Year (1980, 1983, 1986)
1994 Naismith Memorial Basketball Hall of Fame Inductee
2002 Recipient of the Legends of Coaching Award

"I am so proud to support the CF Warrior Project. The CF community is incredible, and they are working hard to make a difference and find a cure or control for CF. These stories are so inspiring because they show that no matter what you're going through, you can overcome it and make the most of your life."

—TENILLE ARTS
Winner of Rising Star of the Year from the
Canadian Country Music Association in 2020
Appeared and sang on The Bachelor in both 2018 and 2020
2021 CMT (Country Musical Television) Music Awards Performer

"One of the most important missions in my life began as I watched my beautiful niece Karine fight her courageous battle against cystic fibrosis. The disease would ultimately take her life when she was just sixteen years old, but I promised her that I would continue to fight this monster of a disease. In that time, I have advocated for newborn screening, oftentimes through public service announcements which has since passed in places throughout Canada. I have also helped secure important funding for CF research and care and have donated several appearance fees from concerts and guest appearances to Cystic Fibrosis Canada.

"The one thing I haven't accomplished yet is the same thing CF warrior, author, and advocate Andy Lipman still wants to accomplish: finding a cure for this disease. In this book, Andy not only documents the inspiring stories of those who fight the disease but also those who fight for those who have the disease. His goal is to raise awareness and funds as well as to raise hope among the cystic fibrosis community. I stand by Andy and all the CF warriors around the world as we continue to search for a cure for this disease that so desperately needs one."

—CÉLINE DION
World-renowned singer and CF advocate

THE

CF

WARRIOR PROJECT

VOLUME 2

THE

CF

WARRIOR PROJECT

VOLUME 2

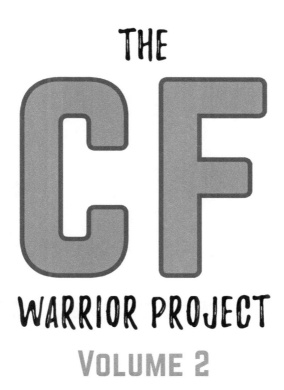

CELEBRATING OUR
CYSTIC FIBROSIS COMMUNITY

ANDY C. LIPMAN

BOOKLOGIX

Alpharetta, GA

ISBN: 978-1-6653-0403-0 - Paperback
ISBN: 978-1-6653-0402-3 - Hardcover
eISBN: 978-1-6653-0404-7 - ePub

Library of Congress Control Number: 2022916809

♻This paper meets the requirements of ANSI/NISO Z39.48-1992 (Permanence of Paper)

093022

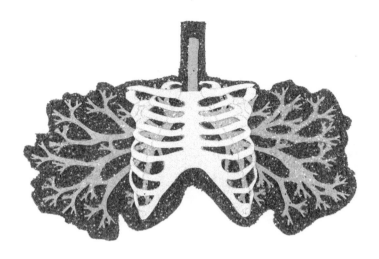

"New Lungs to Breathe," the artwork displayed on *The CF Warrior Project Volume 2: Celebrating Our Cystic Fibrosis Community* cover, was created by world-renowned CF artist, Dylan Mortimer, in 2015. Dylan, a two-time double-lung transplant survivor and one of the many CF warriors whose story is included in this book, describes the piece this way:

> "What would it look like to breathe fully?" asks Dylan. "Here, bronchial tree branches explode through the rib cage, grasping more and more air. This regeneration is a symbol of victory over so many challenges. And offers hope to all."

The CF Warrior Project shares the same optimistic message and therefore we felt it was important to include "New Lungs to Breathe" on our cover. Thank you, Dylan, for inspiring so many with your talents.

CONTENTS

FOREWORD

by Joe Tessitore

ABC and ESPN broadcaster
Cohost of ABC's *Holey Moley*
Two-time finalist for Sports Media Person of the Year
Executive producer of the *30 For 30* films

Truth is I really don't know Andy Lipman; yet I know everything he's thought about. My mother doesn't know his mother; yet she knows her all too well. Our sisters didn't have the chance to know each other. They didn't have the chance to know many. They didn't have the chance to have the lives Andy and I have cherished. Yet because of a gene mutation, something scientists finally discovered in 1989, our families—who never have met—may as well be the closest blood relatives.

With our shared connection to cystic fibrosis, Andy asked me to write this foreword—and one other reason I will get to later—but for now, let me just cover the basics. Andy is a full-on warrior with CF. He battles the disease. He kicks its ass daily. Andy shows more championship mettle than any of the greatest boxers or football players I've lauded on national TV for years. I, on the other hand, am a healthy carrier of the mutated gene that can cause the fatal disease. More important, we were both brothers to little girls who died from cystic fibrosis. We are sons to parents who had to live with the unimaginable horror of burying a child. Our stories are different but both families carry the scars of the capricious genetic lottery.

What lies ahead in these pages is truth, hope, and fight. There are ups and downs to all these tales. There are CF stories that will motivate you. There are CF stories that will have you crying. Some will make you angry about how unfair life can be and some will make you smile knowing the human spirit is nourished best with a healthy dose of optimism and purpose.

Take Beth and Madi Vanstone for example. A mother and daughter team that has taken on CF for years, both with Madi's own personal fight to live and in their unrelenting efforts to help fellow Canadians with CF. This book captures that precious moment so many young CF patients and their parents inevitably all have.

When Madi was five years old, she realized, and expressed, how unjust life can be. Her mom was not quite ready, yet found the right response. Madi stunned Beth when she asked the question that would set the course for their journey:

"Why do I have CF, and the rest of my friends and our family don't?" Madi asked. Beth's response would plant the seed that grew into a giant stalk of effort and advocacy. (They've raised awareness, funds, and offered help.) Beth turned to her young daughter and simply said, "Because God knew you could do this, and you have a family that will always be with you to fight this."

Madi has become a fearless fighter. She presses on for her CF brothers and sisters throughout Canada. She has one tattoo. It reads, "Just Breathe."

Most of the stories in this book are of those who are "just breathing" as strong as can be. In fact, they are breathing stronger than they could have just a few years ago. Drug therapies and the constant funding for cystic fibrosis research have been remarkable. They have been targeted and effective. We understand there is still much work to do but the milestones that have been achieved to this point have been rewarding.

There are many of us who couldn't have dreamed of adult CF patients living this well. I can remember when a headline in the late '80s read: "Researchers Discover Gene that Causes CF." My mother was so happy. Years of never openly discussing our family's loss, of suppressing unspeakable pain, were for a moment not attached to CF but rather replaced with hope.

We thought a cure, perhaps a significant therapy, would be right around the corner. We thought a way to help those battling the disease, which took my sister, Dana, a decade before that monumental breakthrough, was now arriving. That "right around the corner" was further away than we could have ever known. That corner was, in fact, hard to even see, let alone see around it.

We collectively didn't truly turn the corner until October 22, 2019. That is the date that means so much. Interestingly, like so many who have dealt with life-altering family tragedy, you tend to see spiritual connectivity a bit clearer. God has a way of letting you know. On October 22, 2019, that sense of spirituality was obvious. It let me know that the fight, the effort, the long painful road to heal my family by trying to help others with the disease, was all worth it.

That October day of record was a Tuesday. The night before I had been live on-air broadcasting a *Monday Night Football* game to millions of viewers. Tom Brady and the Patriots destroyed the New York Jets that night. That's my father's birthday. My late father's birthday.

Understand this: my father's life was challenging after my sister died from CF. Challenging is a gross understatement. He had great highs and the lowest of lows. He would tell you he was an alcoholic. Sober for the last twenty-plus years of his life, but nevertheless, he would want you to know, forthright and fully, that he was an alcoholic. Or as he liked to say bluntly, "a drunk."

My sister's death unraveled most of his adult life. Booze, recklessness, divorce, financial loss, then gain, recovery, sobriety, newfound parenthood, and joy. Rinse, repeat, hardship, health issues, ups, downs, fickle business troubles, and in 2009, he died unexpectedly. He lived a roller-coaster life that a Hollywood scriptwriter would even shake his head at. My sister Dana's spirit, his prayers to her, his visits to her grave, her medallion, photos of her smiling while hospitalized in Manhattan—those were the inner core pillars holding up his life. On his birthday I always think about that. And for many years I have thought about something that isn't talked about enough with CF, or any fatal genetic disease. It's the ripple effect. How much impact is made on the rest of the family. How the tidal wave of a diagnosis, a disease, a death crashes down on the parents, grandparents. and siblings of a CF patient. How the stats, trends. and anecdotal stories of parents who lose a child are bleak.

The next day was when the news broke that the FDA approved Trikafta. That was the day after his birthday. For CF families, this wasn't just news, this was *the* news. Trikafta was the therapeutic drug we had all been waiting for. The triple combination therapy that helps the underlying causes of CF in 90 percent of patients, the most common mutation of CF. Bottomline, this drug was the best possible answer to the worst possible daily CF battles. Patients could live fuller lives, longer lives. This was the corner we thought we were rounding in 1989.

Fittingly, when the news broke on October 22, 2019, I was with my daughter. She was being recruited to play at Ivy League schools and I was along proudly beaming on campus with her. Yes, my daughter, the niece that my sister never grew up to meet, the granddaughter my father only knew as a little girl but didn't get to see turn into an incredibly impressive young woman. As you read these stories in this book, please think about that. That symbolism. That hope.

In twenty-four hours, the page turned for me. One day I was reflecting on my father on what would have been—should've been—a birthday celebration. I was thinking about his hardships, the grief, pain, and loss that CF struck our family with. When facing so much adversity, my father would always say, "The sun is going to still come up tomorrow." Well, for CF families around the world, it did. And it was glowing brighter than it ever had. That "tomorrow" was indeed the day after his birthday. A breakthrough therapeutic drug, breaking through the dawn, putting away a day reflecting on pain and loss and bringing about hope and victory.

So, you know, I wrote this foreword because I didn't allow Andy Lipman to include the well-written story he centered on me and my family's CF experience. He kindly understood. I decided that our story is too painful, with too many layers that I don't want to tell. Some scabs need to be left to heal over. They are in the past because they allow you to have a future by staying in the past.

My life now is further removed from CF than it once was. Working nonstop throughout with the CF Foundation for years helped ease a lot of pain I had felt for my parents. It brought me great relationships in the CF community and the satisfaction of knowing we helped others. After my father's death, I have decided to have more joy in other ways a little further removed from such loss and the realities of CF. I find much of that joy through my career. My comedy work on *Holey Moley*, hosting on ABC with Rob Riggle, gives that to me. I find it in the football booth on ESPN. I find it calling big fights ringside. And I *always* find that with the spark I see in my healthy children's eyes and the richness of my wife's laughter.

As much as CF has taken from my family, I did feel I needed, and wanted, to write this foreword. To share with you that I know you'll enjoy these CF stories as much as I have. From Terry Wright's tremendous work raising CF awareness for the African American community, to Nicole Kohr, a double-lung transplant recipient. Nicole is an incredible talent as an actress, writer, and now has a CF-based stage musical coming out. These are stories that needed to be told and should inspire many to live their life fully and to continue to fight for the cure.

PREFACE

It was an honor to author the first volume of *The CF Warrior Project* in 2018. So many people wrote me to say how inspired they were by the CF warriors to whom they were introduced. And yet while I, too, found their stories inspiring, I felt the book was missing a crucial element of the CF community: those incredible individuals who make up a CF warrior's support system.

The common understanding is that seventy thousand people in the world live with cystic fibrosis (CF). While this number seems accurate when describing the patients themselves, CF affects more than those who are afflicted by the disease. Like other illnesses, it deeply affects the families, the physicians, and those on the periphery who enthusiastically advocate for the patients' wellness. In this volume of *The CF Warrior Project*, in addition to more inspiring stories of those battling the disease from within, we will highlight people in our small, but powerful, community who help battle the disease from without.

I have been blessed to have people in my life who have played these various roles in my own struggle with CF. To start, there's my wife, Andrea, the love of my life and my best friend, who has vacillated among wife, mother to our two children, and, when I am sick, caregiver. I can't imagine what it's like for her to await my return from a doctor's appointment, wondering if I'll come back with a thumbs-up, all-good, or an IV in my arm and diagnosis of diminishing lung function. In the latter case, not only is she the one who has to, most often, administer an IV in the days that follow, but she also has the unenviable emotional task of relaying my health status to family members because I simply don't have the inner strength to do it myself.

Then there are my children—my daughter, Avery, and my son, Ethan—who are both now teenagers and old enough to comprehend the seriousness of my condition and the part they play in our CF village. In addition to helping their mother, you can imagine the challenge of being teenagers living in a pandemic and having to be that much more mindful of their potential as germ vectors. Plus, difficult as it is for anyone to maintain a social life in this time of coronavirus, they have to explain to friends and friends' parents why I have a vest strapped to my torso, why I cough more than most, and that I am not contagious.

My sister Emily not only had to sacrifice my parents' attention when my health was an issue growing up, but she now continues to help the family by shepherding loved ones in medical need to the hospital and helping me isolate from those who might be unwell—that's in the best of times, let alone during COVID time when respiratory illness is so rampant.

And of course, in addition to the aunts, uncles, cousins, friends, and greater CF community who join me and my immediate family in fundraising efforts, and the physicians, nurses, respiratory therapists, case workers, and nutritionists who each do their best to help keep me living as normal a life as possible, there are my parents, Eva and Charles, who, for me, set the standard for love and care of a CF patient. They not only sought the best medical attention for me from the beginning, but they made a lifestyle of doing postural drainage by slapping my sides, back, and chest to ensure that I could clear the mucus from my lungs. Among those profiled in these pages is my late mom, who contributed to those with cystic fibrosis long before she ever had a child with the disease.

As you turn from one story to the next, I hope you will glean some of the inspiration that compelled me to embark on not only the first volume of *The CF Warrior Project*, but a second, equally packed volume, which includes profiles of a man not diagnosed with CF until his fifties, primarily because of the color of his skin, and a woman who has survived three double-lung transplants before the age of thirty! CF crosses political, economic, and social boundaries, and authoring this book is perhaps, most of all, a document of my life's work—supporting those for whom the purportedly life-threatening condition cystic fibrosis holds within it something very life-affirming.

—Andy C. Lipman

GLOSSARY OF TERMS

Bacterial Cross-Contamination: The possibility of one CF patient passing on a bacterium to another. The Cystic Fibrosis Foundation currently recommends six feet of distance between patients because of this concern.

BiPAP: Acronym for bi-level positive airway pressure, often used in end-stage patients with cystic fibrosis awaiting lung transplantation.

Cepacia (also referred to as Burkholderia cepacia): Bacteria often found in soil and water which is often resistant to common antibiotics and poses more risk to those with weakened immune systems and/or chronic lung diseases especially cystic fibrosis.

CF: Acronym for cystic fibrosis.

CFRD: Acronym for cystic fibrosis–related diabetes, a unique type of diabetes that is common among people with CF.

CFTR: Acronym which stands for the cystic fibrosis transmembrane conductance regulator, which is the protein responsible for regulating the normal flow of chloride and sodium in and out of the cell membranes in the lungs along with other organs.

Cystic Fibrosis: A lung disease that also affects the digestive system, sinuses, liver, and reproductive system. Cystic fibrosis is the deadliest genetic disease in the United States. In order for a child to have CF, each parent must have the CF gene, and then there is a 25 percent chance the child will have CF, a 50 percent chance the child will be a carrier, and a 25 percent chance the child will neither be a carrier nor a patient.

Delta F508: The most common mutation in the gene related to cystic fibrosis (CF).

FEV: Acronym for forced expository volume. This number measures how much air a person exhales during a forced breath. With regard to cystic fibrosis, the FEV1, or the amount of air a person is capable of blowing out in the first second, is normally the most important statistic measured when determining one's lung-disease stage.

Hemoptysis: Bleeding from the lungs and another potential symptom of cystic fibrosis.

IVF: Acronym for in vitro fertilization, a medical procedure done by doctors to attempt to help a family that is having difficulty getting pregnant naturally. Less than 5 percent of male CF patients have the ability to have children without the use of fertility treatments due to the lack of a vas deferens, which is the bridge that moves sperm from the testicles to the urethra. Females can also have a difficult time getting pregnant or carrying a baby full-term due to the effects of cystic fibrosis.

Kaftrio: The trade name for the CFTR modulator Trikafta in Europe.

Kalydeco, Orkambi, Symdeko, and Trikafta: Breakthrough CF drugs (also referred to as CFTR modulators) from Vertex Pharmaceuticals.

Meconium Ileus: A blocked intestine, a common symptom of cystic fibrosis.

Newborn Screening: Public program to screen a newborn to see if he or she has a genetic disease like cystic fibrosis.

Phages (also known as bacteriophages): Viruses that attempt to target and kill certain bacteria and are often used in phage therapy to destroy multi-drug resistant bacteria.

PFT: Acronym for pulmonary function test, which is used to gauge someone's lung function with cystic fibrosis.

Postural Drainage: A procedure where the patient gets into certain positions and either self-administers or has someone else administer therapy to loosen the mucus in the patient's lungs. This is often done by cupping one's hands and hitting the patient's sides, back, and front, until the patient is able to cough up the sputum.

Pneumothorax: When air or gas is stuck in the cavity between the lungs and the chest wall, causing the lung to collapse.

SickKids: The Hospital for Sick Children in Toronto, Ontario, Canada.

Tune-Up: A hospital stay for cystic fibrosis patients that involves IV antibiotics.

TOBI: Inhaled oral antibiotic.

Vest: A device used by many CF patients, often two or three times a day between thirty to forty-five minutes each time, that helps loosen the phlegm in one's lungs.

*** *Disclaimer: Please discuss with the patient's doctor before making any changes to his or her health routine. Everyone's bodies work differently, so what might work for one person may not work for another.* ***

1

THE TRAILBLAZERS: SAVING CF LIVES THROUGH A LIFETIME OF DEDICATION

DR. JOSHUA SONETT

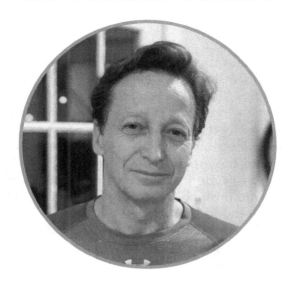

Age: 59

Resides: Ho-Ho-Kus, New Jersey

Connection to CF: Thoracic surgeon

TRANSPLANTING HOPE: MORE THAN A SURGEON

In the early morning hours of November 10, 2009, Dr. Joshua Sonett, Chief of General Thoracic Surgery and Director at Columbia University Medical Center (CUMC), performed Tim Sweeney's double-lung transplant surgery. "The true miracle," Tim says, "wasn't that my life was saved by Dr. Sonett. The true miracle occurred when Dr. Sonett gave my life meaning the very next morning. In the ICU, Dr. Sonett made me a promise that changed everything. He told me that we would cross the finish line at the New York City Marathon in less than a year."

"Collectively, CF patients and the CF community are awe inspiring to me," says Dr. Sonett, who has made lung transplant surgery and care integral to his practice. "So, to be able to help CF patients and [their] families, at a most difficult time—facing a lung transplant—is so important. But in return to the hope and help we offer as doctors, the friendship, love, and inspiration that, in particular, CF patients return to us is immeasurable. So I look forward to always being a part of the amazing CF community, and we can now actually see a future where lung transplant for CF will be mostly historical!"

Dr. Sonett helps many patients with many issues regarding the lungs, esophagus, and mediastinum, giving all patients the chance and ability to live their lives to the fullest potential. "It's what perhaps make me most happy," says Dr. Sonett. "On the way to this journey, I am blessed to be able to be part of many people's lives, on a very intimate level, this is really the core privilege of being a physician."

Dr. Sonett, who says that growing up he enjoyed each person for who they were and how they treated other people—"I never liked being labeled or associated with a particular clique or group," he says, "and preferred moving freely with friends of all backgrounds and interests"—attended Duke University for undergrad and East Carolina University for medical school. His residency followed, beginning at UMass for general surgery before transferring over to the University of Pittsburgh and then Sloan Kettering for cardiothoracic. Lung transplantation would lend even greater purpose to his journey.

"Being part of giving someone the chance for a full life," he says, "looking into the eyes of my patients who are worried about just getting their next breath." His goal with each patient is to help them "get past transplant and fulfill their life goals and passions." And he accomplishes that goal inside and outside the operating room.

In 2001, Dr. Sonett joined Team Boomer. "Jerry Cahill [a CF warrior who works for the Boomer Esiason Foundation] introduced me to Team Boomer," says Dr. Sonett. "The foundation does amazing work and supports and creates an amazing message of fortitude and resilience. The message Boomer [Boomer Esiason, former All-Pro NFL quarterback, who started the foundation] delivers and the help the foundation brings not only uplifts those associated with CF but, frankly, all of us, of all shapes and forms.

"After I got to know Jerry and Team Boomer, whenever I felt like not pushing through a run, I would think, *What would Jerry and other CF patients do?* They would push their bodies mentally and physically to the best they could. It really kept me going on long runs and really made me admire the work of Team Boomer. It is a real privilege to be able to help the foundation's mission and with all the good Team Boomer delivers. The Boomer Esiason Foundation and Boomer himself are all so good and so dedicated to helping all aspects and individuals with CF and educating all. My family is so supportive of [the] time and mental energy I need to devote to my patients, always understanding of my

4

time away. And all have helped or run for Team Boomer, including multiple marathons (three family members have done the full New York City Marathon and one has done the half)."

During the latter part of 2009, thirty-two-year-old Tim Sweeney was given a few months to live due to end-stage lung disease. "At the time, I had a wife and an eighteen-month-old son at home," says Tim. "It was a terrifying time in my life. My future seemed like a small dark room that I was trapped in without hope." Dr. Sonett performed the successful surgery, and the next morning made the fateful promise. "I hadn't run more than a mile since I was twelve years old," says Tim, "but in that moment, for the first time in my life, I had hope for the future. I had a purpose and direction. My dark room suddenly had a bright light that Dr. Sonett had lit."

Tim says that he first met Dr. Sonett at a lecture at Columbia University talking about the future of lung transplants. "I knew his reputation," says Tim. "He was the youngest head of the department in a major hospital at that time, and I knew he had operated on [former president] Bill Clinton. I was attending as part of the pre-transplant protocol," says Tim. "During the class, I asked Dr. Sonett if he was in my shoes, what would he do? Without hesitation he said he would exercise. He told me if I can walk into the surgery, I can walk out. So I thought to myself that I wanted to jog in and jog out of the operating room even though I was not a runner at that time."

After Tim's surgery and Dr. Sonett's pledge, Tim began training. "When you have a doctor with his credentials telling you that you could run a marathon in less than a year," says Tim, "it completely changes your self-image and how you view your own capabilities. Dr. Sonett taught me the value of the right mindset."

Tim ran his first mile a month after his transplant, in December 2009, a four-mile road race to benefit the Cystic Fibrosis Foundation the following April, and completed a half-marathon in June and called Dr. Sonett to tell him once he'd completed the half-marathon. "He then knew how serious I was about running the marathon," says Tim. "We started talking at that point about training and strategies and he invited me to New Jersey to run with him. Dr. Sonett ran with a group of people and they were all preparing for the marathon. Unfortunately, being so far away for me and my work schedule [in Connecticut], I wasn't able to go to New Jersey. So the first time I saw Dr. Sonett after being in the ICU was the morning of the marathon.

"As we approached the finish line of the marathon, I jokingly asked, 'Are you going to let me win?' With a serious expression, Dr. Sonett said, 'No.' I looked over at him. 'We're going to cross the line together.'

"We talked during the race almost nonstop, and we learned a lot about each other," says Tim. "We even had dinner that night with our wives."

What began as a doctor/patient relationship quickly became a friendship of deep admiration. "I was so proud to run with Tim, to hear the crowd cheer him and be able to support him during his run is a life memory," says Dr. Sonett. "And seeing his family, and his son so excited to see his dad run the marathon at the finish line, is a joyous memory that lives with and motivates me."

"Without Dr. Sonett, I would've had my surgery with another doctor," says Tim, who asserts that he would have lived but that "Dr. Sonett gave me something very special that can never be taken away. For someone at their darkest time who was given two weeks to live, my friendship with Dr. Sonett is the true miracle and gift I had prayed for."

Drs. Batsheva & Eitan Kerem

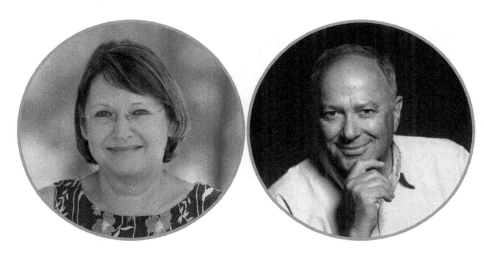

Age: 67	**Age:** 69
Resides: Mevaseret Zion, Israel	**Resides:** Mevaseret Zion, Israel
Connection to CF: Geneticist	**Connection to CF:** Professor and physician

Israel's Dynamic Duo: Husband and Wife Team Take on CF

There are few power couples more important to the cystic fibrosis community than Israeli Drs. Batsheva and Eitan Kerem who have worked in the field of cystic fibrosis for several decades.

Batsheva grew up in Tel Aviv and Eitan in Jerusalem. They both studied at the Hebrew University in Jerusalem. Batsheva was the best friend of the wife of Eitan's best friend, and they were introduced when she came to study biology at the Hebrew University. "It was love at first sight," says Batswheva.

"I grew up in a small, simple neighborhood of Jerusalem, in the early 1950s," says Eitan. "All the neighbors were Holocaust survivors." During his army service, serving in one of the elite Israel Defense Forces (IDF) units, Eitan went to a medic course where he was introduced to the world of medicine. "I was always interested in breathing problems and how to help people breathe easier," says Eitan. "When I was in medical school, I first met a small child with CF and read that these children do not live more than ten years. Later as [a] pediatric resident, I learned that they die as teenagers, and now most of my patients are adults, working and having families. My work was divided between taking care of patients and research in order to understand better the disease to treat it better."

Batsheva, who served as an IDF officer prior to studying biology at the Hebrew University, was "a serious pupil" who grew up in Tel Aviv, Israel. "I was immediately interested in biology," says Batsheva, "particularly in high school. My desire was to learn [about] human molecule diseases." She received her bachelor of science degree in 1979 and her PhD in 1986. Next, she sought out a place to do her post-doctoral fellow in human genetics, so she wrote to several labs in Toronto, which Batsheva says was, at that time, the only place that had good centers for pediatric pulmonology for Eitan and a good department of human genetics for her.

"Lap-Chee Tsui was the first to reply to my letter," says Batsheva. "I met with him and, though I received other letters of interest as well, I was set on going to Toronto to help find the CF gene."

Batsheva, Eitan, and their two daughters moved to Toronto in the summer of 1987. "The start in Toronto was very difficult, until our daughters felt comfortable at school, talked English, found friends, etc.," says Batsheva.

"It was very difficult until we got adjusted and got used to the different culture," says Eitan. "We had two daughters at that time who went to school with no English. Our salaries were very low, and we lived in a very modest way. We had no family around us, but had good Canadian friends whom we knew before coming to Toronto who helped us. Later, we learned how to make the most out of the time there, we traveled, and we had very special and significant time as a family."

"The professional start was also a challenge," says Batsheva. "But after [a] few months, we all started to enjoy [it]. We had a very good time as a family in Toronto."

Batsheva developed a rapport with Dr. Tsui. "Lap-Chee is a wonderful person," she says. "I really enjoyed working with him. My contribution was in genetic analysis and in 'walking,' which means isolating the DNA segments in a region we suspected to harbor the CF gene. I was in charge of the walking itself and of identification markers that are different among individuals to allow us to build a genetic map in the region." Batsheva and the entire Tsui team identified and cloned the CFTR gene in 1989 that they determined was responsible for causing CF. "The results of this part appeared on the cover of the issue of *Science* magazine in which the papers on identification of the gene were published," says Batsheva.

During her time with Dr. Tsui, Batsheva even helped develop the first registry of CF patients' mutations. "The scientific experience for me was unbelievable!" says Batsheva. "I have met many of the patients and their families and I know how important our projects are."

The Kerems moved back to Israel in 1990. "Israel is our home," says Batsheva. "We wanted to raise our children in Israel. Family first, then science . . . But I took back from Lap-Chee's lab the experience of how to motivate students and how to mentor."

"The first thing that I noticed [when we returned to] Israel," says Eitan, "is the lack of comprehensive treatment with a multidisciplinary team. The major challenges were improving nutritional status of the patients, introducing routine treatments with inhalations and physio." So Eitan formed the Israeli CF Society, which includes all the CF teams in Israel. "We have a three-day national congress," says Eitan, "and we meet for an evening, every three months, to teach and learn. Together with Batsheva, we characterized the mutations among Jews, and we published it. Today, all genetic consultations for patients who have Jewish origin are based on our research. We also characterized the disease severity of the different mutations. Later, we collaborated with drug companies that develop treatments for CF."

When Batsheva returned to Israel, she became a senior lecturer at the Hebrew University in 1990 and, soon after, established the Israel National Center for CF Genetic Research before being promoted to assistant professor and, eventually, a full professor at the university in 2003. She has since won the Julodan Prize for Contribution to Medicine in 1993; the Teva Prize for Excellence in Human Genome Research in 1993; the Abisch-Frenkel Prize for Excellence in Life Sciences in 2004; the distinguished Israeli Prime Minister Emet Prize, for contribution to Genetics Research, in 2008; and the ECFS (European Cystic Fibrosis Society) Award, acknowledging her outstanding contributions to the identification of the CFTR gene, in 2009.

Eitan is now developing drug therapies that help CF patients specifically with nonsense genetic mutations (mutations in a DNA sequence that result in a shorter, unfinished protein product), which are mutations that are currently not helped by CFTR modulators like Trikafta. He was, until recently, the head of the Division of Pediatrics at the Hadassah Medical Organization, and he is the founder of the Center for Children with Chronic Diseases at Hadassah Mt. Scopus. He has received many distinguished awards, including the ECFS Award acknowledging his tremendous contributions to CF research. In 2016, he earned an honorary fellowship from the Royal College of Pediatrics and Child Health, UK. In 2020, he was also hired as a senior consultant with Eloxx Pharmaceuticals, a biopharmaceutical company located in

Waltham, Massachusetts, which is dedicated to finding novel therapies to treat those with cystic fibrosis and other diseases specifically with nonsense mutations. Eitan continues treating both pediatric and adult patients at Hadassah University Hospital Jerusalem and, in his spare time, enjoys spending time with his family, hiking in nature, and cycling.

Batsheva continues to make a difference in the CF community today as well. "I am engaged with CF research since we came back," says Batsheva. "I opened my research group in the Hebrew University. I also was the advisor for seven years [2013–2020] to the president of the Hebrew University, for promotion of women in science. I spent a lot of time and energy toward promoting women in science. I recently founded a biotech company for developing drugs for CF patients [called] SpliSense. The company is working on projects that were developed in the lab."

SpliSense is an Israeli-based company founded in November 2016 that focuses on transformative RNA-based treatments for finding the root cause of genetic diseases such as cystic fibrosis and has thus far raised $28.5 million to advance treatments for rare CF mutations. In May 2021, the Cystic Fibrosis Foundation invested $8.4 million in the company as part of their Pathway to a Cure initiative to accelerate treatments for the underlying cause of cystic fibrosis for every individual with cystic fibrosis. In her spare time, Batsheva enjoys playing with her grandchildren and listening to music. "I used to love playing the piano," Batsheva says, "however, I don't have much time for that right now."

Eitan and Batsheva now have three daughters and ten grandchildren. All three daughters have chosen the medical field with the two older ones going into child psychology and the youngest a physician.

Batsheva says that she and her husband can work together, and this has helped their two departments in Toronto and Israel working hand in hand. "We collaborate," says Batsheva. "I do the molecular side and Eitan is on the clinical side."

Eitan finds their working relationship fulfilling as well. "It is very special since we both are interested in what the other does," says Eitan. "We learn from each other, we develop ideas for research together, and we consult with each other when we face challenges."

Dr. Francis S. Collins

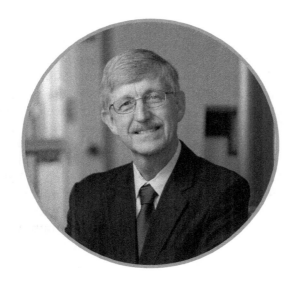

Age: 72
Resides: Chevy Chase, Maryland
Connection to CF: Physician-geneticist

THE SEARCH FOR THE GENE:
THE LIFE AND WORK OF DR. FRANCIS S. COLLINS

Dr. Francis S. Collins served as the director of the NIH (National Institutes of Health) in Bethesda, Maryland—appointed by President Barack Obama, confirmed by the Senate, and sworn in on August 17, 2009. In 2017, President Donald Trump asked Dr. Collins to continue to serve as the NIH director, and in 2021, President Joe Biden asked him to serve again. Dr. Collins thus holds the distinguished honor as being the only presidentially appointed NIH director to serve more than one administration. According to the NIH, before stepping down from his post in December 2021, Dr. Collins was responsible for overseeing the work of the largest supporter of biomedical research in the world, which encompasses everything from basic to clinical research.

Dr. Collins is famous in the world of cystic fibrosis for leading one of the research teams that discovered the CF gene in 1989 while a member of the University of Michigan faculty. "Finding a specific gene causing a disease by 'positional cloning' (a term I made up) hadn't been done before for any disease in the 1980s," says Dr. Collins. "Applying this approach to find the CF gene was extremely challenging. We were traveling through a sea of unknown territory, looking for clues. It took several years and was benefited ultimately by the merger of my lab with that of Dr. Lap-Chee Tsui. We found that we could go faster as collaborators than as competitors. I have lived by that principle ever since."

Dr. Collins remembers the day the gene was officially discovered. "Lap-Chee and I were attending a genetics meeting at Yale, staying in the dorms," says Dr. Collins. "On a rainy night in New Haven, after a long day, we went back to his room, where he had set up a fax machine to receive data from our labs. That was the night where the data about a three base-pair deletion in a previously unknown gene all fell into place. Of course, we had to be sure—and to take care of any loose ends—so the announcement came three months later. But it was that night in New Haven when I was convinced. It was exhilarating; it was a relief after years of work, and it felt like the opening of a door toward new treatment ideas."

Dr. Collins says he now has the pleasure of seeing so many discoveries take place thanks to the discovery of the CF gene. "I am overjoyed to see the introduction of effective drug therapy for ninety percent of individuals with CF," he says. "It was a long hard journey to get here, but when I read stories about people whose lives have been utterly transformed, I can't help but get emotional."

While Dr. Collins is on the "Mt. Rushmore" of physicians who played a role in the CF gene discovery, it is not his only landmark discovery. This physician-geneticist also guided the international Human Genome Project, which, in April 2003, completed the finished sequence of the human DNA instruction book. Dr. Collins served as director of the National Human Genome Research Institute at NIH from 1993 to 2008.

Dr. Collins's accolades and honorary appointments include being an elected member of both the National Academy of Medicine and the National Academy of Sciences; awarded the Presidential Medal of Freedom in November 2007; awarded the National Medal of Science in 2009; elected as a Foreign Member of the Royal Society (UK); and named the fiftieth winner of the Templeton Prize, which honors individuals whose "exemplary achievements advance Sir John Templeton's philanthropic vision of harnessing the power of the sciences to explore the deepest questions of the universe and humankind's place and purpose within it."

Still, there is one thing that Dr. Collins would still like to see with regard to CF. He won't be fully satisfied until there is effective treatment for every single patient with CF. "Now we need to find ways to help that ten percent who aren't benefitting from the new drugs," he says. "Perhaps we'll figure out how to use gene editing to fix the misspellings."

DR. LAP-CHEE TSUI

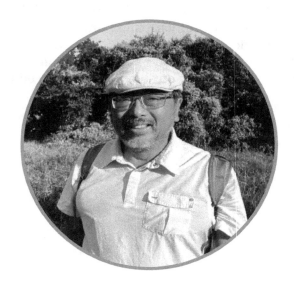

Age: 71
Resides: Toronto, Canada
Connection to CF: Geneticist

THE SEARCH FOR THE GENE: THE LIFE AND WORK OF DR. LAP-CHEE TSUI

D r. Lap-Chee Tsui (pronounced Chui) and his team identified the defective gene that causes cystic fibrosis, which is considered one of the most significant breakthroughs in human genetics and makes him one of the most important persons in the history of the disease.

Growing up in Shanghai, China, Dr. Tsui took to science almost immediately. "I was always full of curiosity," says Dr. Tsui. "The study of science—which is to discover—is therefore very much my favorite subject. Since I grew up with little means, I had to build a lot of toys from recycled materials. Watching tadpoles grow in a jar and seeds germinate were once part of my pastime."

Dr. Tsui's family moved him out of mainland China when he was just three years old fearing that their family would suffer persecution at the hands of the new communist regime, which had taken control just four years earlier. "My father worked in the president's office to edit Mr. Chiang's [a Chinese nationalist politician and military leader who served as the leader of the Republic of China for nearly half a century] genealogy archive," says Dr. Tsui. "So he had a good reason to fear when the communist party came into power. Although both his and my mother's families were rather wealthy in Hangzhou, my father said we arrived in Hong Kong with only two dollars in his pocket.

"We lived on assistance from their family friends for quite some time. Neither of my parents could find jobs in Hong Kong. My father was basically an artist, who did well in Chinese calligraphy, brush painting, and even Peking opera. His handwriting in small characters was well-known in the artists' circle. That was why he got drafted to work in the president's office. My mother did not have to work at all.

"The language barrier was their major disadvantage in Hong Kong: neither of them could speak Cantonese (we spoke Hangzhou dialect at home and Shanghainese with neighbors). We moved from one friend's place to another for quite some time until we exhausted our welcome. My father finally found a job selling life insurance. I recall we moved six times, and I studied in four primary schools. Fortunately, my parents believed in education—I could continue my study without having to work as a child-laborer, as many of my classmates did after primary school."

Interestingly, the person who was almost solely responsible for discovering the CF gene wanted, primarily, to become an architect. "One of my favorite hobbies was to make toy houses and buildings from discarded cardboard boxes, particularly around mid-autumn festivals because there were plentiful of mooncake boxes available during that period of time when I was a kid," says Dr. Tsui. "They were of the right hardness for me to cut with scissors and glue with starch made from rice. I [have] also liked sketching and painting ever since I could get a hold of pencils and paints. That was why I had wanted to be either an art designer or architect.

"Since I studied in the Chinese school stream from the start, there were no such programs available when it came time for me to enter university here in Hong Kong. Science subjects were available, however. I got admitted to studying biology in the Chinese University of Hong Kong because I did well for that subject in the university entrance examination. I joked that perhaps it was my nice drawings got me the high marks. Unfortunately, I did not do well in most of the biology subjects in college because much of the study materials required straight memorization. In fact, biology was regarded as a recording science in those days. Biochemistry, molecular biology, and genetics came much later in my life."

In his mid-twenties, Dr. Tsui had the opportunity to come to the United States. "Most of my college classmates became high school teachers," says Dr. Tsui. "Teaching was a rather lucrative profession at that time because the population of Hong Kong was expanding. Since I only graduated from the college with a Third-Class honor, I was unable to find any teaching post. I could have been a laboratory technician because I was good in carrying out experiments. As fate would have it, I was admitted to a graduate program for a master's degree as an alternate in the biology program of the Chinese University, because the admitted candidate did not show up.

"I did well on my master's thesis dissertation. The study was on a particular gene regulation pathway for a bacterial virus [bacteriophage] called 'lambda.' One day in early 1974, I had an opportunity to speak to a visiting professor named Chien Ho from the University of Pittsburgh after his seminar. It was my turn to tell him what I did for my thesis. Chien was apparently very much impressed by my work. He told me that he had a young colleague in Pittsburgh who was working on the assembly of bacteriophage lambda and was recruiting students to work in his lab. He said he could also help me arrange for an assistantship to pursue a PhD degree there."

Five years later, Dr. Tsui moved on to Oak Ridge, Tennessee, to be a postdoctoral investigator and postdoctoral fellow in 1979. "I thought I should get into a research area related to health and disease," says Dr. Tsui, "because it would be easier for me to find [a] grant should I run a research lab myself. Cancer was an obvious choice. Unfortunately, I discovered that the particular approach I was assigned to study — tumorigenesis in mice — was not a viable one, because I failed to reproduce the early findings in the lab. Basically, the preliminary studies done in the Oak Ridge National Laboratory had not been peer-reviewed. My supervisor was not keen in letting me do anything else. So I had no reason to stay on."

Then fate played a role in the form of the classified ads in an issue of the journal *Science* on May 9, 1980, in which Dr. Tsui was first introduced to an opportunity to work in the world of cystic fibrosis. "My wife noted a job advertisement for a postdoctoral fellow to study the basic defect of cystic fibrosis in the Hospital for Sick Children in Toronto," says Dr. Tsui. "I had no knowledge about the disease other than what I could read from the literature after reading the ad, but I thought I could apply all the molecular biology techniques I acquired from my previous research training to tackling the CF problem. No one had applied molecular biology and gene cloning for CF at the time. I thought I would have a good chance to contribute. Also, my wife thought we could move to Toronto, close to her family who had recently immigrated from Hong Kong." He interviewed for the job soon after in Toronto and, four months later, received an offer from geneticist Dr. Manual Buchwald with the goal to find the underlying cause of cystic fibrosis.

When Dr. Tsui arrived at the Hospital for Sick Children in January 1981, he was still not certain how to determine the CF gene from other genetic mutations, until he read an article in the May issue of the *American Journal of Human Genetics.* "I only read the conceptual paper on using classical human genetic mapping with the newly discovered class of DNA markers by [Raymond] White and coauthors after my arrival in Toronto," says Dr. Tsui, "but I thought it was probably much better than several of the other schemes that I had devised at that time. Since I did not know anything about human gene mapping, I studied the White paper in great detail and learned the statistical methods required to perform human disease gene mapping from reading all the reference materials. It was a rather gratifying experience because I learned everything from first principles so that I had no trouble discussing the nuances of gene mapping with many of the well-known scholars in classical human genetics, whom I met later.

"I was also fortunate that I got my first independent research grant support from the Canadian Cystic Fibrosis Foundation [now CF Canada]. The gene mapping approach was so new that none of the grant-review panel members could understand what I proposed, as the director of the foundation told me years later, but I got the money anyway, because I did not ask for a lot of money. However, I got a huge support from the foundation in a different way—I received the valuable blood samples solicited by the foundation from CF families all over Canada. With the panel of family samples [DNA], I started to conduct my gene mapping studies."

It wasn't just the science that interested Dr. Tsui. "The ultimate objective of the gene mapping studies," says Dr. Tsui, "was to identify the basic defect underlying the disorder so that better treatment could be devised for CF patients. During my gene-mapping studies, I had the opportunity to work with the Canadian CF Foundation to travel around the country to explain my work to family members and patients as well as CF doctors and nurses. I had made many friends across the country. However, while I was confident I would be able to find the gene if given sufficient time—because I knew all the steps that were required to take—I had no illusion that I could find a treatment for CF in my laboratory. In fact, I refused to answer any questions from reporters regarding when treatments would be available."

In late 1987, Dr. Tsui asked Dr. Francis S. Collins (who would later become the director of the National Institutes of Health in Bethesda,

Maryland) about working together since both had their own specific ways to locate the gene. "I once told Francis that he was such a convincing speaker and so eloquent with words," says Dr. Tsui, "that he should run for president of the USA."

Eventually Dr. Tsui and his team reached their first magical moment when, on May 9, 1989, Richard Rozmahel, a member of Dr. Tsui's team, arrived to tell him about a potential CF-gene finding with regard to a three-base-pair deletion.

"What Richard found was a three-base pair deletion in a CF patient sample when compared with the non-CF sample," says Dr. Tsui. "Since three base pairs would correspond to a single amino acid residue in the encoded protein (which was named CFTR subsequently), it was not immediately apparent that it was a disease-causing mutation because a protein could still be made (albeit missing Phenylalanine at position 508). In other words, we had little confidence that it would be the CF gene. The DNA deletion could have been a 'hitchhiking mutation,' whereas the real disease-causing mutation would be elsewhere in the gene. In any case, we would need to sequence the rest of the gene and confirm the finding with additional CF samples."

It turns out that the mutation Delta F508 (F stood for Phenylalanine and 508 was the position where it was found) affects about half of the cystic fibrosis population worldwide.

A month later, it was official, but Dr. Tsui admits he was not jumping for joy just yet. "It was neither a moment of eureka nor a time for champagne," says Dr. Tsui. "What I received with my portable fax machine was just a table tabulating the latest result from the additional CF and non-CF samples we examined. So far, we only detected the three-base-pair deletion in about seventy percent of the CF samples but none of the non-CF samples. We had not finished sequencing the rest of the gene. The story became dramatic, not because of Francis's uncontrolled excitement but because Bob Williamson's [Dr. Williamson was also looking for the gene in the UK] fellow was staying next door to my dormitory room in Yale University where a human gene-mapping meeting was hosted."

Dr. Tsui needed more confirmation, so he reached out to his friend and colleague at the University of Pittsburgh, Dr. Aravinda Chakravarti, who, after investigating a piece of the X-ray film revealing the DNA sequence and calculating the mathematical odds for a few hours, told Dr. Tsui that the odds that they had not found the correct gene was one in 10^{-57}, or one in 1,000,000,000,000,000,000,000, 000,000,000,000,000,000,000,000,000,000,000.

"A highly significant statistical score was anticipated," says Dr. Tsui, "but Aravinda's expertise was required to come up with a credible number. His final offer of 10^{-57} was truly exhilarating! Who could argue with that! However, deep down in Batsheva's [Dr. Batsheva Kerem an Israeli geneticist working in Dr. Tsui's lab], Johanna's [Dr. Johanna Rommens, a Canadian geneticist working in Dr. Tsui's lab], and my minds, we worried that we had the wrong gene because the real gene could be just next door. A statistical number is merely a probability score! It was far from any solid proof. Our anxiety was not erased after the publishing of our papers, but only went away when additional mutations were found in the gene."

On August 24, 1989, Dr. Tsui, Dr. Collins, and a few others held a press conference to confirm that they had indeed found the CF gene. The story was featured in the *Los Angeles Times* and the *New York Times*, among other national publications. Nine years after answering the classified ad in the journal *Science*, the discovery of the CF gene earned them the cover.

Dr. Tsui has been able to see what his team's discovery has meant to those in the CF community by meeting people afflicted with the disease. "Indeed, many times [I have met people with CF]," says Dr. Tsui. "However, while I was happy that I was able to make a significant contribution in fighting CF, I could only encourage the patients by saying that our finding had made discoveries of rational treatments possible for the first time. Now, thirty years on, I am extremely happy that so many lives have been saved with our initial discovery."

A lot has changed for Dr. Tsui since discovering the gene. There is now a bust of him in the Donnelly CCBR building at the University of Toronto. He has received various awards and honors, including the titles of Distinguished Scientist of the Medical Research Council of Canada. He is now a fellow of the Royal Society of Canada, a fellow of the Royal Society of London, a fellow of Academia Sinica, a foreign associate of the National Academy of Sciences (of the USA), and a foreign member of the Chinese Academy of Sciences.

He has also received honorary doctorates from the University of Toronto, the University of Hong Kong, Tel Aviv University, and many others. He also received several awards including the Killiam Prize by the Canada Council for the Arts, the Mead Johnson Award, and the Gardner International Award.

In 1991, he was made an officer of the Order of Canada (established by Queen Elizabeth II, which recognizes outstanding achievement in Canadian society); in 2006, the fifth floor of the University of Toronto's Donnelly CCBR building was named after him; and in October 2007, he was decorated as knight of the French Legion of Honor and received the title of Justice of the Peace from the Hong Kong SAR (Special Administrative Region) Government. In 2012, he was inducted into the Canadian Medical Hall of Fame, and in 2015, Dr. Tsui became a founding member of the Hong Kong Academy of Sciences, at which he is currently president.

Dr. Tsui and his wife officially moved back to Toronto last summer, six years after his retirement from the University of Hong Kong where he was vice-chancellor for twelve years. "I had planned to travel two to three times to Hong Kong every year for the next three years to fulfill my remaining obligations there," says Dr. Tsui. "I got stranded in Hong Kong last February (2020), however, because of the various imposed travel restrictions during the COVID-19 pandemic." Dr. Tsui says he passed the time by walking and hiking along many of the beautiful trails in Hong Kong. "I [spoke] to my wife twice daily via video online," says Tsui. "I also [spoke] to our children and grandchild the same way." Dr. Tsui was eventually able to return to Toronto.

As of this book's publication, Dr. Tsui has over three hundred peer-reviewed scientific publications and sixty-five invited books' chapters, and he has served on the editorial boards of twenty-four international peer-reviewed scientific journals, several scientific review panels, and various national and international advisory committees, but today, while he is proud of the publications, the accolades, and various appointments, one thing means more. "The discovery of the CF gene," says Dr. Tsui, "was definitely on the top of my list."

DR. BONNIE RAMSEY

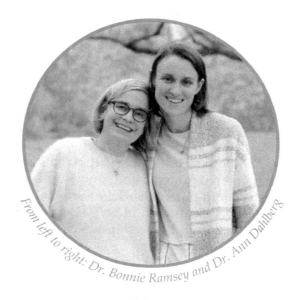

From left to right: Dr. Bonnie Ramsey and Dr. Ann Dahlberg

Age: 71

Resides: Seattle, Washington

Connection to CF: Physician

RIGHT PLACE, RIGHT TIME: A PIONEER THROUGH FATE

There's the old idiom, "Being in the right place at the right time," and that is perhaps the best way to explain how Dr. Bonnie Ramsey has become a trailblazer in the cystic fibrosis community for more than four decades.

Dr. Ramsey, who received her BA from Stanford University in 1972 and her MD from Harvard Medical School in 1976, was doing her residency at Boston Children's Hospital working with Dr. Harry Shwachman (who directed the hospital's clinical laboratories from 1946 to 1971, where he founded one of the largest nutrition clinics in the country).

"We had all the patients housed together in what became known as Division 37," says Dr. Ramsey. "Now, you would not have everyone together. Multiple people were sitting on beds together. Obviously, there was potential for cross-infection. It wasn't until a Burkholderia cepacia outbreak in the late eighties that strict infection control started. I was very interested in treating respiratory bacterial infections, especially with Pseudomonas aeruginosa (Pa) because it required intravenous antibiotics such as aminoglycosides resulting in long hospital stays. Interestingly, the two largest populations of patients in pediatric hospitals in the 1970s were cancer and CF. It wasn't unusual for patients to spend thirty to fifty percent of their lives in the hospital. I got to know these people and their families, and I was very fond of them, but I thought I was going to be a hematologist oncologist."

After her two years of residency in Boston, Dr. Ramsey moved back to her home in Seattle in 1978 with the intention to do her fellowship in blood disorders and cancer but was told that the American Board of Pediatrics had changed the protocol and now required a third year of residency before she could pursue her fellowship, and so she went to complete her residency at Seattle Children's Hospital in 1978. In 1979, she began a general pediatrics fellowship which included working in the cystic fibrosis outpatient clinic led by Dr. (Jack) Docter.

"He was a lovely, lovely man," says Dr. Ramsey. "He had trained with Dr. Dorothy Andersen [the doctor who founded and coined the name cystic fibrosis, originally naming it "cystic fibrosis of the pancreas"] and started one of the first CF centers in the country. He said he needed a physician to work in the CF clinic." Dr. Ramsey, who had spent a great deal of time working in CF centers in Boston during her residency, knew she could make an immediate impact.

"I began attending the clinic," says Dr. Ramsey. "There was a pulmonary physician helping Dr. Docter at the time." For unclear reasons, she resigned without notice during a clinic session, asking Dr. Ramsey to see the remainder of the patients. "I called Dr. Docter and told him 'I'm all you've got,'" says Dr. Ramsey. Dr. Docter was no longer seeing patients since he became medical director of Seattle Children's. "I approached the patients and families in the clinic and told them that their pulmonary doctor had resigned," says Dr. Ramsey, "and that I would now be their physician, and I remember one of the families looking at me and saying, 'So are you going to leave us also?'" Dr. Ramsey did not know what to say. She was now a fellow so that still meant she had limitations as to what she was allowed to do. For example, she could not sign patients' charts without an attending physician signing them.

"I didn't tell them I was only there as a fill-in," says Dr. Ramsey. "It was like this crushing feeling. I can't walk out the door. So I went down to Dr. Docter. He said, 'We'll work this out. I'll sign the charts.'" Dr. Ramsey never envisioned this would be the path that she would take. "It was almost like there must have been a reason this happened," she says.

Dr. Ramsey, who was not a pulmonologist at the time that she took on the responsibility at the clinic, spent the next year learning from other CF centers about how to handle symptoms of patients. After her fellowship was completed, Dr. Docter asked her to become the director of the CF clinic, and she accepted. It was a very exciting time for Dr. Ramsey as she became a mother for the first time in July 1979 after the birth of her daughter Ann. By 1980, Dr. Ramsey was an attending physician.

While she had dreams of being a hematologist/oncologist, her passions steered her elsewhere. "I became board certified in 1991 in pulmonary medicine," says Dr. Ramsey. "I basically had to self-teach and learn from my colleagues. At that time, you could be 'grandfathered' in to take the boards. Now, you have to have an official fellowship."

Dr. Ramsey wanted to make an even bigger difference. In January 1992, she helped to create a report referred to as the "Nutritional assessment and management in cystic fibrosis: a consensus report," an agreement among nutrition specialists and CF caregivers regarding nutritional management for CF patients with the goal to educate clinicians as to the significance of regular assessments and early intervention. "As a clinician, poor nutrition was a severe problem for children with CF when I started in the 1980s," says Dr. Ramsey. "I became a member and then chair of the CF Center Director's Committee. We decided to develop Standard Care Guidelines for CF management. It sounds odd that guidelines did not exist, but it was actually a new concept. We started by tracking nutrition, and I was asked to lead that working group. It was a very productive meeting, and I have always been proud of the outcome." The report would be sent out by the Cystic Fibrosis Foundation to all CF care centers around the United States and would create national guidelines to improve the long-term health of CF patients.

Soon, Dr. Arnold "Arnie" Smith, whom Dr. Ramsey knew from her days at Boston Children's and who had become head of infectious diseases at Seattle Children's Hospital, got her involved with a novel drug called dornase alfa (Pulmozyme) developed by Genentech. "I was involved in the conduct of the Phase 2 study with Genentech," says Dr. Ramsey, "and was the first author on that study. I helped with the study design for both Phase 2 and Phase 3 in the early nineties." The drug would help people to breathe easier and cause less infections. Pulmozyme is still used by a great number of CF patients today.

At the same time of her assistance with Pulmozyme, she was working with Dr. Smith when he told her an interesting story. "He had met an adult patient, and this person had said to him, 'I know this doesn't make any sense, but I've been putting my IV antibiotics in a nebulizer and I think it really helps.' Arnie came home and said, 'As a scientist, this doesn't make any sense to me, but I have to believe this man. I can tell from listening to him that he thinks it makes a difference. We have to determine the best therapy it can be.' He began with laboratory studies to measure the concentration of tobramycin that killed Pseudomonas aeruginosa (Pa) in sputum from patients with CF. He found, because sputum itself is so inhibitory, the concentration of an aminoglycoside like tobramycin necessary to kill the bacteria in the airway would be about twenty-five times the dose required to kill Pa in the blood stream.

"If this high concentration was given by intravenous route, it would be very toxic and potentially lead to kidney damage and hearing loss."

At that time, in the early nineties, there was no FDA-approved inhaled antibiotic, and physicians were prescribing intravenous antibiotic formulations to be given to patients by inhalation through nebulizers which Dr. Ramsey says it could be dangerous. Smith and Ramsey completed the study and found a safe amount to use, and the result after their work together was the breakthrough drug—a new formulation of tobramycin (TOBI) was developed and would be used specifically as an inhalation therapy. The product developed with a startup company called PathoGenesis. The Phase 2 and 3 studies, both published in the *New England Journal of Medicine*, showed a marked improvement in lung function after a month of the drug (> 10% improvement in FEV1). The drug was FDA approved in December 1997.

"I was very pleased," says Dr. Ramsey. "I had families come to me in clinic and tell me how it had changed their lives and allowed them more time out of the hospital."

Soon the CF Foundation was collecting royalties for TOBI, which helped provide the infrastructure needed for the foundation to invest more funds into research, which eventually led to the development of CFTR modulators such as Trikafta.

Dr. Ramsey had a long and productive working relationship with the CF Foundation. "I was asked to join the CFF Center Committee from 1996 to 2007," says Dr. Ramsey. "It was an important time when patient health was improving. We were able to develop adult care centers and standards of care for both children and emerging adult populations. Subsequently, I was asked by Dr. [Bob] Beall [president and CEO of the Cystic Fibrosis Foundation] to lead the Clinical Research Committee (CRC) after Arnie Smith completed his tenure as CRC Chair. Bob Beall is one of my dearest friends and we had an excellent working relationship. While I was leading the CRC, I recommended to Dr. Beall that the CFF consider establishing a national clinical trials network similar to the NCI-supported Children's Oncology Group.

So, in the late 1990s, Bob came out to Seattle, and he sat down and asked me to lead the Therapeutics Development Network (CF-TDN). It was part of his 'moonshot' CF Therapeutics Program leading to the eventual development of CFTR modulator therapies."

The CF-TDN began in 1998 and eventually became the largest CF clinical trials network in the world while completing over 150 clinical studies for cystic fibrosis in a large array of therapeutic areas and is based out of Seattle Children's Research Institute. The goal of the program is to accelerate the clinical evaluation of new CF therapies.

"It is amazing that in Dr. Beall's mind he sat down and put this whole thing together," says Dr. Ramsey. "He said we'll need five to ten years to get this done. I thought it would take thirty years! He gave me some funds to take a sabbatical. I had no idea how to put together a network. I had my research coordinator Judy Williams, who is an RN with a master's in epidemiology, and I found a biostatistician at the University of Washington named Dick Kronmal. We started to put the pieces together. The CFF provided me with start-up funding and the network began with eight large academic centers.

"Over the years, it has expanded to over seventy research sites across the US. We weren't sure whether industry would be interested in us. But the day we opened, industry partners were very interested and continue to be collaborators today. We had growing pains, but the foundation [was of great help]." Dr. Ramsey would take a break from her work with patients to take on this endeavor over the next nine months.

"My partners, Ron Gibson and Susan Marshall, saw patients and Jane Burns, who ran the CF microbiology lab (she is a pediatric infectious disease doctor), covered my clinics," says Dr. Ramsey. "I felt okay about leaving my practice with them. I knew that the TDN would change CF clinical research, and this would be my chance to be part of creating a clinical trials network. TDN was critical in creating a bridge between industry and academic center and the CFF. There is no question this organized approach moved therapies forward more quickly." Dr. Ramsey would eventually go back to being an attending physician while still taking charge of the TDN.

Dr. Ramsey has a great deal of admirers in the cystic fibrosis community. One of those being Dr. Beall. "Dr. Ramsey has been recognized worldwide as an innovator and leader in caring for individuals with CF," says Dr. Beall. "She has played a pivotal role in developing many current therapies and protocols to manage CF. In addition, she was the architect of the Foundation's TDN. The TDN, working with the pharmaceutical industry, has led to accelerated completion of clinical trials critical to the improved outcomes for CF patients."

In October 1999, Dr. Ramsey also played an important role in another venture. She, along with Dr. Beall, a gentleman by the name of Paul Flessner who worked for Microsoft Corporation and had two boys with cystic fibrosis (both were patients of Dr. Ramsey), met with William H. Gates Sr., the father of billionaire and Microsoft founder, Bill Gates, and also the cochairman of the Bill and Melinda Gates Foundation established by his son and his daughter-in-law. "It was a great meeting," says Dr. Ramsey, "and he told us he would support the Therapeutic Development Program." The word "support" was perhaps an understatement as the Bill and Melinda Gates Foundation donated $20 million to the Cystic Fibrosis Foundation with the intent to put those funds toward the development of new drugs to treat cystic fibrosis. "It was really the initial gift that moved the program forward," says Dr. Ramsey.

In 2005, Dr. Ramsey became the endowed chair in cystic fibrosis at the University of Washington School of Medicine. In 2012, Dr. Ramsey was the lead author of a groundbreaking study on ivacaftor, which months later became known as Kalydeco and was the first CFTR modulator to be FDA approved. Kalydeco specifically went to the 4 percent of the CF population who had the G551D gene and increased lung function in patients six and older. Since then, the drug has been used for patients six months and older and approximately thirty-eight genetic mutations. "There have been many patients telling me the incredible impact," says Dr. Ramsey.

Dr. Ramsey was named Seattle's top doctor by *Seattle* magazine three different times between 2012 and 2017 and was named U.S. News Top Doctor in 2012 by *U.S. News and World Report*. In 2013, Dr. Ramsey decided to step down from the TDN, and two years later, she was elected as a fellow of the National Academy of Medicine. In 2018, Harvard Medical School presented Dr. Ramsey with the Warren Alpert Foundation Prize for her remarkable cystic fibrosis discoveries and was director of the Center for Clinical and Translational Research at Seattle Children's Research Institute until 2021. She is also co-principal investigator of the University of Washington (UW) Institute of Translational Health Sciences, which provides clinical research infrastructure across the University of Washington including Seattle Children's Hospital.

In 2019, her role changed. "I closed my clinical practice two years ago," says Dr. Ramsey. "I work mainly with junior faculty at this point in my career. I do a lot of faculty mentoring as I am the vice chair for research for the UW Department of Pediatrics. I lead the CF research program at UW with Dr. Pradeep Singh, so I still work a lot with CF scientists."

While Dr. Ramsey has already had a great impact on the world of CF, she has also had a lot of influence on female physicians everywhere, including her forty-two-year-old daughter, Ann (Dahlberg), the clinical director of the outpatient stem cell transplant clinic at Fred Hutchinson Cancer Research Center, who is now married with two children of her own.

"My mom's work has certainly been inspiring in my career," says Ann. "I didn't fully realize how much she had contributed to the field of CF until I was in residency. I've always thought of her just as my mom. Professional mentorship has developed over the years and really from when I ask for her advice. As I started to take care of CF patients in residency and prescribe the medications she had been instrumental in investigating, I realized the impact she had on the field. I also saw firsthand the special bond she had with her patients. I am very proud of her and awed by all she has accomplished in her career. As her daughter, however, her focus at home was always on us and our activities, so it wasn't until later in medical school and early residency that I really started to understand the impact she had, when I started to see it in person."

Ann also bonds with her patients. "I take care of patients both early and later out from transplant," says Ann. "My research focuses on cord blood transplant for patients with malignancies (leukemia and lymphoma). I certainly derive the most professional satisfaction from the relationships I have the privilege of forming with families throughout the transplant process."

Besides Ann, Dr. Ramsey has a son, Tim, born in 1981, who is an engineer. She also has four grandchildren: Dash (12), Clara (9), Penny (2), and Rosie (4 months).

Dr. Ramsey still remembers her mindset with regard to her young CF patients in Division 37 that she first worked with during her residency in Boston and the struggles many of them faced.

"I wanted to feel like I was doing something to make it better."

DR. ROBERT "BOB" BEALL

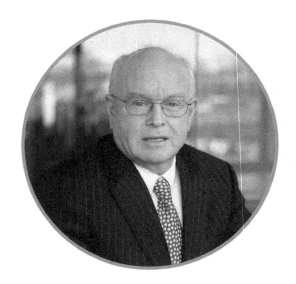

Age: 79
Resides: Rockville, Maryland
Connection to CF: Scientist and former president
and CEO of the Cystic Fibrosis Foundation

BEHIND THE SCIENTIFIC DISCOVERIES:
THE METHOD TO HIS MADNESS

"I did not experience a eureka moment when I decided to be a scientist," says Dr. Robert "Bob" Beall (pronounced Bell), who's considered by some to be the most influential contributor to the success of the Cystic Fibrosis Foundation in the sixty-five-plus years of its existence. Instead, Dr. Beall's career path gradually evolved because of meaningful educational experiences. He enjoyed math and science in high school, and initially, he decided to prepare for a career in dentistry.

"During my junior year in the pre-dental program at Albright College," says Dr. Beall, "I was taught by a gifted professor who changed the course of my career and has continued to be an influential mentor in my life. I was inspired by his enthusiasm for the possibility of discoveries in scientific research."

Motivated by his new interest in scientific research, Dr. Beall's next educational experience was a PhD program at SUNY at Buffalo. Although the graduate studies geared toward research were still interesting to him, he was more inspired by the teaching role of his professors. His mentor was a talented teacher who inspired him. As a result, Dr. Beall decided to pursue a career in academics instead of industrial research after completing his graduate degree. His career continued to evolve at Case Western Reserve University, where he completed a postdoctoral program and taught physiology courses to dental and medical students. Here, his career path took another unexpected turn.

"I had both research and teaching responsibilities while I was on the Case Western Reserve University faculty," says Dr. Beall. "In addition, because of unusual circumstances in the physiology department, I also was assigned administrative responsibilities which would not normally be given to an assistant professor."

Dr. Beall discovered that he liked the "problem solving" aspect of his administrative duties. The next step in Dr. Beall's career took him to the National Institutes of Health, where he was accepted into a training program in health administration and policy. After completing the NIH training program in 1974, he worked in the National Institute of Diabetes, Digestive and Kidney Diseases, where he was involved in implementing the National Diabetes Research and Education Act.

"Initially, I interacted mainly with the diabetes community," says Dr. Beall, "but in 1976, the director of the NIH asked me to administer the extramural cystic fibrosis program. At that time, I hardly knew how to spell cystic fibrosis and knew that I needed to learn more about the disease. The director suggested I attend a Cystic Fibrosis Foundation research conference in San Diego. During this CFF conference, I met scientists, fellows, and clinicians involved in CF research in academic institutions. I was excited by the possibility of expanding the NIH support of cystic fibrosis research. I was inspired by the courage and dedication of the parents hosting the meeting, providing both food and logistics. During informal sessions, I heard the parents' desperate pleas for help to save their children. I realized that CF research needed an infusion of NIH resources to attract new scientists and expand academic research projects. I decided to focus my NIH effort on CF. It was one of the best professional decisions of my life."

While at the conference in San Diego, Dr. Beall met Doris Tulcin, a parent of a child with cystic fibrosis and president of the Cystic Fibrosis Foundation at the time. Doris, along with Bob Dresing who also served as president of the Cystic Fibrosis Foundation for twelve years, would later become inspirational mentors in Dr. Beall's career as they were passionately dedicated to the mission of the CFF, "to find a cure and control of CF."

"When Doris Tulcin's daughter was born with cystic fibrosis," says Dr. Beall, "this inspiring mother began her relentless pursuit of a cure for the deadly disease. She recruited her family, friends, and other CF families to found the CF Foundation with the ambitious mission of 'finding a cure and control of cystic fibrosis.' The first step toward this ultimate goal was the establishment of two innovative programs—the CF Care Center network and the Patient Registry, which collected critical medical data. Doris served in various leadership positions in the foundation for more than fifty years. She was joined by Bob Dresing and Frank Deford, the iconic sportswriter, who both assumed important leadership roles in the foundation."

For three years after his initial introduction to the CF community at the conference, Dr. Beall concentrated on increasing financial support for cystic fibrosis basic research funded by the NIH extramural program. Then, in 1979, Doris Tulcin and Bob Dresing recruited Dr. Beall to be the medical scientific director of the CF Foundation. This was another pivotal decision in Dr. Beall's career as he left NIH to join the CFF.

"I hired Bob Beall from the NIH," says Doris. "I knew from observing him that he was very smart and was interested in CF and its science." Dr. Beall began his tenure at the CF Foundation on January 1, 1980.

"I feel that accepting the position with the CF Foundation was the best professional decision of my life," says Dr. Beall. "Initially, my main goal was to recruit more scientists whose research would add to the scientific knowledge about the disease and accelerate the development of new therapies. We dedicated funds to establish a network of Research Development Program (RDP) centers to conduct multidisciplinary CF research in leading academic institutions."

The first RDP center was established at the University of Alabama at Birmingham (UAB). In 1981, Alabama Governor Fob James made a four-year pledge to match the $300,000 per year commitment of the CF Foundation. Governor James had lost a son to cystic fibrosis and was passionate about building the research center at the university. When the RDP center was established at the University of Alabama at Birmingham, only a few researchers on the faculty were interested in studying cystic fibrosis. However, after the first several years, dozens of scientists at UAB were committed to CF research. By 1983, the CF Foundation had established RDP centers at the University of North Carolina and the University of California at San Francisco.

Eventually, the network was expanded to include thirteen RDP centers, and the number of peer-reviewed publications related to CF increased exponentially.

"The research conducted in the RDP centers and CFF-supported labs in other academic institutions expanded our knowledge about the basic genetic defect in cystic fibrosis," says Dr. Beall. "In addition, the growing community of scientists now committed to CF joined forces with the established care centers, which were a source of clinical trial participants, data for the patient registry, and blood and tissue samples needed for research. This union of researchers, caregivers, and patients increased the momentum in developing new approaches to therapy."

During the early '80s, research revealed that the fundamental defect in cystic fibrosis is the abnormal movement of chloride through the airway epithelial in the respiratory tract. These results provided research teams with a "working hypothesis" critical for developing new therapies. Current treatments (as of 2022) function by correcting the movement of chloride ions across membranes of affected organs and tissues in CF patients.

While some researchers concentrated on the link between the abnormal movement of chloride and the pathology of cystic fibrosis, other research teams worldwide focused on identifying the defective gene causing CF. The foundation facilitated collaboration between many leaders in the field of genetics. Among the essential early resources for genetic research were tissue and blood samples collected from thousands of CF patients and families across North America.

"To accelerate the progress toward identifying the CF gene," says Dr. Beall, "the foundation increased funding, provided tissue and blood samples for experiments, and encouraged collaboration among research teams. Multiple laboratories were now intensely focused on the search for the CF gene. The work of Dr. Francis Collins at the University of Michigan and Dr. Lap-Chee Tsui and Dr. Jack Riordan at the Hospital for Sick Children in Toronto proved to be the most important collaboration in the history of CF research. In addition to frequent contact with the collaborative Michigan-Toronto team, those of us at the foundation were closely following the progress of genetic research in Utah, Houston, NIH, London, Paris, and other locations."

During the summer of 1989, Dr. Tsui, Dr. Riordan (Toronto lab), and Dr. Collins (Michigan lab) were making excellent progress toward identifying the defective CF gene. The CF community eagerly awaited the news that researchers had discovered the underlying genetic cause of the disease. The Michigan-Toronto collaboration team was the first to submit conclusive data to *Science* magazine for peer-review. The data identified the defective CF gene that codes for a protein CFTR, which has a critical role in the movement of chloride across cell membranes throughout the body. Mutations of this gene in cystic fibrosis patients result in abnormal CFTR, which interferes with the chloride movement.

The CF Foundation worked with Drs. Collins, Tsui, and Riordan, and the university communications departments at Michigan and Toronto, and *Science* magazine to plan a joint public announcement in September 1989. The discovery of the CF gene was the most important milestone in CF history at that time. News outlets worldwide covered this groundbreaking scientific event.

Dr. Beall remembers, "It was exciting for our CF community to see Danny Bessette, a four-year-old boy with cystic fibrosis, featured on the cover of the *Science* magazine issue announcing the discovery of the CF gene. Thousands of families bought the magazine and posted the front cover on their refrigerators and mirrors."

Even before the specific defective gene was identified, researchers were exploring the possibilities of gene therapy in which a normal copy of the gene could be delivered to start normal function in the airways compromised by cystic fibrosis. The foundation held workshops with the NIH and FDA to accelerate gene therapy research, an exciting scientific topic in the early 1990s. With support from both the NIH and CFF, scientists created viruses and other molecules to carry the normal copy of the CF gene into the airways of people with CF. However, the body's immune response against the delivery agents made it impossible to effectively deliver the normal copies of the gene into the airways. This initial immune response continued and prevented the reintroduction of the normal copies of the gene needed to sustain function. Unfortunately, these first attempts were disappointing, but the collaborative research resulted in knowledge which, coupled with the utilization of more effective delivery systems, has increased the possibilities of successful gene therapy in the future. Presently, the CFF is supporting a large number of grants in gene therapy.

In 1994, Bob Dresing stepped down as president and CEO of the Cystic Fibrosis Foundation after being an inspirational leader for twelve years. "His business acumen and passionate dedication as a CF parent," says Dr. Beall, "were attributes that made him exceptionally effective in his role."

Dr. Beall continues, "I was privileged to work side by side with Bob Dresing for those years when the foundation developed into a prominent health-related charity," says Dr. Beall. "For more than twenty-five years, Bob Dresing, Doris Tulcin, and Frank Deford, all parents of children with CF, provided dynamic leadership for the foundation. I learned so much from these three amazing people and am grateful to have been touched by their passion.

"After Bob Dresing's retirement, I assumed the daunting role of president and CEO of the foundation. I immediately realized that the foundation needed a dynamic executive vice president for medical affairs. The CF community is very fortunate that Preston Campbell III, MD, accepted that challenging leadership position at a crucial stage in CF history. He was the first physician to join the CFF administrative team. Dr. Campbell recognized the urgency of our mission because he was already involved as the director of the outstanding CFF Care Center at Vanderbilt University and had served several terms on the CFF Care Center Committee. I am incredibly grateful that Dr. Campbell's expertise and perspective guided many crucial decisions during our years of shared leadership. His positive impact was immediate when he joined the CFF team and continued as president and CEO after my retirement in 2015.

"C. Richard Mattingly, Executive Vice President and COO, was our third partner leading the foundation," continues Dr. Beall. "Rich is a gifted person who has an exceptional ability to motivate people. He administered an extensive national network of CFF chapters in which countless volunteers raised millions of dollars to support CF research and expand care programs. During his thirty-year career with the CF Foundation, Rich directed multiple organizational operations with exceptional skill. His leadership provided the momentum for the grass-roots fundraising effort supporting the CFF's innovative programs."

After the defective CF gene coding for the protein, CFTR (cystic fibrosis transmembrane conductance regulator protein), was discovered, researchers began to understand the protein function in CF and non-CF cells.

"In 1999," says Dr. Beall, "the CFF administrative team, supported by the CFF Board, made the important decision to recruit biopharmaceutical companies to join the academic effort to correct the CFTR protein function in CF patients. However, since cystic fibrosis affects a relatively small population, the companies were reluctant to invest in CF drug discovery and development. Therefore, the foundation initiated the Therapeutics Development Program to engage biopharmaceutical companies in CF drug development. The program's two components are the Therapeutics Development Network (TDN) and 'Venture Philanthropy.'

"Dr. Bonnie Ramsey and her amazing team at the University of Washington established the CFF Therapeutics Development Network to provide logistical support for the multiple clinical trials required for FDA approval of new drugs. Under the inspired leadership of

Dr. Ramsey, the TDN has conducted nearly two hundred studies and clinical trials. At present, the TDN includes more than ninety centers around the country."

The foundation initiated the novel "Venture Philanthropy" program, which committed charitable funds as "seed money" to biopharmaceutical partners for CF drug development. The CF Foundation could incentivize the companies to join the CF effort by offering financial support, access to patients for the clinical trials, data from the patient registry, and shared expertise of the CF researchers and caregivers.

To provide funds for this innovative "Venture Philanthropy" program, the CFF had to increase its financial resources. Mr. Paul Flessner, the parent of two sons with cystic fibrosis, was an executive at Microsoft and Bill Gates's friend. He facilitated a meeting with Bill Gates Sr., who administered the Gates Foundation.

Dr. Beall recalls, "Dr. Bonnie Ramsey, Paul Flessner, and I went to Bill Gates's childhood home to present the drug development proposal to his father with a request for $20 million.

"After reviewing the proposal, the Gates Foundation agreed to contribute twenty million dollars to support the collaborative drug development program. Two weeks later, the twenty-million-dollar check arrived in the mail in a regular envelope with a single stamp. The Therapeutics Development Program was initiated because of the generous support of the Gates Foundation."

With the financial support of the Gates Foundation and the Therapeutics Development Network in place, the foundation initiated their bold plan to develop drugs to treat the basic defect, not just the symptoms of the disease. The CF Foundation now requested biotech companies to submit applications for CFF support for research to "identify one or two druggable molecules that could correct the CFTR defect in CF patients."

"We received several applications that were then peer-reviewed by a panel of CF experts," says Dr. Beall. "As a result, the foundation selected Aurora Biosciences as its first pharmaceutical partner. The company was already using high-throughput screening to identify new, potentially druggable targets for other diseases. Because of the Gates award and the monetary reimbursement from the development of TOBI, the foundation now had sufficient funds to commit an initial forty-six million dollars to Aurora Biosciences. The investment was a risky shot on goal, but in the words of Wayne Gretzky, 'You miss one hundred percent of the shots you do not take.'

"Soon after the collaboration began, Vertex Pharmaceuticals purchased Aurora Biosciences. Vertex hired outstanding scientists and physicians who had prior knowledge of CF.

In addition, CFF leadership and consultants from the CF community met quarterly with Vertex to evaluate progress.

"There were memorable milestones during the collaboration," continues Dr. Beall. "I remember celebrating after seeing the first data showing lung function improvement and correction of the sweat chloride defect in people participating in the drug trial for Kalydeco. I remember the call from the acting director of the FDA, Janet Woodcock, congratulating the CFF and underscoring the importance of our patient registry in the approval of Kalydeco. I remember the exciting moment watching Dr. Michael Boyle, now president and CEO of the foundation, writing an Orkambi prescription for a CFF employee as soon it was approved.

"The entire CF community was very involved in the collaborative program in multiple ways. The volunteers raised funds; the scientists conducted research; the patients participated in clinical trials; the caregivers supported the patients. The cooperative efforts of all these dedicated people contributed to the program's ultimate success. This innovative program has resulted in developing three miracle drugs— Kalydeco, Orkambi, and Trikafta. These drugs have the capability to effectively treat more than ninety percent of the CF patient population.

"I am excited to know that these chloride modulator drugs are improving the quality of life for many CF patients. This medical miracle has happened because of the tireless, cooperative efforts of the entire CF community. Outstanding volunteer leaders like Doris Tulcin, Frank Deford, Bob Dresing, Joe O'Donnell, and Catherine 'Cam' McLoud have motivated volunteers and staff.

"I am honored to have worked as 'leadership partners' with talented colleagues like Preston Campbell and Rich Mattingly. I was inspired by the dedication of staff, caregivers, researchers, volunteers, families, and courageous people coping with CF . . . all pursuing the common goal to find a cure for CF. I am proud of the sense of community created during my time at the foundation."

Dr. Beall goes on, "I still keep the CF Foundation very close to my heart. In my home office, I have a chart showing the improvement in life expectancy since the foundation began in 1955 until the present time. I am so glad to have witnessed that improvement that has continued to rise during the years since I retired. It was recently announced that the current median life expectancy is fifty years—an all-time high. I sadly realize that we lost many young people in past decades, but I also can visualize the lives of so many young people with CF who are finally living the dreams we have for all of our children."

"Bob Beall was a force dedicated to people with cystic fibrosis," says Cam McLoud, Chairman of the Cystic Fibrosis Foundation Board for more than two decades, "and he supercharged our journey toward a cure. His leadership was instrumental in creating 'shots on goal' that eventually became life-changing treatments, and his drive was key to the acceleration of CF science.

Dr. Beall and his colleagues created real hope for the CF community, and we are forever grateful to him for his passion for all people impacted by the disease and the impact that he made on all of us."

Today, Dr. Beall enjoys life with his wife, children, and grandchildren. "In the summers, we live at Deep Creek Lake in western Maryland," says Dr. Beall. "We especially enjoy visits from our children and grandchildren, who have grown up coming to the lake. Last year, Mimi and I moved to a senior community near our former home in Rockville, Maryland. We are happy participating in various activities with our new friends there. I am still in touch with friends in the CF community and am always eager to hear news of progress still being made at an amazing rate."

DORIS TULCIN

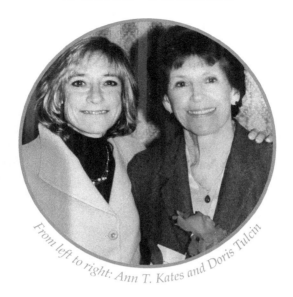

From left to right: Ann T. Kates and Doris Tulcin

Age: 93

Resides: Estero, Florida

Connection to CF: Mother to a CF warrior and former president and cofounder of the Cystic Fibrosis Foundation

THE PERSON BEHIND IT ALL: THE CREATION OF THE CF FOUNDATION

On June 14, 1953, Doris Tulcin's life changed forever. That was the day she and her husband, Bob, welcomed a baby girl by the name of Ann Elizabeth Tulcin at Doctors Hospital in New York. Ann was two weeks late and still only weighed five pounds, four ounces. She was born with a blocked intestine, and three months after birth, still only weighed eight pounds. Cystic fibrosis was rarely tested for then but based on the symptoms, Doris knew something was wrong.

One day, her friend Carrie, who was a nurse who had worked with Ann in the hospital, read an article by Dr. Dorothy Andersen who discovered what she then called "cystic fibrosis of the pancreas" in 1938 (which was later shortened to "cystic fibrosis").

Bob and Doris met Dr. Andersen at Babies Hospital—founded in 1887 and the first dedicated hospital for children in New York City—where

Ann was admitted for tests. She was given a duodenal drainage to collect stomach fluids to see which enzymes were missing. The absent enzyme was trypsin, which is produced by the pancreas and helps the body digest proteins. In babies with cystic fibrosis, blockages like the intestinal blockage Ann had can prevent trypsin from reaching the small intestine. Doris was told few doctors could treat cystic fibrosis and the tools for treatment were virtually unknown. Dr. Andersen told them that Ann would maybe live a year. With this prognosis, Doris and Bob took Ann home on September 21.

Doris developed a resolve that she was going to help Ann beat cystic fibrosis. Not only that, but she was going to make it a cause. Doris's father, George Frankel, who had established the children's ward at New Rochelle Hospital years earlier, went to bat for his daughter and granddaughter. They spoke to Dr. Ruston McIntosh, who was the chairman of pediatrics at Babies Hospital. Dr. McIntosh put them in touch with a group in Bayside, Queens. From there, Doris and her dad started to find doctors at major medical centers around the country. Washington, DC, Philadelphia, Cleveland, Boston, and Los Angeles were their first contacts. Doris was meeting with friends to determine how to fundraise for the disease.

George soon contacted Dr. Wynne Sharples, a non-practicing pediatrician and mother of two children with CF who was already working on the legal framework to start a foundation called the Children's Exocrine Research Foundation to help those with cystic fibrosis. A year later, the name was changed to the National Cystic Fibrosis Research Foundation. After meeting, George was invited to serve on her board of trustees. The new foundation was incorporated as a not-for-profit voluntary health agency in the state of Delaware. With knowledge gained from his time on the board, George helped Doris start her own chapter of the new foundation in Scarsdale, New York, in June 1956, which she ran from her basement.

Doris and her team began forming chapters and having fundraising events. Still, very little was known about CF, and kids were dying very young—many not living to the age of five. George eventually convinced Dr. Sharples to move her office from Philadelphia to New York to help gain visibility.

Meanwhile, as she sought to help a large and underserved population, Doris didn't lose sight of the root of her enthusiasm. "My mom . . . always got me to the best doctors and saw that I had the very best care," says Ann. "She also was amazing when it came to imparting information about CF to me in order to not overwhelm me and helped me to lead as normal a life as any person would, and while she took such care of me, she never made me feel different from any of my friends."

Doris had young moms over for tea to tell them about CF, as these individuals, who were unaffected by CF, were looking for something meaningful to which they could make an impact. The National Cystic Fibrosis Research Foundation was now twenty-one chapters nationwide. Seventy-five thousand dollars was raised with most of it going to research. In spring of 1957, Doris organized a luncheon in Connecticut, where, before more than three hundred women from New York and Connecticut, Connecticut Governor Abraham Ribicoff made a speech while Doris and the newly formed foundation would show a film explaining the ins and outs of cystic fibrosis. Dr. Paul di Sant'Agnese, one of the first known physicians for CF, was a speaker too. Doris also spoke, though she admits she did it impromptu as people had difficulty understanding Dr. di Sant'Agnese's Italian accent, and therefore Doris, who admitted to having a fear of public speaking, followed with a speech of her own to explain all about the disease and its effect on young people. "My first speech was the beginning of many in my long career," says Doris. "Some more meaningful and important than others."

It must have worked because national articles soon followed. National Cystic Fibrosis Week was held in November with a luncheon in Philadelphia. "Growing up, I was aware of my mom working on CF events locally," says Ann, who continued to grow and thrive along with the National Cystic Fibrosis Research Foundation. "However, I didn't participate in any of them, as my mom felt there was no need to involve me. Later in college, I was fully aware of the various roles she took on the national level."

In 1958, while still working out of her basement, Doris hired her first staff person, Katherine Earnshaw, who had been director with the Arthritis Foundation. She eventually moved her office to 110 Mamaroneck Avenue in White Plains, New York. New York Governor Averell Harriman proclaimed their first Cystic Fibrosis Week in May 1958 and Gary Moore, TV talk-show host, became their campaign manager. That week followed with a New York City luncheon sponsored by the Greater New York Chapter and the Greater New Jersey Chapter, which honored Dr. Dorothy Andersen on the twentieth anniversary of her discovery of CF. The event was big, and the momentum helped the cause to make the newspapers. Doris's chapter held its own first large luncheon in New York at the Hotel Pierre and raised $80,000, after which she began doing house fundraising tours that would become more successful with each passing year.

In May 1960, the foundation launched its first national campaign for funds. It was around this time that Doris and her father met with the March of Dimes and decided to start a center program for CF based on the March of Dimes Model. Dr. Kenneth Landauer, Medical Director of the March of Dimes, was hired to set up the program for the National Cystic Fibrosis Research Foundation. In March of 1963, the foundation became more successful than ever due to the abundance of events, including house tours, luncheons, and a movie premiere.

In 1965, with the National Cystic Fibrosis Research Foundation's fundraising success proliferating and research increasing, Doris, along with a fellow parent and her coworker, Kay, helped start a CF center in Westchester, New York. Doris and Kay worked in the clinic as coordinators, helping with all the paperwork needed and to schedule appointments. They also helped find a physician to run the practice. Thanks to their hard work and word of mouth, the clinic grew tremendously.

George Frankel passed on April 7, 1971. "Without my father," says Doris, "I would say that the foundation would have struggled for many more years than it did. He had the vision and the money to make many changes and to move it ahead. He turned down the approach from the March of Dimes to take us over. He felt that we would never become a nationally recognized disease unless we built a foundation that would educate the general public and the medical community on our own. This would be crucial to our development and to eventually finding a control or cure for CF." In late May, Doris became national trustee of the National CF Board.

In March 1973, the foundation sponsored its first international conference in Washington, DC, and that summer, the Association of Tennis Professionals (ATP) adopted the National Cystic Fibrosis Research Foundation as its national charity. Doris was a big tennis player, but the relationship was espoused by legendary sportswriter Frank Deford who not only knew the head of the ATP but whose daughter Alex also had CF (and would sadly pass away in 1980). All the big tennis players signed on. Arthur Ashe and Cliff Drysdale were honorary chairs for the Westchester Chapter's event, "A Day and Evening at Forest Hills." Tickets were sold for tennis matches, cocktails and buffet, and a chance to meet the players.

In May 1974, the National Cystic Fibrosis Research Foundation moved from New York to Atlanta, allegedly for simply cheaper office space, and Doris was elected vice president. In May 1976, and coincidentally on Mother's Day, Doris was elected president, and soon she and her team shortened the name of the foundation to the National Cystic Fibrosis Foundation (CFF). Her first initiative was to hire a new national director of the CFF.

During this time, Ann was leading a relatively normal life and began her adult journey in college. "Whatever treatment was suggested," says Doris, "she complied one hundred percent." Ann married in the fall of 1976.

In December 1976 *People* magazine did a major article on Doris and her work at the CFF, which at the time was raising $8.5 million and was composed of three hundred local chapters. Doris and her executive VP and good friend, Bob Dresing, knew that they had to move the CFF out of Atlanta because of lack of visibility in the public sector. They especially wanted more attention from the NIH, which would play a big role in research funding. It took them a while to convince the trustees but eventually they got their wish and moved the CFF to Washington, DC, with a board meeting approval in May of 1977.

As national president, Doris received her first appointment to the Advisory Council of the National Heart, Lung, and Blood Institute (NHLBI) of the NIH. During this year a study called "Cystic Fibrosis: A Plea for a Future" commenced because of the severity of CF as a medical and socioeconomic problem and requested that a study be carried out to assess current and future opportunities for improving care through research. Doris had her eye on Dr. Bob Beall and knew that once they moved the foundation from Atlanta nearer to Washington, DC, he would be interested since the foundation would be much closer in proximity to the NIH. Fortunately, she had a lot of help from her Vice President Bob Dresing.

"Bob Dresing became my most valuable partner working with the foundation for over thirty years," says Doris. "I never could have moved the foundation from Atlanta to [Bethesda, Maryland, which is within twenty miles of Washington, DC] without his support and drive. When he was the CEO [Bob Dresing would take over as CEO following Doris in 1983], in those twelve years he changed the foundation from an ordinary, hardworking, voluntary health organization to a thriving business enabling growth of activity nationwide, increasing it by millions of dollars. He literally put the CFF to the top of other competing agencies."

Bob Beall took the job—as Doris predicted when they were able to move the foundation—and began working January 1980. "In becoming our medical director," says Doris, "[Bob Beall] completely enhanced our medical and scientific programs, starting with the RDP [Research Development Program]. His approach to partnering with the NIH for additional funding, including his unconventional development of partnerships with the biomedical and pharmaceutical companies, opened the door for the breakthroughs leading to the modulators of today."

The fall of 1980 was the CFF's introduction to building the Cystic Fibrosis Foundation's Research Development Program. It was clear the CF medical world knew very little about the basic science of the disease. Doris and Bob Dresing actually got turned down by the NIH for funding, so they went to Bob Beall to ask him to put together a Research Development Program. They met with the University of Alabama at Birmingham (UAB) in what would be the first capital campaign attempted by a voluntary health agency, setting a goal among their trustees of $15 million over ten years.

In the spring of 1982, Doris was honored in Chicago by the CFF Board of Trustees for her six years as president. Bob Dresing took the reins. Doris became chairman of the Research Development Council that would be responsible for the capital campaign to support the RDP. She recruited members of the corporate world the next year to raise the money and the first starter million-dollar gift was from a generous donor of the Palm Beach Cystic Fibrosis Foundation Chapter.

In 1983, the first four RDPs applied to become official centers. First, UAB—supported by a two-million-dollar gift from Governor Fob James. Second, the University of North Carolina at Chapel Hill (UNC). Third, the University of California, San Francisco (UCSF). Fourth, Baylor College in Houston. Doris said they felt the mysteries of the disease would come from the centers where, for the first time, young investigators under senior directors were looking at CF full time. To hit their fifteen-million-dollar campaign goal, Doris was setting up regional councils in locations where the approved RDP centers had opened. They also wanted to make their presence felt in Washington, DC, the home of the NIH. They would do this with a social venue, a children's ball that would invite the support of the White House. Joan Clark, wife of President Reagan's National Security Advisor William Clark, became their first chairperson. In early summer, over $28 million was raised in the RDP campaign. Twelve RDP centers were established.

"I was aware of her traveling to start the Center program throughout the country, where she began to work on R and D in conjunction with taking care of patients," says Ann, "and I was very proud of what she was doing to help the CF community."

The Board of Trustees established the Doris F. Tulcin Research Award. The first one going to CF patient and scientist Paul Quinton for his work on sodium absorption. Doris was also honored for her volunteer work at the National Health Council where she served fifteen years. By May of 1987, she was finishing her second appointment at the NIH on the NHLBI Advisory Council.

In January 1988, Doris began working at the CF Foundation in the New York office as she worked on major gifts. Doris wanted to raise more money than was already being raised so she became the executive director of the Greater New York Chapter—a position she held for eighteen years.

"I [officially] retired [from the CFF in 2005] at the age of 78," says Doris who, at age ninety-three, is the CFF Chairman Emeritus, serves as a member of the national board, supports CFF's agenda, and is still an active supporter of her local chapter. In 2008, she wrote *Memoirs of a Monarch* in which she revealed her incredible journey to making a difference in the world of cystic fibrosis. "I enjoy my family, my friends, and playing cards," says Doris. "I moved to Florida just four years ago along with Ann and her family."

Doris's contributions to the CF Foundation are immeasurable. "I am grateful for all the wonderful volunteers and staff that I have worked with over fifty-five years with the CFF," says Doris. "My greatest accomplishments were trying to find ways to save lives, moving the foundation from Atlanta to Bethesda to be closer to the NIH, creating the care centers, but most importantly, the creation of the RDP centers where the gene was discovered, supported by the first capital campaign ever undertaken by a voluntary health organization."

"My mom," says Ann, "has several extraordinary assets: perseverance, determination, vision, and not accepting the status quo, and intelligence. Those exceptional traits were put to good use with regard to the CF Foundation in developing various medical advancements, including CFTR modulators."

"We both were thrilled when the gene modulators became available," says Ann, who began Trikafta upon its approval in the fall of 2019. "With the approval of Trikafta, my mom and I were absolutely thrilled as it represented the culmination of all of my mom's and her colleagues'—including doctors, scientists, and CF staff and volunteers—extraordinary commitment to helping CF patients lead better lives and longer lives."

Ann just turned sixty-eight and has been married to her husband Dave for forty-five years. "As a woman who has CF, who is now in her late sixties," says Ann, "I am eternally grateful for the extraordinary research and care of the CF population that the foundation has provided throughout my lifetime. I am appreciative of the vision that my mother had with the support of her family in starting the foundation, as they believed that people with CF could lead productive lives. I have been fortunate in having outstanding doctors who have enabled me to access the pipeline of medications that tame infections and activate the CFTR protein through the generation of gene modulators that have been developed. I hope that others have experienced the positive results that I have in my life."

Ann continues inspiring Doris as an educator while raising her own family. Both of Ann's children have graduated college and start-ed families of their own—making Doris a *great*-grandmother. "As grandmother and great-grandmother, [Doris] is incredibly loving and devoted and generous," says Ann. "She is always present for her grandchildren, and she enjoys visits from her great-grandchildren when she sees them."

While cystic fibrosis brought a lot of difficult times and hard work to her life, Doris knows her life would not be the same without it. "My life has been extremely meaningful and positive as a result of CF entering my life, as I have met so many wonderful people along the way," says Doris, who still speaks frequently with her "good friends" Bob Beall and Bob Dresing. "To see the results of my work over the years has truly been amazing. I am astounded at the lega-cy that the CFF will leave not only for all the patients and families but for all the other disease organizations who are struggling to gain the successes that we have. It's truly a miracle. The CFTR modula-tors have caused life-changing results for those who are eligible. Still more work to be done for many others."

2

TELLING MY STORY: THE VALUE OF TRANSPARENCY

LIAM WILSON

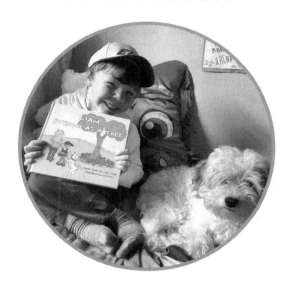

Age: 6
Resides: Milton, Ontario, Canada
Age at Diagnosis: 3 weeks

STRONG AS A TREE: THE SIX-YEAR-OLD AUTHOR'S STORY

Six-year-old book author Liam Wilson was born on Valentine's Day 2015 at Oakville Trafalgar Hospital. Labored breathing and a concerning amount of weight loss over his first three weeks led doctors to test for CF. The test came back positive. "We were shocked and heartbroken," says his mom, Deana. "But we vowed to be proactive."

Liam needs medication with all his meals to help him digest food, regular airway clearance to bring the mucus up, a prescription nebulizer he inhales twice a day—more when he's sick—and postural drainage, which Deana administers morning and night. "I don't always like doing it," says Liam of his treatment, "but I know it makes me better." Deana also had the support of her father, Wane, Liam's grandfather, who he referred to as "Grandpa." "My dad was prouder than punch of Liam," says Deana. "He was his whole world. Everything revolved around [his grandson]."

Liam is already a big advocate for CF awareness. His first year of the Walk to Make Cystic Fibrosis History in Milton, Team Liam raised $10,000. "Liam is a superhero," says his proud mom, who continues to lead the fundraising efforts and hopes to pass the torch to Liam as he gets older. "He shows strength and perseverance as he overcomes all these obstacles, and he continues to do it with a smile. His war is one that we hope will never take over his life, so I fight as his mother to do whatever I can to find a cure."

At the age of four, Liam announced that he wanted to explain his condition to his friends. "I never want to be any different than anyone else," says Liam. Deana remembers her precocious son telling her, "I want them to know my story." So he and Deana looked for an age-appropriate book that might help them communicate Liam's experiences. Since they couldn't find a good CF children's book, Liam suggested to his mom that they make their own.

Deana immediately thought of her aunt Leesa, who is an illustrator and joined their editorial board right away. Then she searched for publishers around Toronto and found Iguana Books, a non-traditional Toronto-based book publisher that considers the author's vision and, if publisher Meghan Behse and her team are excited about the potential for a fruitful partnership, will help the author to budget for the making of the book and advise on how to finance the project—namely, crowdfunding. If the book can be financially supported, Iguana will help the author—in this case, author and illustrator—begin the act of creation and publish and distribute physical copies. So Deana launched a Kickstarter campaign on Liam's birthday, which quickly resulted in the sale of two hundred books, enough for Iguana to agree to fully participate and send it to press!

The result would translate into a children's book titled *Liam, Strong as a Tree*.

"A big tree in our backyard inspired the metaphor for our experience," says Deana. "Trees need lots of oxygen from the air, just like Liam's lungs. And trees need food from the ground, just like Liam's stomach. At times, our actual tree has gotten sick, so Liam and I have had to give it special food and extra love, leading it to grow big and strong again. I tell Liam it's just like when he takes his enzymes."

Deana says Liam was so excited when he was finally able to hold the actual book. "See, Mommy?!'" she recalls him exclaiming as he held up the book, "I will never give up on anything!" With little marketing, *Liam, Strong as a Tree* has sold more than eight hundred copies. Fifty percent of the proceeds from the book go to Milton District Hospital.

"They loved it!" says Liam about his friends' reaction to the book, which depicts Liam showing all his peers and teachers his enzymes and his mask on the first day of kindergarten. "I want them to understand me and know I'm no different than them," he says. "When I'm sick, it takes longer for me to get better, but I just do things differently than them."

About being a published author, Liam says, "It feels amazing! I'm so proud."

Among Liam's favorite activities are bike riding with his friends, bouncing on his indoor trampoline, and playing with his cockapoo rescue therapy dog, Chloee, who's been especially comforting during the pandemic. But nothing captures his attention like his Toronto Maple Leafs and favorite player Auston Matthews. Matthews advocates for the SickKids Foundation, one of Liam's patient support systems and an organization for which Deana put together a fundraising event called, "SuperStarrs 2 SuperHeros," which was attended by seven hundred kids and parents who were invited to dress up as their favorite superhero (Liam dressed as The Flash). "[Liam] always yells at the screen when Auston scores or almost scores," Deana says, laughing.

Liam's health, to this point, has been pretty good, having avoided hospitalizations since his three-week stay when he was born. Liam switched over to SickKids in Toronto in June 2021 and has become one of the hospital's ambassadors. His mom was concerned because CF patients in Canada were still fighting for access to Trikafta, a life-changing CF drug. "He doesn't like his cough and he wants me to take it away, and that broke my heart as his mom knowing there was medication out there and we didn't have access to it." Thankfully, in October 2022, Trikafta was finally approved in Canada, though Liam will still have to wait a little bit longer, as the drug has not been approved yet for his age group. "I have waited his whole life to be told there is this miracle drug, and he can get his hands on it," says Deana. "It was the most amazing day of our lives."

Deana says that she tries to build confidence in him as he slowly grows up. Deana says Liam's many supporters around town call him "Milton's Little Superhero." "We have instilled in Liam that he can never give up. He's already proven that he's a fighter and a champion. Every single day he surprises us with the way he looks at the world and deals with this awful disease."

Liam's future aspiration is to become a police officer, but his more immediate goal is to publish the second book he's currently working on, which is about the passing of his grandpa to whom he lost just three days prior to his sixth birthday from his own chronic lung issues and to whom he credits his resilience. "Never ever give up on anything," says Liam. "My grandpa told me that."

JESSICA FRANKLIN

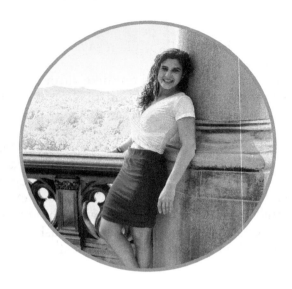

Age: 27
Resides: Tampa, Florida
Age at Diagnosis: 3 ½

BREATH OF LIFE: JESSICA'S CF JOURNEY

When Jessica Franklin met fellow CF warrior Colette Bleistine, Jessica was twenty pounds underweight and wearing an IV in school. She was in the eleventh grade and says that it was the first time her friends saw her as "sick." "I never looked 'sick,'" says Jessica. "And I always considered myself healthy. Before then, I had an outstanding FEV1 ranging from 90 to 111. If I was at ninety, I was hospitalized or on IVs, but I considered myself one of the lucky ones without a harrowing survival story."

Jessica's mom, Valerie, admitted that when Jessica was diagnosed, she had never heard of cystic fibrosis, but she knew something was wrong with her daughter because she was suffering from malabsorption. "I constantly battled our pediatrician's lack of concern that there was something wrong," says Valerie. "He finally agreed to a stool sample test and that lead to the sweat test at three and a half years old." On July 1, 1998, Jessica's parents would meet at a hospital conference room with the chief of pulmonology and his assistant. "The chief confirmed the sweat test results, and we were numb and in disbelief," says Valerie. "How could this be? There was no family history of the disease." But she and Jessica's father, Michael, educated themselves quickly and immediately helped her develop a healthy daily regimen.

"Each day, I'd wake up at 5:30 in the morning to put on her oscillating vest, feed her a pill, having cleaned or sterilized the nebulizing tools the day before to make sure they were germ-free the next time she uses them," says Michael.

As Jessica grew up, Valerie and Michael not only helped keep Jessica organized with her medications but they also strongly encouraged physical activity. They showed up to cheer her on at all her softball and soccer games, and Michael even created special workout routines for her.

"I woke up every morning at six a.m. before high school and ran for thirty minutes or reluctantly wore my vest if the weather was bad," says Jessica. "If I was too tired, I would push and work out at night. If my knees ached, I'd bike instead."

"Jessica was always an active child," says Michael. "We encouraged her to play sports. Our pulmonologist encouraged exercise as part of Jessica's daily treatment and stated that a vest treatment could be replaced with a vigorous exercise session. That's what helped inspire Jessica to incorporate exercise as part of her life."

Jessica eventually transitioned from team sports to running. "I realized I was only playing to benefit my lungs. I wasn't good at the 'sport' but rather good at just the running part. In college, that transpired to joining the running club and truly only competing against myself. Running was like breathing to me. The more I did it, the longer I would live."

As Jessica got older, she also began taking more of a leading role in the CF fundraising arena. Jessica began volunteering for the Cystic Fibrosis Foundation when she was just eight years old. "I spoke at small events—walk-a-thons, carnivals, and rock shows," says Jessica. "I also did a commercial when I was twelve to promote Great Strides across the country."

Both pairs of Jessica's grandparents have been together for more than sixty years. "That synergy evolved into giving back," says Jessica. "They played an integral part in our fundraising to help their own grandchild and others just like me with CF." The family was constantly doing events to raise money for the Cystic Fibrosis Foundation Delaware Valley Chapter, beginning two months after Jessica was diagnosed with an event they created called "Jessica's Carnival of

Fun." The event was held at a local park and brought together the community to promote awareness and raise money for CF research. The event went on for several years and cumulatively raised more than 250,000$. "Money buys science, and science saves lives," says Valerie who says she has learned that from working with the CF Foundation. Valerie and Michael played an integral role in the Philadelphia Eagles black-tie fundraising events at which the team's players would show up in support. All told, Jessica figures that during their twenty-year tenure supporting the Cystic Fibrosis Foundation, her family has raised over $10 million.

Up until her junior year in high school, Jessica seemed to be on a good roll, flying by without too many consequences from her chronic disease. To that point, she was maintaining a 4.3 GPA, was a member of the National Honor Society, and was partaking in numerous productions from musicals to plays from fifth grade up through high school. But suddenly, her CF symptoms started to flare up and interrupted her life. Over several years to come, she underwent six grueling sinus surgeries. "My cavities were impacted with thick, rock-hard, emerald-colored mucus that settled near my brain and created constant pressure."

While she kept up with her two and a half hours of treatments a day, not to mention an intense exercise regimen primarily consisting of daily runs or bike rides, Jessica spent many days of her crucial junior year of high school in and out of the hospital. "I was able to maintain my GPA, but my standardized college test scores suffered tremendously during bouts of my illness."

Then, she met Colette. Colette was the "hero" speaker at the Breath of Life Gala in center city Philadelphia, an impactful CF fundraising event. Jessica was supposed to be at a dance with her boyfriend that evening; however, due to a snowstorm, the dance was canceled, therefore, allowing her and her boyfriend, already dashingly dressed, to join her family at her first CF gala. Her parents were always reluctant to permit Jessica to be around too many people with CF due to bacterial cross-contamination. Because of the blizzard, her family was notified that there was likely only one other person with CF in attendance—that being Colette.

"My mom mentioned to me in the car that the hero speaker could be very sad," says Jessica, "but I told her I was strong." Jessica listened to Colette captivate the audience. "I didn't cry until the very end. I ran to the bathroom and bawled my eyes out," says Jessica. "Then I saw Colette when I returned. We carefully maintained a safe distance apart when we met, instantly bonding over our mutually shared life challenge—our dreaded disease. I realized right away how tiny her arms were when comparing my body to hers. Even though she was dressed to the nines, you could see there was something wrong. Her cheeks were puffy. Her arms and legs didn't have much meat on them. She was very poised though. I congratulated her, and we talked."

Maintaining the six-foot-apart rule, they conversed while discovering that they had a lot in common. It turned out the two shared the same gene mutations, experienced many of the same adolescent and physical issues and were seeing the same doctors. "Honestly, it felt like fate meeting her at the time that I did," says Jessica. "I needed an angel to guide me in the right direction for my health and for my sanity. She was the only one who understood what I was going through." They exchanged numbers and in the ensuing days "texted constantly."

The rest of the evening, Jessica was so impressed by Colette's positive outlook on life despite everything she had experienced. It changed Jessica's perspective on seeing CF as an obstacle.

Colette told her to be proud of her CF and not to be ashamed of displaying IVs and anything else CF-related. "She always had some solution to fix my issues and how to overcome something with a positive outlook," says Jessica. Colette encouraged Jessica to switch her gastroenterologist, which Jessica believes helped her not only avoid a g-tube, but it may have even saved her life. "I never thought a twenty-year-old could know more than a doctor," says Jessica. "She had solutions that many of us wouldn't even think of. Doctors didn't even think of them."

Colette inspired Jessica to tell her own story, so Jessica ended up creating a documentary. She entered 2 *People in 1 Body* into the WHYY Film Awards in October 2013 and took first place. "I was ecstatic," says Jessica, "but Colette was the first one to come to my mind when I won."

Sadly, within a short period of time, Colette lost her battle to CF. She was the one person Jessica deemed her go-to CF buddy and her loss still digs a hole into her heart every time she thinks of her. Colette, who was on the transplant list, lived only twenty-two years. "She wasn't healthy, even when we met," says Jessica. "I came home one day, and my mom was in tears and told me that Colette had passed away, and I hyperventilated. I could not breathe."

"I never felt such a pain in my heart," says Jessica. "Losing Colette was worse than any breakup I could ever go through. I couldn't understand. I lost my sense of faith in God." And yet, while Jessica only knew Colette for nine months, "she made the most impact on my life," says Jessica, "how I looked at life, how life should be lived, and how struggles should be overcome." Jessica says that while she questioned how she could still be alive while so many people she knew with CF had passed, she eventually came to the conclusion that her reason for living was to tell their stories. That included Erin McKenna, whom she met in 2019.

"I was working with ABC and NBC and produced a piece regarding the movie *Five Feet Apart*. I produced the piece from my desk while I sent a camera guy to film her. Later, we ended up video chatting and talking about everything. With Colette, I could not do anything to help. I truly had no idea how quickly she had gone downhill. With Erin, I was able to send care packages to help her gain weight. I would write to her on a weekly basis. She was there for me while I was there for her . . . until she passed away in 2020. Colette and Erin have become my angels," says Jessica. "I don't turn to a higher power. I turn to those I knew. All the symbolism in my life leads back to those who have made it and those who haven't."

Jessica eventually attended Drexel University in Philadelphia where she became a sister of Delta Phi Epsilon whose charity, ironically, just happened to be the Cystic Fibrosis Foundation. Jessica helped coordinate the Deepher Dude event, a male beauty pageant, which raised over $75,000 in one year to benefit the CFF. While putting together this big event, Jessica decided to honor Colette's memory. She made chocolate-covered pretzels, called "Coletezels," and fundraised selling them outside in the freezing cold to students—something she'd also done in high school during intermissions for school musicals and plays.

On her last day of college, Jessica made her college cap with Colette's saying written on top of it . . . "Your problems are never bigger than your purpose." There was also a picture of Colette who had never had the opportunity to graduate. "I wanted to give her that recognition to show the world how much she accomplished even after she died," says Jessica.

In college, Jessica's battle with CF was getting more challenging. "I was in and out of the hospital in college," says Jessica, "getting IV meds and more sinus surgeries." Jessica never gave up on her goals and dreams though. "I graduated Drexel with a 3.8 GPA (honors), a major in TV production and a minor in film and business, all while taking care of my health and taking on a multitude of internships during my studies." Jessica went on to work for local affiliates at ABC and NBC News from 2015 to 2019. At the end of 2019, she moved to Tampa where she got her feet wet working in real estate. Recently, she took a job close to heart as she works for the St. Joseph's Hospital Foundation doing marketing and communications to assist in fundraising for special equipment for the hospital.

On November 14, 2019, Jessica's life changed. "I received Trikafta," says Jessica. "This drug did miracles for me. Hours after taking it, I was able to smell again, after four years of not being able to. After a month of taking it, I was able to get off every nebulizer, vest treatment, and puffer. I received two and a half hours back to my day! It has been a little over a year since I have done these treatments, and I have maintained a 106% FEV1 lung function, just by exercising. I was able to put that time to good use with working harder and being able to achieve my five-year goal of buying my own place at the age of twenty-five. And for the first time in my life, I am truly planning my future for a 'normal life.'"

Jessica says she is also putting some of the added time to her day to work out five to seven days a week. She now wakes up between 5:30 a.m. and 8 a.m. most mornings and does jump training, runs three to five miles, Zumba, yoga, boot camp, barre, tennis, and weight training. She has competed in 5Ks, 10Ks, and even half-marathons. "When I race, I think about all of those who have lost their lives and their battles to CF, and I run not only for myself but for those who have perished."

Jessica continues to contribute to CF awareness in her spare time. Years later, she was asked to speak at the Breath of Life Gala in Philadelphia, and she helped raise over $1,000,000 in one night where she honored Colette. Coincidentally, the event was at the same location where Colette and Jessica had met several years prior. Soon after, Jessica traveled to the Capitol to march on the hill and individually speak to the House of Representatives in regard to requesting increased funding for the NIH. Jessica served on the Youth Advisory Board of CHOP (Children's Hospital of Philadelphia) for eight years representing the CF community while helping to change hospital policies.

"We helped create and pick out the interior for new buildings," says Jessica, "making them kid-friendly. We got to help create pajamas for the patients that were fashionable and worked based upon their medical conditions. We designed and created an entire kid-friendly café that allowed everyone to choose options based on their diets." Jessica is now the face of Genzyme Pharma for those with cystic fibrosis. "I worked for them as an intern and traveled the country to tell my story. I sat on the board for a women's group in regard to adult CF symptoms. I also sat on the board for a CF research study to help collect data across the USA."

Jessica currently volunteers for the CF Foundation, as well as the Make-A-Wish Foundation. She plays the guitar and even wrote a song about CF called "65 Roses" that raises money to benefit those with CF.

Jessica's motto is simple. "If you focus that negative energy and do something positive for someone else, it will help minimize your pain and improve your mental outlook on life."

NICK KELLY

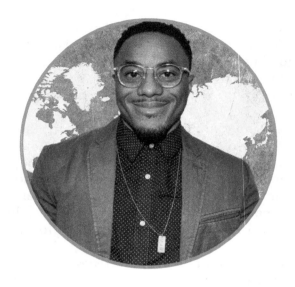

Age: 34
Resides: Cleveland, Ohio
Age at Diagnosis: 3 months

BRIDGING THE GAP: UNITING CLINICIANS AND PATIENTS

Nick Kelly is a person of many passions. He is a dietitian, motivational speaker, professional dancer, poet, advocate, teacher, and former TEDx presenter. He is also one of the rare African Americans living with cystic fibrosis.

Only one in sixty-five African Americans are carriers of the CF gene compared to one in twenty-nine Caucasians. Nick says his CF journey started at three months when his mother, Sheila, had to diagnose him because, "thirty-four years ago people didn't believe African Americans could have this disease." Nick's mother did the research, learned the symptoms, and managed to identify what was wrong with him.

"My mother's relentlessness, drive, and curiosity are elements that have carried on and resonated throughout my life," says Nick. Growing up in Cleveland, Ohio, Nick describes his childhood as relatively normal, but might jar the average reader when he unflinchingly adds, "despite having CF and open-heart surgery when I was five." Nick spent six months in the hospital after the ASD (atrial septal defect) repair surgery (fixing a hole in his heart). He adds that he currently lives with liver disease, kidney disease, CFRD, and several food allergies. "Otherwise, I felt like any other kid."

He also says that being African American and having cystic fibrosis, while rare, did not make him feel different. "It doesn't feel like anything," says Nick, "as I have always been unique and an outlier, thus this was just one more example of that. I have CF, true; I am African American, true; but I never felt the need to specifically intertwine the two past my initial diagnosis story. I am aware when I meet other African American [people with CF], because it is less common, but it stops there for me. Yes, every now and again people will be surprised when I tell them I have CF, as it always comes with a 'Really? You? Hmm, I didn't know that was a thing . . .'"

Nick says that growing up, he did not talk about his CF much. "I was open to answering questions," he says, "for example, when kids asked why I took enzymes or needed a chest protector when I played baseball. However, even that was few and far between because I did all I could to be seen as normal. I knew I had to take medicine, but it was incorporated into my life. I had a lot of support from my friends and family. I wasn't treated differently because I had CF. I was held to the same standards, and I had the same opportunities. I pretty much did all the same things my siblings did [Nick has an older sister, Gabe, and a twin sister, Nicole, and neither has CF]. I did not want special treatment, and I never got it. Everything was expected and thus everything was earned. My parents made sure of that. I was not allowed to use my disease as an excuse. My family even made games out of my PD (postural drainage) time. One of the games we had was who could hit Nick the hardest. My cousin Allen always won. He seemed to have a whole lot of pent-up aggression toward me. I even made games out of taking my pancreatic enzymes. As a kid, I would see how slyly I could take them, like a secret agent."

Nick continues, "I got to travel and play competitive sports and even managed to be All-State in wrestling and baseball. I started playing baseball when I was six years old. My dad was my coach. By the time I was thirteen, I was playing in international competitions against teams like Mexico. I was recognized as a top standout. By the time I was sixteen, I tore my ACL, and my baseball career ended. I started wrestling at the end of eighth grade. I was about ninety-two pounds. My friend Donte asked me if I wanted to wrestle because they kept forfeiting that weight. Little did anyone know, I took to it. By my freshman year, I had a stellar record. I started to get ranked. I went up two weights my sophomore year for health reasons. My junior and senior year I was ranked number twenty-five in the state and beat four people ahead of me, including the number four wrestler in the state of Ohio."

When Nick was fourteen, he was in GI discomfort and had fifteen endoscopy procedures in the span of six months. "During the last one, I went to the hospital and one doctor said we were going to try something different so we can try and get different results. Another doctor came in. We started talking. His energy was off, like he didn't want to be there. We were talking about my symptoms. He says 'I've got to go' in the middle of me answering his questions. He set down his binder. I asked my mom, 'Am I allowed to grab that?' She said that it was my chart so why not. I've never opened my chart before. The first thing I read is 'I believe Nick is a hypochondriac and that this is a ploy for attention.'

"I had never been so crushed by anything. The idea that someone who was supposed to be caring for me didn't believe I was having these symptoms because they couldn't find anything. He came back in. I said, 'You know what? You can go.' I handed him his binder and said, 'I believe this is yours.' My actual doctor came in later and we discussed what happened. They eventually found polyps that were hidden in the lining of my intestines which was what was causing me so much pain." While Nick admits the situation with the doctor was traumatic, it inspired Nick to become a clinician, or as he refers to himself, "a professional patient with clinical training."

Despite all the GI problems, Nick tried not to let these things dim his spirits. He preaches, "The world will not care if you are different but will notice if you are extraordinary."

While Nick adjusted to his physical symptoms, he had difficulty adjusting mentally to the realities of CF. And it was more than just the GI discomfort. "I was sixteen the first time I realized how scary CF could be," he says. "Prior to this, I had never viewed CF as scary; it was simply a normal part of my life. However, this all changed when I lost my best friend Nick Statford." Nick says he, his friend Nick, and their friend Michele Held, who he also referred to as Shelly (all of whom had CF), were inseparable. Nick understands the six-foot rule is something that is widely accepted in the CF community, and he knows that not everyone is in favor of going against it, but he says things were different when he was growing up.

He met Michele Held and Nick Statford in CF camp prior to concerns about bacterial cross-contamination. "There was more risk for me *not* knowing those people than knowing those people," says Nick. "I understand infection protocol and the need for infection control. I understand that there is a choice and as long as you're educated about said choice then that's what matters. I don't knock anyone for going the other way if they don't knock me for going my way. For me, I'd rather have people with CF in my life than not have them. I learned more from my CF friends than I learned from my clinicians collectively."

He says of Michele and Nick, "We were the three musketeers. They were both a few years older than me. Nick meant so much to me. He gave me confidence to be an artist. He was the first person to support my desire for poetry, which is my first love. He wrote an absurd poem for camp. He said, 'See all this? Tell your own story and people listen.'" To this day, when Nick writes poems, he refers to himself as Samuel Vincent. Samuel is his middle name and Vincent was Nick Statford's middle name. He enjoys paying homage to his close friend.

Nick Statford passed away at the age of nineteen. Michele would pass away at age twenty-seven. "There was no separation between us," says Nick. "When Nick passed, I went into depression. I didn't really want to do anything. It took me a long time to navigate. Wrestling was a great distraction at that time. After the funeral, I went to my wrestling meet. People asked me why I was there. I needed something different. I'm a huge competitor. I'm so competitive that I hate losing more than I love winning. Being around that spirit is what I needed. That experience was rock bottom. When Nick passed, it was like, 'Wow, CF is a real thing. This can happen.'

"This was the first time I truly lost someone to this disease," says Nick. "This, coupled with the fact I was with him weeks before his passing, shook my understanding of CF and forced me to see the gravity of this disease.

"With Michele," says Nick, "I had spent twenty years with her versus only twelve with Nick. So, when she died, that broke me in so many pieces, and I still haven't put them back together, and it has been nine years."

Nick Statford and Michele Held sadly were not the last friends he lost to CF. "Losing person after person is trying," says Nick. "Some of the most important parts of me are a direct result of the mark they left. I have experienced extreme highs and devastating lows around this disease. I have met some of the best people I've known and lost some of the best people I've known because of this disease. I say this to let people understand the totality and gravity of this disease. Allowing people to understand the weight of the statement, 'I wouldn't trade it for anything.' Cystic fibrosis does not define me, but it has shaped who I've become."

Nick says that like Nick Statford, Michele played an integral role in his success even after she was gone. "Michele always told me, 'Nick, tell your story. You have a good story. You have a way of telling it. You can help people.' I didn't want to do it. When she passed, I found myself in such a broken state; in order to work through things, I told my story as a healing process. The irony was when Michele told me to tell my story because it would help someone, I never thought it would be me I would end up helping. That's how I became a public speaker. I started speaking at small events like Great Strides. No one is immune to the trials and tribulations of life but all we can do is to try and find the best way to navigate it."

After high school, Nick went to college at Bowling Green State University with his sister Nicole where he completed his undergrad in dietetics and his master's in food and nutrition. "I actually went for computer technology," says Nick. "The second I got to Bowling Green, they got rid of computer technology and changed it to computer science. I wanted to transfer to a school that had computer technology. There were only four schools that still had the program I wanted. Most of those were on the West Coast. I always wanted to move west. I didn't want to do it at the beginning of the semester, so I planned on leaving after the first semester.

"My sister was a biology major. She had to take this nutrition class. She asked several times that I take the class with her. She even said she'd do my homework for the class. I finally agreed. The professor was Dr. Julian Williford (Dr. Joe). The way he talked about nutrition was the greatest puzzle I needed to solve. The class was so fascinating. After one day I called my mom and asked her, 'How do you feel about me being a dietitian?' I changed my major the next day.

"College provided me with my first real test at managing my care," says Nick. "I have always felt I was given the tools to succeed versus shortcomings that lead to failure."

After college, Nick became a registered and licensed dietitian. He even wrote a book called *No Need for Seconds*, a high-calorie cookbook. However, nutrition was only one of Nick's interests. "One of my most notable passions is dance," says Nick, who has been a professional hip hop dancer for twelve years. "I first started dancing when I was thirteen at a skating rink. I had no rhythm. As I got further into it, at the age of sixteen, I started doing my wrestling warmups in clubs and people started doing it with me. I got invited to clubs to dance, and I even got paid to do so. I did that until I was twenty-one. I ran into an organization called 'I Am D.A.N.C.E.,' and I would eventually join the board. Seeing the difference between what I could do and what those dancers did showed me that while I had gotten paid, I was not a professional dancer.

"I decided to elevate my training; I took classes at the Broadway Dance Academy in New York. I started understanding musicality. A year later, I now felt like a peer and that I could truly call myself a professional dancer. I started commanding payment for my performances and got paid enough that it could be my sole income. I've been blessed enough to travel the country. I've opened for national recording artists such as Juicy J, Kirko Bangz, MGK, and Teyana Taylor at venues for ten thousand or more fans. Dance has connected me with so many people and unbelievable opportunities. I eventually retired from it after practicing and performing for years."

Nick continues, "I still put a lot of time in public speaking. I'm like a professional athlete because I watch my speeches like game film. I did thirty-four speeches in 2019. I already had booked four speeches in 2020, and then the pandemic happened. That derailed my speaking. I'm now trying to navigate back."

Nick's success in so many diverse skills brought him back to his greatest passion: publicly advocating for those suffering with CF, specifically by bridging the gap between clinicians and patients: "By presenting information on both sides," he says, "and showing examples of how we can better communicate and better blend. Say we have a fifteen-year-old girl who is not taking her enzymes because she doesn't want anyone to know she has CF. It is our job as clinicians to fix the question that was asked and not answer the question that we feel should be answered. What I mean by that is the answer shouldn't be 'Well, I understand what your concerns are but they're eventually going to have to know about your disease, and if they care for you, taking medicine shouldn't change that.' However, that's not the question that was asked. The question asked is, 'How do I take my enzymes where I still don't have to disclose to my friend that I have CF?' The answer you should give is, 'What I suggest is you keep them in your pocket and when dinner is arriving, tell your friend you have to use the bathroom, take a sip of water, and when you get in the bathroom, swallow your pills and go back to the table. Now no one has to know, and you got your medicine in. It's up to you when you want to tell your friends.' It's my job to answer the question that was asked and not provide an answer for the question we think should be asked."

A big year for Nick was 2019. He was a special guest on *The Jim Rome Show* for the Super Bowl in Atlanta where NFL football star and CF advocate Jarvis Landry, who lost his high school sweetheart to the disease, surprised Nick with two free Super Bowl tickets on national TV for Nick's work with the Cystic Fibrosis Foundation. He gave a TEDx Talk entitled "Healing through the Human Experience," in which he explained the nature of cystic fibrosis and the importance of improving communications with an emphasis on the patient-clinician dynamic. He spoke with the FDA on behalf of patient advocacy. He also became the author of *The Adventures of Miss Messy Suzie McGoo*, the story of a little girl with CF who lives for adventure while navigating the special lung therapy that helps her remain healthy and strong.

But on April 9, 2020, Nick's work would come to an abrupt halt when he was diagnosed with COVID. "COVID broke me," he says. "It didn't physically break me. It tried, but it mentally broke me. Physically, it ravaged me. I thought it would last a few days and be over with, but instead I spent fourteen days in strict isolation in the University Hospitals in Cleveland." Nick's symptoms would flare up and subside during that period, and he would often require oxygen. "One day after my positive test, I had my first acute respiratory distress (ARD) episode," he says.

"I was resting most of the day and within twenty minutes of answering the phone, walking to the door, and talking with nurses and doctors, I went from being okay to feeling as if I was hit by a Mack Truck. I was exhausted, with chest tightness and difficulty breathing. I was able to sleep it off after several hours and started to feel like myself again. Fast-forward to Saturday, where similar to Friday, I was resting, on the phone with my cousin Josh—who was helping me take my mind off stuff—we got off the phone so I could do my treatments and boom, this time within ten minutes, Mack Truck. However, the difference was this time I didn't just need sleep, I needed oxygen (two liters)."

Nick was able to communicate. He was just exhausted with the same symptoms as before. However, this episode lasted well into the night, much longer than Friday's ARD. Onto Sunday where he was laying down and barely got up. "It was a lazy day, just some TV and me," he says. "I remember sitting up to make a call for dinner and *boom*! I started experiencing a pain I had never felt before. I couldn't breathe, I couldn't speak, and the pain was so intense, I began to dig my nails into the tray table in front of me as my eyes filled with tears and claw marks appeared on the table. In two-point-five seconds, I had gone from calm and peaceful to something I had never experienced. Understand, I've been through a lot but never this. This felt like someone was pouring hot lava down my throat and into my lungs as someone else tried to rip my lungs out from the front and back simultaneously.

"I had to use my phone to type messages, as I had to savor each breath. I had to be carried to the bed a mere two and a half feet away. In a matter of minutes, my respirations more than doubled to thirty-eight, my pulse ox [O_2 saturation] dropped to the lowest I have seen in my adult life—ninety-two, that's bottoming out for me. I was placed on over four liters of oxygen so I could complete half sentences. I was given lidocaine through a nebulizer all with the efforts to ease my struggles. A code white was also called [the hospital rapid response team]. This ARD lasted well into the next day, making the pattern of what seemed to be daily ARD episodes longer and [more] intense with each one. The physical toll these events took on me are one thing, but the mental toll was just as severe, if not worse.

"All told, I was in the hospital sixty-seven days from April to June due to COVID symptoms. It wasn't until October that I was able to get off the couch for seven days in a row. It drained me to a point that I was questioning everything."

Nick never gave up, though, and eventually he was COVID-free and living his life again, though he admits "it is too difficult to say where CF begins and COVID ends" with regard to his symptoms. He credits that to not only his doctors and a terrific support system but also his outlook. "Success is not a goal to be reached or obtained; it is merely a by-product of the hard work put forth" is Nick's mantra.

Nick threw a party for himself when he got out of the hospital. "Getting out of the hospital was exciting," says Nick. "I was really small. I had lost all my muscle mass. I lost twenty-four pounds, going from 145 down to about 120 pounds, but eventually gained the weight back. I chronicled my time in the hospital. I've been in the hospital a bunch of times. This was different. I wasn't able to be around anyone. They set a food tray down, they knock on the door, and you have thirty seconds to grab it because it's a pressurized room. There were a couple of good nurses and doctors working with me, and they could slap me on the face tomorrow and I still wouldn't recognize them."

Now that Nick has turned the page on his harrowing COVID chapter, he is back to being a spokesman regarding cystic fibrosis. Nick's ultimate CF advocacy goal is to dispel a little bit of darkness that surrounds this disease while educating and helping people understand. "I want to shine some light and goodness on the disease," says Nick. And he has a vision of how he would like to do it.

Nick has other pursuits as well. "I have things I want to do outside of my CF work," says Nick. "For starters, I want to visit all fifty states before my thirty-fifth birthday." With less than a year to go, he's at forty. Nick plans on making Hawaii his fiftieth state and celebrating his birthday on March 16, 2022.

"I try not to use the word 'goals' or 'objectives,'" says Nick. "Those are things you're hoping happen. I'm not hoping it happens. I'm doing it."

STACY CARMONA

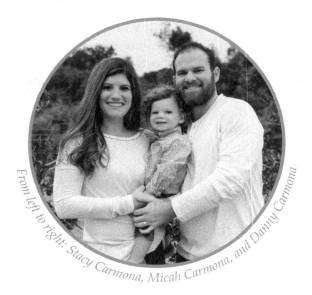

From left to right: Stacy Carmona, Micah Carmona, and Danny Carmona

Age: 35
Resides: Orange County, California
Age at Diagnosis: 3 months

BEYOND THE NUMBERS: THE ULTIMATE UNDERDOG

Stacy Carmona's story isn't about achieving one major milestone or accomplishment. It's about overcoming a lifetime of obstacles that cystic fibrosis placed in front of her. Stacy is the ultimate underdog, and her story is a lesson in fighting for what you want.

"My life has been about defying the odds," says Stacy. "I have to work harder for everything in my life, but that makes my accomplishments so much sweeter." Stacy has lived a life defined by numbers. "According to my doctors, I was supposed to be dead seventeen years ago. Eighty is the number of weeks that I have spent on IV antibiotics. Twelve is the number of surgeries I have had. And I am part of the ten percent of people with cystic fibrosis who don't have a therapy to treat the cause of our disease."

The first indication that Stacy had CF was when she presented with meconium peritonitis, an intestinal blockage that burst, spilling poison into her abdominal cavity *before* her birth. Her mom, Debbie, had an emergency C-section a month before Stacy was due. At less than a day old, the doctors removed half of Stacy's small intestine. "I was diagnosed a few months later and spent the first six months of my life in the hospital," says Stacy. "My parents were told that I would unlikely reach my eighteenth birthday. They remained hopeful, but they did not expect that I would go to college, get married, or have children."

"When the doctors told us our baby daughter had cystic fibrosis, they said, 'Love her and cherish the time with her, but don't expect her to live to be an adult,'" says Stacy's dad, Paul. "The first time she coughed, my stomach tied in knots, and from three months old until now that's the way it has been."

"My family immediately got involved in the fight to give me a better life through their involvement with the CF Foundation," says Stacy. "And they also immediately got involved with my daily care. I remember my parents taking every breath alongside me when I took breathing treatments as a kid. My grandparents sat in the waiting room during every surgery I had. My sister Lisa (who is three years older and does not have CF) had sleepovers with me in the hospital. My relatives across the country have been putting on events and fundraising for the CF Foundation for years. My family is passionate about keeping me healthy and they continue to be my motivation."

Growing up, Stacy, a shy child who was still dealing with the scariness of having a chronic disease, had one friend with CF. "Her name was Sarah Kanofsky," says Stacy, "and she was my only friend with CF at that point in my life. Our families were close and would often get together as this was before we knew how dangerous it was for people with CF to be near each other. Sarah was speaking to large audiences at CF events at the age of nine. I remember being in awe of her abilities and feeling proud that she and I shared the same illness. When she passed away at the age of twelve awaiting a double-lung transplant, it was devastating on many levels. Not only was she a friend and the first person I knew to die, but she was the only other person I knew with CF. That was a difficult time for my entire family as it showed us firsthand the realities of CF."

At the age of ten, Stacy was faced with life lessons that were far beyond her years. "I was attempting to grieve and also reconcile my fears that Sarah and I shared the same disease," she says. "I will never forget the moment when I looked up at my dad and asked him, 'Is that what is going to happen to me?' My dad assured me that my life journey was unique. But when Sarah passed away, CF quickly went from being a nuisance to me to being a nightmare."

"Looking back on it, my childhood was often defined by my limitations," says Stacy. "I lived within the constraints of what CF would allow. CF didn't allow me to sleep over at friends' houses because it was too difficult for me to do my demanding medical regiment outside of my home. CF didn't allow me to go to fifth-grade science camp or to play with my friends when I had an IV in my arm. It was difficult to make plans or to dream for my future. I spent many days in the hospital and even more at home on IV antibiotics. I had medical procedures and surgeries often and missed many days of school due to doctors' appointments and not feeling well. Stomach aches, chronic sinus infections, lung infections, and nights of endless coughing were my normal. I longed to fit in and do things like my peers, and I lived in fear of my lung function declining."

Stacy had her first sinus surgery when she was six years old. "After that, I rarely went a year without sinus surgery growing up," says Stacy. "I had another stomach surgery when I was twelve to repair a hiatal hernia. By the time I was eighteen years old, I had become all too familiar with being put under anesthesia in the operating room."

Growing up, Stacy didn't like to tell others about her CF. "I felt a deep sense of shame and embarrassment about my disease," she says. "I wanted more than anything to feel 'normal' and fit in with my peers. I would go to great lengths to hide my disease from others. I would hide my medical equipment when a friend came over, I would go to the bathroom at lunch to take my enzymes, and when I eventually was able to have sleepovers, I would take my treatments in the bathroom while running the blow dryer so that friends couldn't hear. I always made up excuses why I was absent from school, and I was constantly made fun of by the other kids for being so thin and for missing so much school. I didn't want to be labeled as the 'sick kid' and that drove me to a level of secrecy that was ultimately very damaging to me."

Stacy started to come "out of her shell a bit" at the age of fifteen when she became an advocate for CF. That was the year she made her first speech at a CF event. "I was inspired by my dad who told me that he believed my purpose in life was to bring out the goodness in others," says Stacy.

Though she was in and out of the hospital and probably missed more days of school than she had attended, Stacy graduated high school with a high GPA and was accepted into almost every college to which she applied. She selected the University of California, Santa Barbara (UCSB). "When I went away to college, it was both an exciting and scary time for me," says Stacy. "I was free to become the person I wanted to be, and I was feeling more comfortable sharing my

CF story with others. On the flip side, I was now completely responsible for my care and was not always prioritizing my health over other, more desirable activities."

During her sophomore year, she had to take a semester off because she had pneumonia and wound up in the hospital and on IVs. "I quickly learned that I had to make my health my number one priority," she says. "I was devastated to leave my friends and my new life, but I was determined to get my health back on track so that I could get back to school as quickly as possible. There I was, nineteen years old and dependent on oxygen for the first time. I remember pleading with whatever higher power there was to help me get back to health. That was my much-needed wake-up call to become my own advocate and to assume complete responsibility for my care. And that life lesson has stayed with me ever since."

Stacy continues, "When I returned to school for the second half of my sophomore year, I was coming back physically weaker but mentally stronger. I had seen how quickly my health could decline, and I was committed to my medical regimen above all else. I made sure to schedule classes with enough time to do treatments in the morning. In fact, treatments became the first thing I did when I woke up. That way, if I was running short on time, something else would have to give, not my treatments. I also made treatments a part of my getting-ready routine at night before I went out with friends because I knew that I wasn't going to do them when I was coming home late and tired. I mastered the art of multitasking as I took breathing treatments while simultaneously straightening my hair and putting on makeup. Luckily, I was able to recover fairly quickly from that health scare and take full ownership of my care. But even the strictest of adherence does not guarantee that things will be smooth sailing with CF."

Stacy decided to spend her junior year of college studying abroad in Sydney, Australia. On her first day there, she ended up in the emergency room with an intestinal blockage. "I was completely alone in a foreign country that was clear across the world and my parents urged me to come home," she says. "But I chose to stay and face my fears. I'm so glad I did because that year in Australia was one of my most challenging and happiest times." In fact, Stacy went back to live in Australia again a few years after she graduated college. Traveling abroad with CF can be tricky, and Stacy loves telling the story of when her treatment machine set off the fire alarm in her hostel and the Australian fire department burst into her room. It was an embarrassing scene, but as Stacy jokes, "How often do you have hot Australian firemen in your room?"

Stacy took on a greater-than-full course load each semester

thereafter so that despite her sophomore-year absence, she could graduate on time. Not only did she walk with the rest of her class, but she also graduated with honors while majoring in communications and minoring in educational psychology.

After graduating from UCSB, Stacy worked at the Cystic Fibrosis Foundation as a special event manager. "The job was worthwhile in more ways than one as it led me to my soul mate," says Stacy. "Some people live their whole lives and never find their soul mate. I was lucky enough to meet mine at the age of twenty-one. Her name was Leslie.

"We met at a CF event and became fast friends. We connected on a level that I had never experienced with anyone. And our connection went much deeper than our shared experience of having CF and relating to each other's struggles. It was as if our souls recognized each other from another life.

"To know Leslie was to love her. She had an infectious smile and confidence that lit up the room. She had such a unique and beautiful way of viewing the world, and she taught me countless life lessons, including how to focus on gratitude. She significantly changed my perspective on having CF, making me less afraid of what the future could hold. Leslie didn't let anything stand in her way and she normalized CF struggles that had always scared me deeply. But perhaps, most importantly, she taught me to believe in myself and to believe that anything was possible.

"She encouraged me to take better care of myself and motivated me to start exercising, something I had never done up until that point. She showed me by example how to fight and how to get back up when I was knocked down.

"I would visit her often when she was in the hospital. We would sit across from each other in the lobby where I took comfort in just being near her. We would look into each other's eyes and we were so overwhelmed with emotion that we would often cry. We cried because we wanted so much more for each other in this life. And we cried because we were so happy that we found each other.

"Leslie taught me that I should not fear death, but rather an unlived life." Very sadly, Leslie passed away in 2011.

Yet CF still presented Stacy with challenges when it came to her social life. "It was always very difficult for me to tell guys I was dating that I had CF," says Stacy. Then, at twenty-five, Stacy met Danny.

"I knew on the first date that Stacy was the girl for me," says Danny.

"I feared that he didn't know what he was signing up for when he asked me to marry him," says Stacy.

"And that didn't make sense to me," he says, "not to continue the relationship. That something bad could happen. I had an equal amount of hope that something *good* could happen." They were married June 25, 2016.

At thirty, Stacy decided to take on the challenge of the CF Foundation's Xtreme Hike fundraising event in Mammoth, California, a twenty-five-mile hike with significant elevation gain. "Any form of exercise has always been more challenging for me, as it makes breathing more difficult and I tire easily," says Stacy. "About ten months before the event, I started participating in training hikes to prepare myself for the big day. After my last training hike, several weeks before the event, I felt confident that I could complete the twenty-five-mile trek. But as life with CF goes, you can plan all you want, but CF does not follow suit."

A few days before the Xtreme Hike, Stacy got really sick. "I had put too much work in to quit," she says, "so I stubbornly insisted on attempting to climb that mountain. Amazingly, I was able to complete twelve miles with a fever, body aches, and chills. My sister-in-law was driving me back from the hike and asked if she should take me to the hotel or straight to the hospital. I was so disappointed that I was not able to complete the hike and sadly, I did end up having to be hospitalized afterward. I wish I could say that this was the only time something like this has happened to me, but life with CF is all about uncertainty. One step forward and two steps back. When things like this happen, it is really hard to continue to dream and set goals, because there is no way to predict when CF will knock you down. But I will never let CF stop me from trying." Stacy would need this attitude for her next life venture.

"I never imagined that starting a family would be so difficult," says Stacy. "But the three-year journey to my son, Micah, was perhaps the most difficult one I've endured so far." It was challenging to find an obstetrician that would take her case, but eventually, she found a doctor who committed himself to helping Stacy make her dreams come true. "He did not seem fazed by the potential challenges with my pregnancy," she says, "which made me even more confident."

In 2019, after three IUIs (Intrauterine inseminations), five rounds of IVF (in vitro fertilization), two transfers, a miscarriage, and three different fertility clinics, Stacy finally became pregnant. "I was ecstatic, but also in disbelief," says Stacy. "It took both Danny and I a long time for us to believe that I was really pregnant. When we heard our baby's heartbeat for the first time, I broke down sobbing in the doctor's office."

On March 14, 2020, Stacy and Danny welcomed Micah. "There are no words to describe that moment. After all of the heartache and devastation, we never gave up hope. When Micah was born, I felt complete for the first time in my life. Being a mom is the greatest joy of my life, and I do not take a single second for granted. And how many people get to say that they witnessed a miracle?"

There are still many hard days with CF, and adulthood came with its own set of challenges, such as CF-related diabetes, CF liver disease, and several multiresistant bacteria in Stacy's lungs, "but I make the choice every day to fight." For the past twenty years, the once shy little girl is now a motivational speaker, fundraiser (Stacy's family has raised millions of dollars for CF research), volunteer, and advocate. In 2015, she gave a TEDx Talk to over two thousand people about breaking boundaries. She is a peer mentor, a patient representative for the FDA, cochair of the Adult Advisory Council Alumni Group with the CF Foundation, and she was recognized by *OC Metro* magazine as being one of ten women making a difference in her community. And, in honor of her friend Leslie, who died from CF nearly a decade ago, a team leader for Great Strides.

"It had always been [Leslie's] dream to raise one hundred thousand dollars in one year for CF, and before she passed, she asked me if I would take over her team. So I spent the year after her death devoted to planning and fundraising for walk day, at which friends and family gathered to honor her memory. I'm proud to say we raised one hundred and fifty thousand dollars that year. There aren't many people we come across who change who we are," says Stacy, "but she changed me to my core. It has been ten long years since Leslie passed away, but not a day goes by where I don't remember her with deep and profound gratitude. I will never fully recover from the loss of my soul mate. But I know her spirit lives on in me, and I am more determined than ever to beat this disease for her."

It is important for Stacy to use her experience to help others. She has been working as the director of patient advocacy for a CF specialty pharmacy for the past ten years. Today, at seventeen years past her life expectancy, Stacy stays healthy by adhering to her treatment regimen and being a regular attendee at Orange Theory Fitness. Because of her commitment to exercise, she recently ran her first 10K. "I learned a long time ago if you don't feel good, nothing else really matters," says Stacy. "So, although it is a great deal of effort, it is important to take the best care of ourselves as possible so that we can enjoy our lives."

And Stacy doesn't have to look far for incentive to take good care of herself. "Each day when I look at my husband, Danny, and my son, Micah," says Stacy, "I am given new strength to continue to overcome all of the challenges that CF brings." Stacy admits that there is at least one positive thing about having cystic fibrosis. "I have learned to see the good that CF has given me," says Stacy, "such as a unique perspective and deeper appreciation to live life to the fullest, closer relationships with loved ones and strength and resilience that I would have never thought possible.

"Despite an immense number of challenges, I am living a fulfilling life and have accomplished much of what I always dreamt of," says Stacy, who has eaten sushi in Japan, been skydiving over the Great Barrier Reef in Australia, swam with sharks in the Bahamas, and explored the ruins in Italy. "But I still have a bucket list of dreams for my future, including: I want to run a half-marathon, I want to write a book, I want to have another child and see my kids grow up, and more than anything, I want to be here to celebrate the cure for CF."

STEPHANIE STAVROS

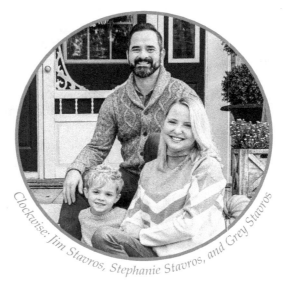

Clockwise: Jim Stavros, Stephanie Stavros, and Grey Stavros

Age: 38
Resides: Toronto, Ontario, Canada
Age at Diagnosis: Birth

CF GETS LOUD: REVEALING STEPHANIE'S SECRET

S tephanie Stavros was diagnosed with cystic fibrosis in 1983 right after her birth, but it would be thirty-four years before she revealed it to anyone else, and by doing so, start a nationwide movement.

"The day that Stephanie was born she was rushed to the Hospital for Sick Children (SickKids in Toronto, Canada) for emergency surgery," says Stephanie's mom, Judi Hayford. "I was upset that I couldn't be with her and terrified that she wouldn't make it through the operation. She was only five hours old and so very tiny. She was a month premature and weighed less than five pounds. After the surgery, the doctor phoned us to say, 'She made it through the operation. She's okay. She's a fighter.' He said that meconium ileus was a classic sign of CF, but they could not be sure that it was CF until they did a sweat test and that could not be done until she was over three months old."

Stephanie was in the hospital for nearly three months and had one more operation to reverse the ileostomy — a surgical procedure where a piece of the ileum, which is part of the small intestine, is diverted to an artificial opening in the abdominal wall —she had done on her first day. "On the day we brought her home," says Judi, "I kept hoping that the doctor was wrong and that she would be fine."

Judi took her back to SickKids a few weeks later for the sweat test, and when they told her the test was positive for CF, "it was like a punch to my gut," says Judi. "I didn't know what the future would be or if I could do everything she would need me to do. I had done a lot of research in those three months, and I was hopeful but very afraid for Stephanie's future. I just kept reminding myself of what the doctor first said, 'She's okay . . . she's a fighter.'"

Stephanie says her parents treated her the same as her older sister and brother (neither has the disease), and that growing up, her sister, Lisa, was the closest person in her life.

"[Stephanie] is my best friend, my biggest supporter, and the person I look up to most in life," says Lisa. "She's always been like a second mom to me [though Lisa is the older of the two sisters, Stephanie says Lisa considers her younger sister to be wise beyond her years]. From an early age we did everything together. All the normal sister things, but also with all the things that she went through, we were always there for one another. While our biggest wish was for CF to be a thing of the past, one of my biggest wishes was that she never lose her fight. Selfishly, I wouldn't know what to do without her."

"When I was young," says Stephanie, "I always had deep concerns about my health, and I worried that I wouldn't be able to be a mother. My sister promised when we were barely teenagers that she would carry my child for me one day. It was a beautiful, youthful dream to look forward to."

Stephanie recalls, "I had to take digestive enzymes and eat a high-calorie diet but beyond that, life was very 'normal,' until age eight. That's when I started to culture the bacteria pseudomonas in my lungs, and my weight started to drift downward off the charts. Slowly, my height followed. My lungs started to decline, and a routine of inhaled treatments was introduced. It was at this time that I started to notice the difference between my routine and other children's routines. As a kid, I never wanted to feel different from my peers. I slowly began to hide aspects of my CF, and it snowballed from there. What started off as a need to normalize my disease became an obsession to hide it."

"From a very young age, Stephanie did not want CF to define her as a person," says Judi. "I understood and respected that decision. She want-ed to be the same as all her friends. One day she came home from school and happily told me that she had a friend that coughed a lot like she did. He had asthma. So from that point on, asthma became her 'go-to' answer if people asked why she was coughing. Asthma seemed to be a common condition that didn't require an explanation to anyone."

Stephanie remembers the first time she heard the dreaded words "life expectancy" and "cystic fibrosis" in the same breath. "In 1989, when the gene for CF was isolated, I remember the news reporter talking about life expectancy being thirty-two years, and I just broke down and cried thinking it could not be true," she says. "I was six years old, but I remember understanding the gravity of a shortened life. It was a moment where I thought, *I don't want to be known for that.* I didn't want to be a poster child for CF and actually resented those CF kids on the posters."

It didn't get easier for Stephanie as she got older. While she was reticent about her CF, she wasn't *as* closely guarded as she would become. "As a preteen, when we learned about genetics in grade seven, kids in my class bullied me saying that my life was half over," says Stephanie, who adds that in that same year, a boy who she had a crush on was giggling behind her and teased, "Hey, Steph, is it true that you have this crazy disease that means you're going to die when you're thirty?"

Stephanie says that was a pivotal moment in her journey with CF. "I felt that if this is what I will experience with people that find out about my CF, well, then no one will ever find out again," she says. "I needed to hide it and protect myself from an experience like that. I never wanted to feel like that again."

As a ninth grader, Stephanie had to get a GI feeding tube because she was unable to absorb enough calories even though she was eating much more than kids her age. She still hid it from her peers, often by wearing an oversized hooded sweatshirt. In high school, she was taking enzymes covertly in the public bathroom and someone saw her and asked what they were. "I said they were for my lactose intolerance," says Stephanie. "The girl said, 'My friend takes something like that but it's for cystic fibrosis and her life expectancy is nineteen.' That was a punch in the gut."

Stephanie says that for thirty-four years she lived in denial. Friends and even some family didn't know about her disease. She would have nightmares of people finding meds or a nebulizer in her house and revealing Stephanie's secret identity as a CF patient. And then there was dating, which she didn't have much of a problem hiding her disease. "I feel that people with CF have this superhuman way of suppressing their coughs in certain environments," says Stephanie. "But the process of hiding and pushing down this illness from the public eye was incredibly self-destructive. In a big way, I was living a lie. I can remember countless stories of being out in public and having to escape to the washroom for a coughing fit or to take a handful of pills.

"One evening in particular, I was walking by the waterfront of Toronto for a romantic after-dinner stroll when, all of a sudden, the cold air hit my chest, and I could feel blood bubbling up in my throat. I swallowed the blood, excused myself, and popped into a nearby coffee shop. In the washroom, my lungs gushed more blood, and I was worried that it wasn't going to stop. Minutes felt like hours, and the bleeding slowed, then stopped. I washed the blood from around my mouth, gargled some water to flush the blood stains from my teeth, scrubbed the blood spatters from the public sink, and headed back outside to continue the date as if nothing happened. It was as if I was living a double life."

Then she found Jim. "He and I met on the beach in cottage country here in Ontario," says Stephanie. "We were dating for a few months when I opened up to him about CF. I had big walls up, but this man was able to knock them down quickly through laughter and vulnerability. At this time in my life, I could count on two hands how many people in my life knew about my disease. From my perspective, telling Jim was a huge gamble. A big part of me thought that it would send him running . . . but he stayed. He listened and he learned. I felt so comfortable around him, and for the first time as an adult, I started taking care of myself. I stopped hiding and skipping my treatments. His acceptance helped me with my own acceptance of my disease. Everything that was hard to handle, we tackled together. For over a decade, Jim kept my secret safe. On our wedding day, even his own family didn't know about my illness. My secret became our secret. Jim was never ashamed—he deeply supported the way I handled my disease in that season of life."

Over the years, Stephanie's health declined, and her illness became more difficult to hide. "Even then, Jim remained patient with my need to keep a sense of control over my disease," says Stephanie. "Jim is the strongest man I've ever met and because of that, sometimes the both of us forget that he, too, needs a support system."

"I was entirely in favor of Stephanie sharing her CF," says Jim. "For years I had privately hoped that Stephanie would be able to find the self-acceptance and willingness to let people into this aspect of her life. When Stephanie and I started dating, she chose to share with me her health story only after she felt she could trust me and my ability to keep this element of her life private. Stephanie was very clear that she was to have complete control over this domain, and she decided who could be brought into her circle of trust. For a decade, I kept my commitment to the trust she put in me. However, the ability to keep Stephanie's CF hidden became more and more difficult when her CF began to manifest in more obvious and troublesome ways. The years of trying to keep Stephanie's health private was beginning to take its toll. Regardless, we would soldier on, and I would do my best to be the rock that Stephanie needed."

Lisa wanted her little sister to open up too, but she understood that would not be easy. "As soon as I started working downtown, I began to volunteer at the Cystic Fibrosis Canada Toronto Chapter," says Lisa. "I would help organize events and our family would attend as many as they could. I can remember watching all of the key speakers who have CF tell their stories of what it was like to have CF, the challenges, the wins, and the losses. I was inspired by each of them, but if Steph was in the room, she would excuse herself during the speech so that she didn't hear them. I understood. Steph didn't want to have their story. She didn't really say it, but I know she didn't want people to feel sorry for her, didn't want people to look at her as sick. The thought of getting up at that podium was terrifying for her."

Stephanie and Jim married in 2011 and began planning a family. "When Steph and Jim got married, naturally the topic of babies came up again," says Lisa, "and I again said I would happily carry their baby, but I wanted to be married at the very least. It wasn't too long after that that I met my husband, and we got married. After my first son was born, Steph's health started to decline, and she was hospitalized for several weeks."

Stephanie still thought about Lisa's promise to carry a child for her. "My sister had her first baby the year after I got married," says Stephanie, "and I was there for most of the labor experience. It was then that I understood the gravity of what she had offered. I witnessed her go through the most tremendous pain and realized that I couldn't ask her to do that for me.

"I wanted to carry the baby myself," says Stephanie, "but around that time, I had a major health setback. While I was at work one Thursday afternoon, my left lung collapsed. It was so severely damaged that it spontaneously suffered a pneumothorax. The road to recovery was long and complicated. My lung would inflate and deflate several times during my six-week hospital stay. I was eventually transferred to another hospital that specializes in thoracic surgery to 'glue' (as they described it) my lung in place. The doctors told us that after my lung collapse, I would have a fifty percent chance of it happening again within the next two years. We decided to wait on starting our family."

Stephanie continues, "During that stay, waiting for surgery, my mental health spiraled. After weeks of very little sleep, hospital delirium started to set in. One night, I had the most intense dream. I woke up with my pillow drenched in tears and felt very shaken. I had dreamt that two nurses were standing outside my hospital room re-viewing scans of my uterus on a monitor. One kept saying the words, 'Someone has to tell her,' while the other nurse kept saying, 'She's going through too much right now, she can't handle that.' They were talking about cancer. I was disturbed by the experience but even more confused. Why would I be worried about any area of my body other than my lungs? The thoughts of the intense dream lingered with me, but I chalked it up to the state of my anxiety."

Lisa tried to help her sister with her mental anguish. "I would bring my son into the hospital," says Lisa, "and Steph would light up when she held him or tended to him."

Stephanie tried to rebound but sadly her recent nightmare turned into reality, and it wasn't just her lungs she had to worry about. "I was diagnosed with cervical cancer," says Stephanie. "I had an annual physical exam with my family doctor and everything appeared to be going well. One afternoon, I was at my office when I answered the phone, and I heard the words 'cancer cells' from my doctor. They were sending me to a women's hospital to have further biopsies done. This, once again, put a massive roadblock in my plan. This felt like a sign that was hard to avoid—perhaps I truly wasn't meant to be a mother.

"Jim and I knew we had to prioritize my health and that for me to carry would be too risky," says Stephanie, "so we began searching for surrogates."

"Steph's cervical cancer diagnosis launched her into a deep dark hole," says Lisa. "I have never seen Steph so absolutely defeated."

"At the specialist office," says Stephanie, "I learned that I had ex-tremely aggressive cancer on my uterus lining. I immediately thought of my surreal dream while in the hospital. I've never made sense of this coincidence but it felt like some sort of divine intervention. The doctor immediately booked surgery to remove three sections of my uterus lining. During the wait for the surgery, it felt like my universe broke in half. All at once, my dreams to become a mother were ruined, and I now had a second disease threatening my life. I described the feeling as being chased by two murderers—cystic fibrosis and cancer. I was beginning to feel defeated. During that time, my sister offered to carry my baby for me. She was ready to step in and help, and we were ready to accept her incredibly gracious offer."

"I would call her or visit with her," says Lisa, "but when you looked at her you could see her soul had dimmed. It was the scariest thing I have witnessed. I remember driving her up to our parents' place to have tea with them, and Steph was in the passenger seat, slumped onto the door and staring blankly off into the distance. The air was thick, and I had no words . . . or I thought I had no words, but when

I opened my mouth, I said, 'Well, once your surgery is over, I guess your next big decision will be when you will be getting me pregnant!' Probably not the time for that statement, but I needed Steph to have something to hold onto, something to look forward to. I needed that positivity that she always had to return, or I knew I would lose her.

"I remember having a deep conversation not too long after with our mom about whether or not I could have Steph's baby for her. At the end of that conversation, we both agreed that if Steph needed a lung, a kidney, a liver, or anything else, either one of us would sign up without hesitation, but in this case, Steph needed purpose. She needed hope and she needed to be a mom, and I needed to share motherhood with her and have our kids grow up together."

Stephanie had the surgery in October of 2014, and the doctors felt confident that the boundaries of the areas that were removed looked excellent, and she did not need to have chemotherapy. "A mere four weeks later in November 2014," says Stephanie, "I had a second surgery to have an egg retrieval procedure and start the journey of surrogacy with my husband and sister."

In 2015, Lisa carried and nurtured Stephanie and Jim's child in her womb for thirty-eight weeks. The result was a baby boy born August 4, 2015. Stephanie and Jim named him Grey. "Many people would look at these health roadblocks as signs against being a mother," says Stephanie, "but I refused to let fear drive the direction of my dreams. My son is my inspiration and my reminder that miracles are possible."

Grey is now six, and Stephanie is truly thankful for her little boy. "Grey is the most incredible gift," says Stephanie. "His birth story changed the way I look at the world and is a constant reminder to dream big. He's an old soul with a big heart. He is wise beyond his years and dreams of being a doctor one day. Being his mom helps me fight and push harder to stay healthy."

Lisa still comes over to spend time with her nephew. "Lisa holds a special place in his heart," says Stephanie. "We call her Auntie Roo because she carried Grey and kept him safe like a kangaroo. She treats him like one of her own and her boys feel like siblings to Grey. Six years later, I'm still wrapping my head around how I got so lucky to have a sister like Lisa.

"My sister is my hero," says Stephanie. "She assisted with my CF care for my entire life and has been my best friend through all of the ups and downs. My CF forced her to take on heavy responsibilities at an early age, and she never complained. Lisa used to do my physiotherapy after school, help me set up my inhaled antibiotic treatments, and attend my hospital appointments and be there to remind me how brave I needed to be." The sisters even lived together as adults.

Stephanie says her sister has always been her best friend and their bond has grown even stronger. Stephanie knew that it was time to demonstrate her own courage.

"This *new* bravery shifted the world as I knew it," says Stephanie. "It showed me that anything is possible. Through discovering my new role as a mom, I found myself. I found self-acceptance and shifted my view of my health. When my son was born, I felt transformed. This child represented so much hope. I needed to fight back to stay with him as long as possible. I would do anything necessary to fight." After the birth of her son, Stephanie did some intense soul searching to find her way back to the reality that she had admittedly abandoned. "Through therapy, mindfulness, long chats with friends, and stacks of self-help books, I found my way back to me—the full version. The raw struggle and the beauty. Jim was there every step of the way. When I was ready to tell my story to the world, we cried happy tears together and felt a large weight lift off of us. We were free. We were finally able to accept support from others."

When she was diagnosed with cervical cancer in 2014, she decided to be open with it. She noticed that she was getting so much emotional support. "People were calling me a warrior," says Stephanie who adds it was like an audition of what it would be like to introduce her CF. Finally at age thirty-five, she shared her struggle with the world and a weight was lifted. She started to share her story and raise awareness for CF.

Jim laughs at the irony. "It took Stephanie a lot of deep introspection and work on self-acceptance before she felt that she could share her story," says Jim. "However, in typical Stephanie style, she made sure she did it in a fashion that guaranteed her control over the information. She decided to share it on social media for everyone she knew to see. There were so many questions. How would her friends and peers view this new info? Would their relationship with her change? Would it be better? Would it be worse? I remember clearly the look on her face and the nervous excitement we felt right before she hit 'send.' The outpouring of support was overwhelming. This is exactly the reaction I felt would be waiting for her. The relationships with our friends strengthened. Our relationship strengthened. There was an entire village behind us, offering a helping hand whenever we needed it. I felt an enormous weight lifted from my shoulders. When challenges arose, I could turn to friends for the support I needed. I no longer felt like Stephanie and I were battling her CF alone."

Thankfully, Stephanie's openness about the disease happened just in time. "In my mid-thirties, my health started to spiral," says Stephanie. "My lungs were bleeding. I was constantly on IVs. I was no longer able to fight off infection, my lung function was in the twenties, and I was being evaluated for a double-lung transplant. My health was slipping away." Just when she was at rock bottom, Trikafta got approved by the FDA. "I was at a fork in the road," says Stephanie. "I could go down one of two routes and one of them needed to happen soon—I would list for lungs or I would try to get my hands on Trikafta. Canada did not have access to Trikafta at the time, so my only hope was to gain access through the manufacturer."

Carrying the words of author and research professor Dr. Brené Brown, who said, "When we deny the story, it defines us. When we own the story, we can write a brave new ending," Stephanie began to campaign for her life to be saved on social media and in the news. "I had hundreds of women write letters on my behalf, pleading for my life to be saved," says Stephanie. "I was relentless. On January 8, 2020, I was the first patient in Canada to be granted Compassionate Care for Trikafta. I felt like I won the life lottery. At that moment, I knew that this medicine was my only hope and my second chance at life. This was a gift to not only me but my son and my husband."

"When Steph became truly ill and was at end-stage lung disease, we were all praying for a miracle," says Lisa. "No one was more shocked than me to see that the miracle came in the form of a social media post of Steph 'outing' herself. I could not be more proud. Steph wasn't going to wait around for a miracle, she was going to create it. I *love* telling the story of her 'getting loud,' and I truly believe that she saved her own life. Steph found a way to advocate for herself in a new way and discovered that there was a village ready to stand by her and call out to anyone who could help along with her. She found a way to be on the podium and tell her truth and have people see strength. Every single time that life has thrown something at her, she has found a way to get through it and inspire those who were lucky enough to be by her side along the way."

"When [Stephanie's] health was declining, and she was raising her son amid IV poles and hospitalizations, she didn't give up," says Judi. "Instead, she fought harder to get the medicine that could save her life."

Stephanie took her first dose on Global News, the same news station that had captured her plea to her country to save her life. "I was weak and overwhelmed with joy," says Stephanie. "I had envisioned this day so many times, right down to the finest detail. I had even described it to the media. I knew what chair I would sit in when taking the first dose. I knew what glass I would fill with water, and I pictured the condensation that would form on the ice-cold cup of water. I pictured what the pills looked like and the emotions that I would feel, holding them in my hands. Every detail was accounted for . . . and was astonishingly accurate. The experience unfolded just as I had dreamed. I took those two perfect pills, then hugged my son and husband while crying happy tears. I said to my four-year-old son, 'What day is it?' to which he replied, 'It's a miracle, Mama.' I'm so grateful that the moment was captured on camera."

It became profoundly apparent to Stephanie how much this moment meant, not only to her but to those Canadians with CF fighting the same uphill battles. "It was one of the best moments of my life," says Stephanie. "Months of envisioning the moment in perfect detail, experiencing the emotions and profound sense of gratitude, manifested into my reality. My story went viral in the Canadian CF community. Everyone wanted to know what this med was and how they could gain access. There was a gap in knowledge about this medicine and why Canada did not have access." During the Global News interview, Stephanie stated that at least 90 percent of Canadians with CF need access to this medication and "I will not stop until we all have access."

Stephanie was inundated with messages from across Canada from families wondering what this new breakthrough medicine was and how they could obtain it. The volume of messages was overwhelming. Two of her CF friends offered to help get back to all of the families searching for answers. "At the beginning, it was just the three of us, tethered to IV poles, trying to help," says Stephanie. "We started off with a simple email address, and now we have created Canada's largest CF grassroots movement, CF Get Loud."

Alongside Canada's most seasoned CF advocates and passionate families, the movement has grown to represent a community of over four thousand people across the country, all fighting for access to life-saving medications. "Our goals are to educate, empower, and elevate the voices of CF patients. CF Get Loud hosted educational webinars with guests such as Cystic Fibrosis Canada, the Canadian Organization for Rare Disorders (CORD), and the CF Treatment Society. We have created waves in the provincial and federal government by halting regulations that would negatively impact rare, precision medicine from gaining approval in Canada. As a community, we are stronger together." CF Get Loud just celebrated their two-year anniversary.

"We have made big changes in Canada, as we are working on a non-partisan level to create positive change in our healthcare system," says Stephanie. "We will continue to fight for all patients with CF and other rare diseases."

Stephanie has learned a lot through her campaign. "Accept all of the support that is offered and then ask for more," she says. "CF patients are so brave but can also be stubborn. We feel compelled to put on a brave face, help others feel comfortable with our decline in health and not seek help from our support system until we are at our breaking point."

Stephanie's lung function has increased since she started Trikafta, her FEV1 going from 28 to 41percent. "Within hours of taking it, my body began to transform," she says. "Within seven days, I gained back years of lost lung function. Within three months, I gained thirty pounds after my body had been malnourished for thirty-six years. Within six months, I gained back a decade of lost lung function. For the first time as an adult, I have normal liver levels, my sense of smell and taste returned, and my lungs feel brand new." Incredibly, Stephanie's salt chloride, which was ninety-eight when she started Trikafta, is now at twenty-three after only six months on the drug and therefore she now tests negative for CF when she takes a sweat test. Anything under thirty is considered negative for CF, though she does still have the disease. The other terrific news is that for the first time in her adult life, she is able to take "deep, full breaths."

Stephanie says that Trikafta has allowed her to sleep peacefully, become an active mother for Grey, and, another first, she is going running. She has even witnessed her family's fear for her life turn into "joy and reprieve."

"My parents never limited me, and I love and respect them so much for that," says Stephanie. "I was a child with big dreams *and* a CF patient—not just a patient. My parents have never given up their commitment to my health, even at [my age of] thirty-eight years old. In a heartbeat, they are at my home, helping me out. My parents live in Florida for the winter months but will fly in when things get tough. CF parents are, simply, angels."

Judi is proud of her daughter for coming out and helping the CF community. "Now Stephanie is still fighting," she says. "She is fighting all day, every day to get lifesaving medicine for everyone suffering with cystic fibrosis. Her CF Get Loud movement is truly trying to pay it forward. I am unbelievably proud of her!"

"How many dads can brag that their daughter, along with the help of others, has changed the lives of thousands of Canadians? I couldn't be more proud," says Stephanie's father, Gord.

Stephanie has raised money for Cystic Fibrosis Canada her entire life, and now she dedicates her time and talents to CF Get Loud to be able to gain approval for Trikafta, a breakthrough gene modulator, in every province and territory in Canada, including her home province of Ontario, which holds the greatest number of CF patients at approximately 1,500.

On November 9, 2020, the manufacturer submitted Trikafta to Health Canada, Canada's equivalent to the Food and Drug Administration in the United States. On June 18, 2021, Health Canada approved the use of Trikafta for patients ages twelve and up, and Trikafta officially received a drug identification number (DIN). The next step was for the drug to go through Canada's Health Technology Assessment (HTA), which typically takes twelve months or more to evaluate the quality of a drug and gives it a positive or negative rating. The HTA sets criteria recommendations for coverage that is followed by both the public and private sectors. Due to the breakthrough nature of Trikafta, an Aligned Review—a process designed to support timely access to effective new therapies and must be applied for by the manufacturer—was approved to proceed with an expedited timeline.

The HTA gave the drug a positive recommendation in only six months and made Canadian history when it only took one day after the completion of the HTA for the provinces to start approving it and adding it to their public formularies. On September 24, 2021, Ontario became the first province to approve Trikafta and agreed to fund it. Alberta and Saskatchewan followed that same day. Eventually, all the provinces approved the drug and the private insurance companies followed.

On April 20, 2022, Health Canada approved Trikafta for children between the ages of six to eleven. As of the publication of this book, this age group is still awaiting public and private funding. Currently, the CF Get Loud team is fighting for wider, unrestricted access to Trikafta and sharing the lessons learned with other rare disease communities that are fighting for change. They vow to not leave anyone behind, including the ten percent of CF patients that are not candidates for current gene modulators. For the CF Get Loud team, this work is a marathon, not a sprint.

"It feels incredible!" says Stephanie. "I've spoken to parents and patients across Canada who are crying tears of joy. To be a part of that win fills my heart and soul to the brim! I feel truly honored to have been a leader and a voice in this fight. It has changed my perspective immensely and shown me the power of community."

Currently, Stephanie dedicates her time to leading the CF Get Loud movement, advocating for rare disease access to medicine in Canada, doing speaking engagements, and sharing her personal journey on her blog called *Rosie Life with Grey*.

For someone who spent thirty-four years hiding her disease, Stephanie has made up for lost time. "My biggest dream was to use my voice to make a difference for CF families in Canada. I feel like I am accomplishing that."

3

TEST ME:
TALES OF LATE DIAGNOSES

Dr. Miriam
Frankenthal Figueira

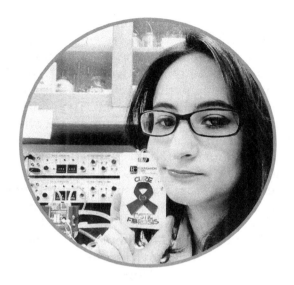

Age: 34
Resides: Chapel Hill, North Carolina
Age at diagnosis: 13

FROM BRAZIL TO THE USA: A RESEARCHER'S FIGHT

Miriam Figueira first *feared* cystic fibrosis at twenty-three years old when she was diagnosed with pancreatitis. "I felt terrible pain and had to lose many classes during my master program staying at the hospital," she says. "Not too long after that, while at Stanford doing part of my PhD in 2015, at the age of twenty-seven, I found out I had the dangerous bug Burkholderia and that my glucose homeostasis was not normal anymore. All of those experiences redefined my disease in my mind and are still a constant threat for my health."

Miriam was born in Rio de Janeiro, Brazil, with symptoms of a chronic cough around six months old. She was misdiagnosed with bronchitis, asthma, and allergies. She says that over the years, as her symptoms worsened, doctors would give her numerous allergy shots to try to keep her symptoms at bay, but at thirteen years old, when her weight plateaued at approximately twenty-eight kilograms (sixty-two pounds), her mom, Viviane, took her to the pediatrician and insisted he look deeper.

"The doctor noticed my cough and took an X-ray, where they found an alteration," says Miriam, "so he prescribed me antibiotics and asked us to come back in two weeks." Viviane, a psychoanalyst and MD, decided to ask for another X-ray after two weeks. "The X-ray showed mucus condensation and hyperinflation," says Miriam. "The radiologist was the one suggesting it could be CF. The pediatrician thought it wasn't CF, but he referred me to a pneumologist who then ordered my sweat test. The pediatrician was dismissive in regard to ordering a second X-ray, so my mom ordered it." Soon after, Miriam's sweat test came back positive.

Miriam's parents were scared and stressed by the news, so her father, Ivan, attended a CF conference in Brazil and eventually went to San Francisco to meet some CF researchers, physicians, and scientists out of Stanford University. "'Have hope,' my father said, because scientists were working to treat my disease in the United States and around the world," says Miriam. "Hope led me to becoming a scientist and eventually to the United States."

Miriam's journey into science, and specifically into cystic fibrosis, began when she learned from her father that there was optimism with treating and maybe even curing the disease. "Since I was a little girl, I was curious when it came to matters related to science," says Miriam, "however, what actually defined my academic path were my experiences with cystic fibrosis."

Miriam's mother soon joined her father in learning about the happenings with regard to treating cystic fibrosis. "My parents proactively connected with CF researchers around the world," says Miriam, "and I learned from them that many scientists were working to find new treatments for CF. This made me hopeful and awakened in me an interest in meeting these scientists and becoming one of them. Ultimately, I developed a will to help hope emerge in other people's lives."

Miriam still remembers being diagnosed at the age of thirteen. "I felt overwhelmed and frightened," she says, "and found myself surrounded by other individuals' stories of their battles against CF and many other diseases. These stories had such a deep impact on me. At first, I experienced an immediate empathy that made me feel powerless. Over time, this feeling transformed into the inspiration to enter a full-time career in biomedical science."

Gradually, over many years, Miriam's dreams to help others became a reality.

"My pathway started with my undergrad degree in biomedical science," says Miriam, "then I obtained a master's in biological science at the Federal University of Rio de Janeiro (UFRJ) in 2013, with a focus on renal physiology, and had the opportunity to work with the Cystic Fibrosis Transmembrane Regulator (CFTR) and other transporters in the kidneys.

"After that, I decided to apply the knowledge I obtained from my master studies to focus on the airways. I pursued a PhD also in biological science but now with a focus on lung physiology. After so many years of research, I completed my PhD in biological sciences (physiology) at the Federal University of Rio de Janeiro in 2017, my hometown. I also spent one year of my PhD at Stanford University in the Cystic Fibrosis Research Laboratory. My PhD work was focused on Prostaglandin E2 effects on ion transport in airway epithelial cells, with the ultimate goal of understanding the differences between normal and cystic fibrosis airways."

Miriam continues, "I was very shy growing up and only spoke to my close friends about my CF diagnosis. I did not become more vocal until my mid-twenties or so, when I was compelled to." Miriam says that being more outspoken is crucial, especially in regard to getting drugs in her home country. "CF drugs are not covered by health insurance companies in Brazil and no pharmacy sells these medications, as they are all produced abroad," she says. "So the only way to get CF medications is from the Brazilian government. The medicines are all for free, but the distribution can be inconsistent. In addition, due to governmental bureaucracy, new CF medications take too long to arrive in Brazil, in some cases we have an eight-year delay compared to the US."

As a result, CF parents' associations have to do as Miriam and her family have done and face constant legal battles to make sure the medications will still be available.

"Having a rare disease such as CF is a huge challenge," says Miriam. "Being born in Brazil with this disease can be even more challenging. Here, a late diagnosis such as mine is common, and it is also common to fight your entire life to have access to new and regular CF medications. I use the inhaled antibiotic Cayston and do well on it; however, the drug is not yet approved by the Brazilian Regulatory Agency. In this case, the company that produces Cayston is not interested in coming to Brazil. In order to receive the drug, my only option was to file a lawsuit against the government and renew it every six months. My mother has helped immensely in that endeavor. It's a constant threat for anyone with CF to live with such a broken system and it breaks my heart."

In 2018, Miriam returned to the US to work as a postdoctoral research associate scientist at the University of North Carolina at Chapel Hill, studying how CFTR modulators and mRNA therapy affect mucus properties in CF while working on the Cystic Fibrosis Foundation–funded project "Efficacy of CFTR Modulators on CF Airway Mucus Hydration." She also began exploring other novel therapies, such as inhaled reducing agents that can be combined to reduce the effect of increased mucus concentration in CF.

In 2019, Miriam spoke at ResearchCon for the Cystic Fibrosis Foundation and received a grant from the foundation for two years to continue her work. Miriam has two rare mutations (1717-1G>A and G85E) and therefore was not thought to be a candidate for any of the current CFTR modulators like Trikafta; however, she learned that the G85E was similar to the Delta F508 and so the G85E mutation was approved for Trikafta at the end of 2020, and she began using the new medicine in January 2021. "I felt a big difference," she says. "Less coughing. Less mucus accumulation. I feel more energy and better in the mornings."

Miriam is now thirty-four and her lung function is good, though she still often needs antibiotics and exercise to keep her lungs stable. She has already begun establishing herself in the US, as she is a board member of the Cystic Fibrosis Foundation Central/Eastern Carolinas Chapter as well as a chair member of the Tomorrow's Leaders Program through the same chapter. She also wants to start a family while continuing to advocate for Brazilian CF patients by telling companies with which she meets about the problem of getting medications in her home country. She currently volunteers for the largest nonprofit organization in Brazil, the United for Life Institute, or Instituto Unidos Pela Vida.

"Although she does not live in Brazil, [Miriam] is always concerned with the reality of her country, and she helps us with our competency, work, and research," says Instituto Unidos Pela Vida CEO Verônica Stasiak Bednarczuk, one of Miriam's closest friends and herself a cystic fibrosis patient. "She is taking Trikafta and is getting better every day, but she is still worrying about us and about all CF patients in Brazil. She is a great advocacy partner."

"My goals are to help more patients have access to transforming medications," says Miriam. "I wish then to continue working on science progress and advocacy."

Fluent in both Portuguese and English, she also spends her time translating and creating relevant scientific texts for the Brazilian CF community, "with the ultimate goal of bringing scientific awareness to patients and their relatives."

Miriam looks back and remembers her dream of becoming a scientist to help patients like her to have hope. "Today, I am part of the world of scientists. I am familiar with the thousands of obstacles I had to overcome, and I am proud of it. I wrote many papers and theses about cystic fibrosis and other diseases that helped to spread more knowledge. For me, knowledge is the exchange currency for scientific development and, consequently, for the development of new treatments. I dream of even better treatments that stop the progression of this disease for me and for other people with CF. I will continue to spread information and fight until that happens. I don't know how many weapons I will use for the years to come, but I know that I'm well equipped for this battle."

Miriam admits that being a scientific researcher while having a chronic disease is not the easiest path to navigate due to the fact that she works so closely with her own disease. "I often have to remind myself to separate the scientist in me from the patient," says Miriam, whose entire research portfolio is related to diabetes, kidney disease, and CF. "But it's the patient in me that inspires me to continue my career as a biomedical researcher."

TRAVIS SUIT

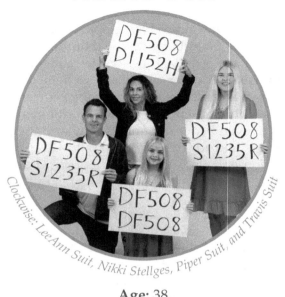

Clockwise: LeeAnn Suit, Nikki Stellges, Piper Suit, and Travis Suit

Age: 38
Resides: West Palm Beach, FL
Age at Diagnosis: 37

PIPER'S ANGEL: A FATHER'S LOVE FOR HIS DAUGHTER

"When my daughter Piper was diagnosed with CF at the age of four, I experienced a seismic shift in consciousness that began with a dark night of the soul, launched me into a journey across an ocean, and birthed me into a community of individuals whose light, courage, and love have inspired me to advocate with a passion as eternal as my love for Piper," says Travis Suit. "I consider it an honor to bear witness to the lives and legacies of every CF warrior. They have been my greatest teachers."

Travis grew up on a dirt road in a rural part of West Palm Beach. He has three siblings—his sister LeeAnn and his brother, Jeff, were from his father's first marriage, and his sister Nikki, who, along with Travis, was from his father's second marriage.

"I got my first BB gun when I was five years old and spent nearly all my extra time walking the pinewood trails near my house, exploring the unknown expanses of wilderness," he says. "I played every sport under the sun, with football being one of my favorites. I was very fortunate to have loving parents who empowered me to cultivate my athleticism and leadership at a young age, and these early lessons of teamwork continue to show up in my life and work today. In eighth grade, I set a school record for the 1600 meters at 5:46; this was one of my earliest and most proud accomplishments. My adventurous and daring nature taught me a lot about myself and facing my fears, especially when I got caught in precarious situations. I said yes to almost everything, which sometimes got me in trouble but also showed me how to push the boundaries of what's possible."

Travis's positive attitude would never serve him better as when his daughter, Piper, and sister LeeAnn both received diagnoses of cystic fibrosis—approximately one year apart—and then just three years later his sister Nikki was diagnosed with the disease. "When LeeAnn [diagnosed November 2010] and Piper [diagnosed November 2011] were diagnosed, it was very confusing at first, because our family didn't know anything about cystic fibrosis," says Travis. "There was a long period of grief over the realization that our family members had this disease. On the other hand, it was relieving to some degree to know what Piper was facing, and why she had been consistently on this roller coaster of sickness. Piper's symptoms [Piper's mutations are two Delta F508's] from the time she was eighteen months until she was four years old were chronic lung infections and eventually walking pneumonia."

LeeAnn's symptoms covered a broad spectrum. At about fifteen years old she started coughing heavy mucus and had a few cases of pneumonia. X-rays showed bronchiectasis and very abnormal lung tissue. "There were no expectations ever given for reoccurring symptoms," says Travis. "She was treated with antibiotics and nasal saline breathing treatments. It persisted for years, progressively getting worse. [LeeAnn] began treatment at the Mayo Clinic after a diagnosis of postnasal drip from a local physician. Mayo Clinic's team did her first sweat chloride test, and it was negative. They decided to treat her with the same protocol for CF patients, which was years of antibiotics in eighteen-month rounds at a time. They would not knock back the aspergillosis, but it was wreaking havoc on her lungs, and she was still vomiting lots of mucus. She had heavy mucus and ran fevers, sweat heavily at night with severe fatigue, only weighing eighty-five pounds."

"I was not able to be diagnosed with CF until the genetic testing was available," says LeeAnn, "because I had a negative sweat chloride. The sweat chloride was the method of diagnosing patients for years. I had every classic symptom of CF for decades so the physicians decided to follow all the protocols that CF patients were treated with because they were so helpful.

"I was forty when the genetic testing became possible for me," says LeeAnn. "I had already undergone a left lobectomy (in 2000) due to significant infections and advanced disease. That would have never been done if they knew about the CF. At the very same time, I was being sent to Colorado for removal of the left lung when I was offered the genetic screening for CF, and it came back positive [LeeAnn's two mutations are the Delta F508 and D1152H]. I was then transferred to the CF clinic teams for all future care. We would then do all we could to preserve the left lung. This was a great relief to finally know why I was so sick for so long."

"Today, LeeAnn is still very sick and facing an array of complications," says Travis, "but she is getting treatment from her CF care team."

Nikki, on the other hand, was born six weeks early in 1981 and was rushed to another hospital with a collapsed lung and in need of surgery to reinflate it and be on oxygen. She was given the last incubator in that hospital. After twelve days in the NICU, she was able to go home, minus a cystic fibrosis diagnosis.

It wasn't as if Nikki didn't have CF symptoms. "As a young child," says Nikki, "I often dealt with coughing. At the time, my mom thought it could be whooping cough, but the doctor said it was not and it was assumed it was allergies.

"I really did not have any other indications of any major health concerns after that," says Nikki, "until I tried to get pregnant and, with various other symptoms, was diagnosed with Hashimoto's disease, an autoimmune thyroid disorder. Then, when I was twenty-nine years old and partway through my first pregnancy in November 2010, I found out, through testing suggested by the doctor, that I was a carrier with the Delta F508 gene, and that cystic fibrosis could be a concern for my unborn child. It was extremely coincidental timing that this was the very same week I had been told by my sister LeeAnn that she was diagnosed with cystic fibrosis. This was not something I had ever heard of until then. Not long after that Piper was diagnosed as well. It was a life-changing experience to learn that cystic fibrosis would impact our family in so many different ways.

"My husband, Gary, decided to be tested and thankfully he was not a carrier. A few months after my son was born, I got really sick. I was treated multiple times on oral antibiotics but was not getting better. It took treatment of a very strong antibiotic, and I spent three days coughing up blood. I felt nervous and decided, due to the knowledge now of cystic fibrosis in my family and the digestive symptoms I had been dealing with for many years, along with this struggle to get over a cough for several months, that I would pursue testing.

"In November 2012, I tested in the positive range with two sweat chloride tests and was diagnosed with cystic fibrosis. The original genetic testing done was not comprehensive enough to identify my second gene. My sister was being treated at Shands and recommended her clinic. They were able to do additional genetic testing for me and, in December 2013, it was confirmed that I had a second gene, S1235R. My sister and I have different biological mothers so we both have a second gene that is different from each other, but we have in common the Delta F508 gene as does Piper, which was passed from Travis. Our only other sibling, Jeff, does not have cystic fibrosis. My symptoms have mostly been comprised of digestive issues, sometimes sinus, and testing showed moderate pancreatic insufficiency. Mostly, my lungs—that I am aware of—have not been affected in the same ways others with cystic fibrosis are; however, I always feel the question of what the future holds for my health. I know that cystic fibrosis is different for everyone and unbelievably challenging for most, and it also brings a perspective on life that is very unique."

Travis, on the other hand, had his own journey to diagnosis. From a young age, Travis dreamed of being an entrepreneur. After attending the University of Central Florida in Orlando, he founded his first company to produce lifestyle events and, like others committed to striking out on their own, had experienced both success and failure in his business ventures. But his determination was never stronger than when his daughter, Piper, was diagnosed with CF.

"As a newly diagnosed CF parent, I found my purpose in the expression of my dedication to Piper and the community we had just become a part of," says Travis. "I wanted to do something that showed the depths of my commitment to honoring their fight, something that would get people's attention and put CF and its warriors in the spotlight so that the world would see what I saw: love and life persisting, even through the darkest of nights."

When Piper was eight years old, she had several long-term hospitalizations. One night in the hospital, around midnight, Piper was asleep in her bed, and Travis was lying on the cot next to her, when she suddenly woke up with tears in her eyes, and looked at him and said, "Daddy, my lungs are burning."

"I called the nurse, who immediately came in and calmed Piper down," says Travis. "She increased the pain medication through her IV, and Piper eventually fell back asleep. I walked out into the hallway and leaned against the wall and collapsed into an emotional wreck onto the floor. It was this experience and this moment that truly pushed me to a new level of desire to help the CF community."

As Travis began to learn more about CF and the needs of the community, he says his heart was filling with a new purpose as he realized his ability to apply his talents and experience to the nonprofit world through the Cystic Fibrosis Foundation. "After many years of volunteering and leading fundraising campaigns and events," Travis says, "I created my own fundraising event in 2013 called The Crossing For Cystic Fibrosis, which is an eighty-mile paddle adventure from the Bahamas to Florida across the open ocean." Travis—who didn't know how to paddleboard or surf prior to Piper's diagnosis but, after discovering the incredible healing benefits the ocean has for people with CF, wanted to be able to teach Piper—says the event was life changing. "Up until then, I had never experienced so much unconditional love and support from complete strangers, which was truly remarkable and inspired me to continue to dream bigger about ways I could make a difference." The most recent annual event included 150 paddlers and 50 support boats and raised a single-year record $675,000 for a cumulative total of over $1.7 million. "The Crossing For Cystic Fibrosis also turned me into an avid waterman," says Travis, "and gave me and Piper a new bond. We have since surfed in Florida, Hawaii, and Costa Rica."

The event also became the catalyst for creating a new nonprofit in 2017 called the Piper's Angels Foundation. "The vision of the foundation is to support and improve the lives of families in the cystic fibrosis community through grassroots advocacy and socially innovative programs," says Travis, referring to the company's mission statement, "raising awareness through education, offering life-expanding activities, providing urgent financial support, and funding critical developments."

Travis says that they have grown the organization to serve CF families throughout the US. Since inception, they've impacted hundreds of families through their different program offerings, which include grants for financial assistance, scholarships for participants in saltwater activities, and mindfulness training for mental health, care packs for hospitalization, and peer-to-peer support. In 2019, they launched Warrior Wednesday, a global day of activism for the CF community which features a video and photo contest to promote awareness.

"I've learned very valuable lessons from Dad," says fourteen-year-old Piper, "and I love that I get to grow up with a community who loves me and be able to help others. I enjoy all the people and friends

I've made from [the foundation] and just getting to see other people with CF and relate to them."

Travis says that his support system has been instrumental in advocating for those with CF. "My family has had a tremendous influence and impact on how we support my sisters, LeeAnn and Nikki, and my daughter, Piper, with their lives with CF," he says. "They've really taught me the value of simply showing up for those we love. It's amazing how profound feeling the compassion of others is for persevering through hard times. Our family is the bedrock of strength behind our drive and purpose to live our best lives possible, despite the challenges of CF."

And then there's the support of Piper's mother. The two never married and are not romantically involved, but they remain close today. "She became a nurse primarily to benefit Piper's care," says Travis. "We had someone early on tell us that having a child with a chronic illness can either tear a family apart or bring them closer together; I am eternally grateful that, for our family, it has brought us together in ways we could have never imagined. We have always kept Piper's health as our number one priority and focused on empowering her to live the greatest life possible."

"I honestly don't really think about CF that much," says Piper. "It's just something unique about me, and it's really amazing how I get to see other people with CF and help them. I think it just gives me more of a reason to live my life to the fullest with the time I have."

Piper has recently started Trikafta, the benefits of which are already presenting themselves. "I have a pretty normal life for the most part because of the new Trikafta medicine," she says. "I don't really get sick like I used to, but I try to find the cool and fun parts about having CF, which sounds weird but there are a lot of perks to it. I take Trikafta in the morning and at night, along with my enzymes with every meal, and I do my Pulmozyme breathing treatment when I get home from school every day." Piper also takes time speaking to her aunts about the disease they share. "It's really nice having someone in the family who understands having CF," says Piper, "because people are either dramatic or pity you, but when talking to them, we can really be realistic with each other."

LeeAnn, who participates in many clinical trials to help others with CF, including Piper, has conflicting feelings with regard to having a niece with CF. "I think one of the hardest things for me now is my feelings for Piper as my niece," she says. "The bond and love are great. We share the common CF diagnosis, but at my age, I have felt the decline and have had many difficult times in life that have felt awful, mentally, physically, and financially. Every aspect I have had to face has been abundantly challenging. I have witnessed so many CF patients do very poorly and even die way too young. I physically feel pain and uncontrolled emotions privately when my mind drifts to these dark times when I think about Piper. I don't want her to ever suffer. I will never allow her to see me in this state, and I rise from that to remain strong and positive about life and CF. I have experienced many things she has to and will face as she ages with CF.

"While I have great gratitude for the advancements for us as CF patients, we do not have a cure and we are far from being free of the constant challenges we are going to face. I feel great comfort in the support Piper has from Travis. His entire life's mission is to ensure she has every need met to be successful in every aspect of her life. He has rallied an army not just for his own daughter but for us all, patients and families. This has been one of the most impactful things I have witnessed and felt in my life. The connections we have made in life, because of our journey with CF, have been an incredible blessing. I personally would not change any part CF has played in my life. Many great things have arisen from my diagnosis. I hope to share my examples, in the way I chose to live, [so] Piper can see [how they] served me well. Perhaps she follows some of these ways as she journeys with CF too."

In November 2021, Travis decided it was time to find out if he may have cystic fibrosis too. "As crazy as it sounds," he says, "I was finally tested and also diagnosed with the same two genes that my sister Nikki has: Delta F508 and S1235R." Yes, Travis, too, has cystic fibrosis, and strangely enough, Piper, LeeAnn, Nikki, and Travis were each diagnosed in the month of November but in different years.

"Over the years since Piper and LeeAnn's diagnosis, as I learned more about CF and how different the symptoms are for every person, I started to become suspicious about some of the physical symptoms I was experiencing myself," says Travis. "My entire life I've had digestive issues with stomach pain, bloating, and processing of certain foods. I always believed it was just something normal I had to deal with and possibly diet related. I tried every diet under the sun to ease the abdominal pain I would get after eating, and although some things helped, like eliminating dairy, nothing ever seemed to work. I was actually hospitalized once with abdominal pain, thinking I had appendicitis, and it turned out to just be caused by gas. Also, in my mid-twenties, I had a girlfriend comment to me about how often I seem to cough and spit. Again, I thought it was normal, but after she pointed it out, I became more aware of the mucus production. I've been an athlete my entire life and had a focus on good health, so my lungs have always been exercised and in good shape. I experienced one episode of severe bronchitis in my twenties that the doctor said seemed abnormal, but other than that, I've never had any major lung infections.

"So when Piper and LeeAnn were diagnosed, and I began to understand the symptoms of CF more, over time it became apparent that my symptoms also might be related to having a CF gene. Once Nikki was diagnosed, I realized it was possible that I would have the same two CF genes, and I had a deep-down intuitive feeling that might be the cause of my symptoms. But because, for the most part, I've fortunately been very healthy, I didn't see the necessity to get tested right away. However, over the last few years, I noticed the mucus production in my sinuses and lungs has progressed, and it was weighing on my mind, so I finally scheduled an appointment at Shands where both LeeAnn and Nikki are seen. The sweat chloride test came back borderline. I was one point away from an immediate diagnosis without the genetic test, but the genetic screening was the final determinant, and it was positive for both CF genes. This diagnosis wasn't a surprise. After all we had been through as a family, and knowing that it was very likely that was the cause of my symptoms, I was relieved to know what was at the root of it all. There was some peace of mind around knowing the truth."

Travis continues, "My symptoms over the last few years have been very light but noticeably increasing. Mostly digestive issues and a steady production of mucus in my sinuses. The Delta F508 gene is what we all have in common, but because Nikki and I have a different mom than LeeAnn, that is where the difference in the gene set comes in. Because my CF is so light, the doctor at Shands has classified me as having cystic fibrosis–related disease.

"The news of my positive test was not surprising to anyone in the family. I had communicated that I was going to get tested, and they were all aware of the symptoms I had been experiencing. It was kind of one of those situations where the writing was on the wall. [The medical team] suggested pancreatic enzymes and a nasal steroid, and that we would keep an eye on the mucus production, and if it progressed, it might be helpful to take Trikafta down the road. Nikki and I are extremely grateful that our symptoms are light compared to many on the spectrum of CF severity. Most people would never imagine I had CF based on my health and athleticism, but that's the strange nature of this disease. With so many genetic variations and different circumstances, everyone's path is different. All of this made me realize, though, there are probably a lot of people living with cystic fibrosis, with light to moderate symptoms that have gone undiagnosed.

"My journey with cystic fibrosis is long term and bittersweet, because for as many times as it breaks my heart, it breaks it open and forces me to fill it with more love and more light," says Travis, who, along with his partner, Dani, welcomed a new member of the family on December 17, 2021, with their son, Hawkins. Dani tested negative for the CF gene and at the time of this book's publication, the family does not believe Hawkins will be diagnosed with cystic fibrosis.

"I've held my daughter's frail eight-year-old body while she cried because her 'lungs burned,'" says Travis, "and I marveled at the delight and wonder in her face as she surfed her first wave. Life experienced in contrasts like these has shown me just how deep my gratitude runs—gratitude for every breath, every sunset, every wave, and every beautiful human fighting to shine their light against CF odds."

Debra Mattson

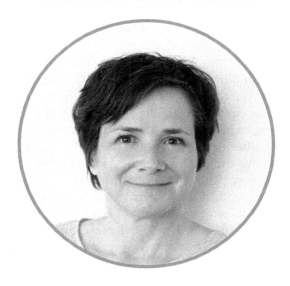

Age: 50
Resides: Whitby, Ontario, Canada
Age at Diagnosis: 6

SERVING HER COMMUNITY: A LIFETIME OF LEADERSHIP

"**H**ere I am," says Debra Mattson, "send me."

This sums up Debra's philosophy of service to the CF community. "I know that I'm lucky health-wise and that not everyone with CF has the ability to give as much time as I can," she says. "I'm in a unique position as well, emotionally, in that I do have a very serious and chronic disease but I have not truly suffered as so many of my friends have. So I walk that line between 'belonging' to a group but not yet truly understanding the struggles. It's for that reason that I give back."

Debra was diagnosed with CF at six years old. "After spending many years 'failing to thrive' without doctors knowing what was wrong," she says, "I was diagnosed at SickKids in Toronto. Growing up, I always knew that I had a deadly chronic disease and never expected to make it past twelve." Debra remembers vividly having a CF Canada fundraising poster in her room with a child on it. The caption read: "Julia just turned six. She just reached middle age." Debra says the poster gave her the feeling that she should worry about dying.

"The poster wasn't all bad," says Debra, "and actually had special meaning because of the other person on the poster was Mila Mulroney. She was Canadian Prime Minister Brian Mulroney's wife and our champion at CF Canada [then known as the Canadian Cystic Fibrosis Foundation]. She was the biggest celebrity to go to bat for us, to even know about CF for that matter. And she was so pretty! So as a kid, it was really exciting to be a part of that community with her leading the way in getting us attention. She was in the picture with the young girl with CF. That's why the poster was up. That age of survival number haunted me in a way, but it was also a challenge to me to beat the odds, so I think, overall, it was a positive thing to look at. It gave me hope, that she was helping us and that I could beat that number."

Debra says she felt like she was more emotionally mature or 'older' in a sense because "I had an acute awareness about my mortality from a very young age," says Debra, who says some of that came from her CF camp experience. "My CF friends were made solely at summer camp—a camp for kids with CF called Camp Couchiching, in Orilia, Ontario," says Debra. "I still have friends to this day from that camp, although most of them have passed away. This was before they knew about infection control, so, yes, cabins full of kids with CF. It was incredible. All of us together, taking our pills openly, coughing, doing all our treatments—everyone just like me, it was one of the greatest experiences of my life. We were in cabins with bunk beds. I remember realizing very early on that there were some very sick kids at camp—lying in bed listening to the phlegm gurgle in their lungs.

"Mostly we just hung out like all kids, canoeing, kayaking, sailing, doing arts and crafts, playing games, eating together, etc. But there was an awareness among us that we were 'different' than others yet the same as each other for those few short weeks every summer. It was easy to make friends because we were together all day and had so much in common. It was just a matter of 'being there' and taking part in activities.

"I would go on to visit one friend in particular, Teena, outside of camp, and my parents drove me down south to see her so we had a few days together. I remember her mom calling one night, and I answered, and she asked to speak to my mom. My mom was busy, so Teena's mom said, 'Well, it's you I should be talking to anyway. Teena died, I'm sorry to tell you.' That was my first CF friend death, and I remember saying 'I'm sorry' and then not really knowing what else to do. I simply processed it. I think with CF we learn at a really young age that death is inevitable and more of a 'matter of fact' than a deep, dark tragedy. It's a cynical attitude for a young person, but it's probably a defense mechanism; I mean, every summer we went back to camp, we would gather and review who didn't make it."

Debra says that cystic fibrosis played a role in who she became. "I think CF matured me quickly and made me strong. I do remember plenty of fear of dying and asking my dad one night when I would die. He assured me it would not be for a very long time." Debra also remembers her time in the hospital, when she was being diagnosed, as both scary and fun. "Scary because I was alone most of the time. My dad was up north at home, working, and my mom could not stay in the big city of Toronto every day, so they were probably gone for most of the time. In fact, I remember my friend's mom sitting with me during the old sweat tests (the ones with many wool blankets over you, needles in your back). But *fun* because of the friends I made!"

Debra says she specifically remembers one friend, Elizabeth, whose mom sat with Debra during the sweat test. "No, she didn't have CF," says Debra, "and I was so young I don't really know what her hospitalization was for. However, I remember we were fast friends, running around the hospital and getting in a wee bit of a trouble for it! I also remember distinctly that we both got in trouble for taking ice cream. I guess there was a communal fridge, and we took a couple of those little ice cream tubs with the wooden spoons that they used to give out in the seventies. It wasn't that we stole the ice cream, it was that I ate it without my [enzymes]—because I forgot that I needed to take them whenever I ate something; and Elizabeth had surgery the next day and wasn't supposed to eat anything. So we were scolded by the nurse." Debra says she doesn't remember what happened to Elizabeth, but she certainly made her hospitalizations tolerable.

Despite the challenges that made it difficult for her parents to be available in those early days, Debra says her parents were always positive and supportive about her CF. "They attended chapter meetings and supported other CF parents," she says. Her mom was also very vigilant about Debra's treatments and, perhaps most importantly, she taught Debra to never be ashamed of CF and to share openly. "I do remember, though, when my best friend 'found out,'" says Debra. "As a kid, you don't really make an announcement or tell your friends 'I have something to tell you,' so I hadn't really mentioned it to my friend. We were quite young, and she came knocking at my door while I was doing a treatment. I had the mask on and the steam coming out of it, and she came in the house while she had a grape popsicle in her mouth, and I remember seeing her mouth wide open with the grape all over it. She must have been shocked to see me like that. I imagine we had a good conversation about it—as much as two young kids could."

Debra began making presentations at her school. "I used to bring in all my meds and percussor and masks, etc. as a show and tell," she says. "My symptoms were mostly bowel related. All my friends knew I had CF throughout my life. I always remember telling them. It is always risky and scary when you tell, so that never ends, up to this day when you decide to tell an employer or colleague. But of course, it always works out and feels better than concealing. I'm quick to reveal it now."

As the years went on, Debra began to imagine a longer future. "Though, I slacked a bit in college and in the years after," she says. "When I was in my twenties, I coughed up blood and went to the emergency room. I had not been doing anything for my CF until that point because I was so healthy. This was a wake-up call to start physiotherapy and medication. I also remember, around this time, attending a support group, and I realized the gravity of the situation and what CF could mean for me—I was very frightened of the future and getting sick. I knew then that even though I was okay, I had to step it up and start taking CF seriously. Despite being very healthy, the truth is that CF can turn on a dime and turn against you quickly. I [may] never know when I will lose lung function, so I need to be vigilant about everything. Hope for the best but prepare for the worst, always.

"Now, here I am at fifty and thriving," says Debra. "I've never been hospitalized for CF and have managed to stay healthy." Debra attributes much of her good health in midlife to running. "I started, eight years ago, participating in my first official 10K run in 2013—the Toronto Waterfront Run—and have now completed a handful of half-marathons. I run five times a week to exercise my lungs and control my CF-related diabetes. I know I've been lucky too, and I use that health and energy to volunteer every minute I can to help raise awareness and funds to find a cure."

Debra began her two-decade-long service with Cystic Fibrosis Canada at the age of twenty-four. "My first instinct to get involved was a bit selfish," says Debra. "I wanted to make friends after I moved across the country to British Columbia (BC) from Ontario. So I approached the CF adult clinic in Victoria, BC, about putting up a poster asking if CF people wanted to get together to share experiences, sort of like a support group. I only got two responses. One person was more aware of infection control than I was, and he was very cautious, but we did meet. Another woman became my good friend, Yvonne. We never did have a support group, but it was my first step in putting myself out there in a new place, as a leader."

Debra continues, "Soon after that, I started writing articles about my life with CF for the Victoria Chapter newsletter. That may have had a selfish edge too, as I wanted to write and grow my portfolio as a writer. But as I did that, I started to go to chapter meetings and just saw so many things I could do and had the desire to do. It was fun; I don't know if it was altruistic. I met great people, learned a lot about CF and my community, did fun tasks, grew my résumé, expanded my skills—I mean, it was all so positive. I think it also had to do with feeling really powerless about CF and not knowing what the future would hold. At least this way I was in control of what I did and how I helped and contributed. I couldn't just do nothing. How could I sit around watching TV or doing silly things when this horrible disease was screwing up and taking away so many lives? At least if I was fund-raising, I was helping to drive the fight for a cure or control. How much regret would I have if I was suddenly sick and hospitalized and felt like I hadn't done anything to fight?"

Debra started as a representative for CF adults on the national CF Adult Committee in the province of British Columbia and continued in this capacity when she moved back to Ontario eleven years later. During her time in the Victoria Chapter, her team won the national Volunteer Development Award for their increase in volunteers, and during her time as Durham CF Chapter President (Ontario), her chapter was awarded the provincial Chapter of the Year Award.

She's represented CF Canadian adults at two international conferences, one in Germany and one in Italy; became editor of the national CF Adult newsletter; chaired many committees for special fundraising events from walks/runs to gala dinners to princess balls; spoke at various conferences and public events about her life with CF; appeared on radio and television to promote CF awareness; and participated in the Royal Commission on the Future of Health Care in Canada, a federal government investigation into how best to offer a national health care plan. She's also had a letter she wrote about her life with CF and saying good-bye to so many CF friends used in a direct mail campaign with CF Canada.

Most recently, she received a national volunteer award from CF Canada called the Summerhayes Award—named after Doug and Donna Summerhayes, who founded the Canadian Cystic Fibrosis Foundation in 1960—which honors an individual with CF who has demonstrated an exceptional commitment of national impact to the cystic fibrosis cause.

"I never take a moment for granted as I never expected to live this long," says Debra. "I have written letters, met with my member of Parliament, and met with my member of Provincial Parliament, and now, most of all, I want to see access to Trikafta for Canadian CF patients [which finally occurred in September 2021]. My vision for the CF community is that we will one day expect to live well into our senior years without pain and suffering . . . without having to exhaust ourselves fighting for insurance, prescriptions, treatments, and benefits. That we could at least have an easier life than those who've gone before us. And that our lives aren't just about getting by and making it to the next day but thriving and enjoying our existence."

CAROLINE HEFFERNAN

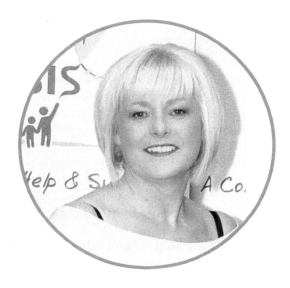

Age: 51
Resides: Tuam, County Galway, Ireland
Age at Diagnosis: 13

IRELAND'S ICON: A CF IRONMAN . . . AND GRANDMOTHER

C aroline Heffernan, who is from the small town of Tuam in Ireland, which has less than ten thousand people, was thirteen when she was diagnosed with CF.

"Two years previous to diagnosis I was getting very tired [and] falling asleep during the day," says Caroline. "My teachers thought I was lazy because I always had my head propped on the desk to rest." Then Caroline got a recurring chest infection that she couldn't shake. "I was X-rayed and diagnosed with TB. After another year, they decided to do a sweat test as I wasn't responding to treatment for TB." That is when it was finally revealed that Caroline had cystic fibrosis.

Though she was likely misdiagnosed at age twelve with TB, Caroline says the CF diagnosis was shocking, "because I was rarely sick as a child. Now I was being told by a doctor that I'd be lucky to reach twenty."

Caroline says her family remained strong despite the diagnosis. "When I was diagnosed, you can imagine the devastation [for] my parents," she says. "But I remember overhearing my mum say, 'If Caroline isn't going to live a long time, she is going to laugh every day and enjoy the time she has.'" After her diagnosis, Caroline was put on enzymes and antibiotics—eventually she would also start using nebulizers and inhalers and, much later, Kalydeco—"but I still think to this day that laughter is the best medicine."

After the initial shock of CF, Caroline's family continued on as normal. Caroline stayed active during this time, predominantly by swimming as a teenager. "CF didn't stop us from doing all the things we did before," says Caroline. "I think this is important, as we recognized it was only a part of our lives. I learned to live every day to the fullest. My glass is always half full. I will do whatever I can to help friends and strangers. I believe life is for the living and not a gift to be thrown away lightly."

Not long after Caroline's diagnosis at the age of thirteen, a girl from the same hometown, who happened to be the same age as Caroline and who was also living with CF, began visiting her either at her home or at a local park. "Denise and I became friends," says Caroline, who points out that back then it was not a concern to have two people with cystic fibrosis within six feet of each other. "She taught me everything there was to know about CF."

Denise passed away shortly after their friendship began, though in that short time, Caroline gained a shared experience that made the loss that much more devastating. "Our physical friendship was brief as Denise was very sick and spent a lot of time in [the] hospital, which was the other side of the country," says Caroline. "We were young teenagers; Denise having lived a much tougher life than me. We both loved animals, and Denise was very good at horse riding. I believe Denise knew she hadn't long for this world and very gently prepared me for the harshness that is [or] was the world of CF. I remember sitting in the back of the church at her funeral crying and not being able to move.

"There is an instant bond when you have something like CF as the common denominator. Sometimes it's the unspoken that's more important. I can't explain the impact of Denise in my life apart from saying I've carried her with me in spirit and always wonder what she would have achieved in life if given the opportunity. I hope if she is looking down on me, she is proud of what I've done for both of us.

"Denise showed such strength and determination that I promised myself I would live the best life possible for both of us. It was very much a defining moment for me."

Caroline is married to Fran, her childhood sweetheart of thirty-five years (married for twenty-six years). Together, they have two beautiful children: a son, Jamie, twenty-three, and a daughter, Anna, nineteen.

"After Jamie was born, I realized I wanted to live more than anything else in the whole world," says Caroline. "By the time he was a toddler, I realized I couldn't just live with CF. I had to work hard to get fit so I could keep up to him as he became active." That's when Caroline began her journey to get in shape. "I exercised with more structure and determination, stretching out walks and started to jog a little bit," she says. "I also went back to swimming. Soon, I was able to kick the ball for longer periods of time. I could jump and fool around more with my toddler without becoming breathless.

"After my second child, Anna, I had a pretty bad year," says Caroline, who admits that breathing got difficult at seven months during each pregnancy, which required her to be hospitalized and undergo IV antibiotics until each child was born. "Lung function in the forties, feeling horrible the whole time, no matter what I did. It took all my strength to fight CF and accept help during this time."

Caroline admits that asking for help is a must when you are physically worn down. "When you don't feel well," she says, "every little thing can be a big deal. I was at home with the kids but couldn't look after them on my own because I had no energy. I relied on my parents and in-laws to help out when Fran was at work. Sometimes, I couldn't even set the open fire but had to sit and watch while someone else did the job for me. It is getting through tough times that you realize that it's okay to get help." With regard to getting fit once again, Caroline says she "had to do the same as after Jamie, [my] starting point was much worse. So I had to [endure] a lot more IV antibiotics during the first year after Anna, with each set of IVs causing a setback."

Caroline worked hard to stay in great shape, and in 2008, she set a goal of completing the New York City Marathon. "I trained hard with a few setbacks for eighteen months," she says. After completing the marathon, things got more difficult for Caroline a few years later. "I started to really struggle with my health when I entered my forties," she says. "I was actually admitted on my fortieth birthday, but I was thrown a lifeline when I was given a second chance at life, receiving Kalydeco as part of a trial in 2016 at the age of forty-six. It completely changed my life." Caroline jokes that it was Botox for her lungs. Her lung function went from the fortieth-percentile range during her hospitalization to now hovering around the seventies and eighties. "Within ninety minutes [of taking my first dose of Kalydeco],

I walked up my stairs for the first time in four years without being breathless and having to stop at the top," says Caroline.

Caroline decided she needed to do something epic with her new-found energy and improved lung function, "so I joined a CF Ireland Fundraiser and cycled Malin [most northern point of Ireland] to Mizen [most southern point of Ireland] on a tandem for the Malin 2 Mizen Cycle 4 CF, for Cystic Fibrosis Ireland," she says. Caroline completed the four-day cycling event, averaging eight hours per day, and returned the following year to ride her own bike without the support of a pilot. She has now cycled the full length of Ireland—640 kilometers—for CF Ireland to raise money on five different occasions.

Caroline has also completed several sprint triathlons around Ireland, including the Joey Hannon in Limerick and the Galway Sprint in Galway City. In 2018, she finished Ironman Barcelona, a full-distance triathlon with a 3.8 kilometer swim, a 180 kilometer bike ride, and a 42.2 kilometer marathon. According to the *Irish Examiner*, she became the first Irish person with CF to complete an Ironman, and she had signed up for another Ironman in Cork for August 2021 before it was canceled due to the global pandemic. She still plans to climb Mount Fuji in July 2022 and Kilimanjaro in early 2023.

"I think every day that I get up and challenge myself is an accomplishment, especially on the bad days," says Caroline, who currently does nebulizers in the morning, followed by Kaftrio (which she began taking in January 2022) and Kalydeco, exercise for physiotherapy throughout the day, and nebulizers again in the evening. "My exercise tolerance is different every day. I have wonderful friends who go with the flow if it's a fifty-five-minute, five-kilometer walk or a thirty-two-minute, five-kilometer jog. We take it day by day."

Caroline has worked for CF Ireland as a patient advocate for the last fourteen years, and before that she was a tutor for children with learning difficulties. "I chat with families with CF," she says. "I particularly love talking to new families, telling them how old I am and reminding them I'm a 1970s baby—completely different world of CF than what we have now—feeling them smile over the phone, realizing [having] hope is such a good feeling." Caroline was also part of a small committee which raised $1.3 million over five years to build a specialized outpatient unit in their local hospital for CF. "I feel very proud when I walk through the doors for a port flush knowing a lot of my blood, sweat, and tears went into making a difference to our local community."

Caroline says that she has lived her ultimate dream by seeing her children grow up. "I also have the added bonus of playing with a grandchild!" she says of her grandson, Milo, now two and a half years old. Caroline also admits that she is now in better shape for Milo than when her son, Jamie (Milo's dad), was a toddler. "I still want to see my children live well into their adult lives, happy with their jobs and partners, and not only watch my grandchildren grow up but be able to run around the playground with them!"

Caroline says that her approach during the difficult times is accepting that there will be hard days and not letting it define her as a person. "I also believe," she says, "that if I didn't have CF, I wouldn't be the strong, independent, determined (stubborn) woman that I am today."

TERRY WRIGHT

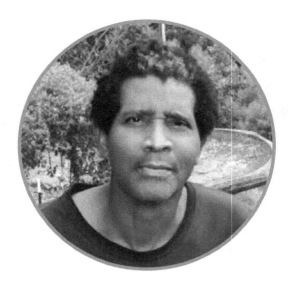

Age: 60
Resides: North Little Rock, Arkansas
Age at diagnosis: 54

FINDING ANSWERS AND LOVE: CHANGING THE FACE OF CF

Michele Wise had been on a few blind dates when she met Mr. Wright on November 1, 1999. "It was my *first* blind date," says Terry Wright who was set up by one of his personal-training clients, and it was love at first sight.

"The moment I laid eyes on her, I called her Butterbean, and she has been my Butterbean ever since. She was and still remains the most beautiful woman I have ever seen in my life. I always tell her that when I count my blessings, I count her twice! This remains the case twenty-two years and counting later. I am fully confident that I would not be alive if it were not for my wife's support, strength, pharmaceutical training, and relentless pursuit of reaching beyond the diagnosis."

"I waited until the third date to fall in love with him," Michele jokes.

Michele and Terry's story is not just about how they met but what they have done to make a difference in the cystic fibrosis community. While approximately one in twenty-nine Caucasian Americans are carriers of the cystic fibrosis gene, the likelihood of someone of African American descent carrying the CF gene is far less likely—approximately one in sixty-five African Americans—which is why many African Americans are diagnosed much later if at all, and why Terry, though he had been hospitalized and seen by a number of health care practitioners throughout his life, wasn't diagnosed until he was fifty-four. So, in 2019, Michele and Terry established the National Organization of African Americans with Cystic Fibrosis (NOAACF), a 501(c)(3) organization, with Terry as president and Michele as board chair.

The mission of NOAACF is to engage, educate, and raise CF awareness in the African American community and to help bring valuable resources, knowledge, empowerment, and support to CF patients, families, healthcare professionals, and the community. Through widespread involvement, partnerships, and outreach, NOAACF's program scope is to ensure that the cystic fibrosis diverse community is educated, informed, and made aware of CF's existence, prevalence, and impact on underrepresented communities. NOAACF's goals are to connect, help build diverse communities, and raise CF awareness in the African American community and beyond through its national platform. The organization engages with a variety of individuals and groups, including the Cystic Fibrosis Foundation (CFF), the Cystic Fibrosis Research Institute (CFRI), the Bonnell Foundation, the Attain Health Foundation, the Cystic Fibrosis Foundation Arkansas Chapter, among others as part of their ongoing community outreach strategies and initiatives.

"As a child, I was extremely sickly," says Terry. "This was due to an array of symptoms including extreme gut pain, GI issues, nausea, asthma, wheezing, coughing, pneumonia, sinusitis, migraines, vision and hearing problems, and breathing difficulties. Although I was not shy, my health issues often kept me isolated, as I missed a lot of school and spent a lot of time home sick during my entire school education from age five (kindergarten) to age eighteen (high school). This unknown genetic disease has literally impacted me my entire life and since the time I can possibly remember. However, because of my unique muscle build and physical activity, I was not skinny. Playing a variety of sports and being active proved beneficial to my health both mentally and physically.

"I am a sixty-year-old African American male CF patient who has spent a great portion of my childhood at Arkansas Children Hospital and a significant amount of adult life in and out of hospitals and on multiple operating tables. I have been near death on numerous occasions, never realizing the true underlying cause of my sufferings until I was finally diagnosed with cystic fibrosis at the age of fifty-four in spring 2017. When I was finally diagnosed with CF, I thought to myself, *Now I know why I was suffering all these many years with so much illness*. Everything finally made sense and the dots finally connected."

Terry continues, "I always knew I was different, because I did not have the normal sickness and health issues that other children had like chicken pox, measles, etc. So to finally receive an answer after fifty-four years of pain and suffering with barely any answers was a very welcomed event. It is painful to think about how long it took for me to get diagnosed, especially since it was based on biased diagnosis and stereotyping my symptoms. For instance, I walked in a clinic about twenty-one years ago for what would have turned out to be double pneumonia, but after being examined, the clinic physician informed me, 'If you were not African American, I would say you had cystic fibrosis.' That would be the last time I would hear the words 'cystic fibrosis' until seventeen years later at the age of fifty-four. It is heartbreaking when I reflect back on all the doctors who did not diagnose me appropriately because of assumptions made on my race."

Terry realizes that while his diagnosis took much longer than it should have, he is fortunate to be alive today. "You must ultimately forgive to heal," he says. "My Butterbean, alongside my mama, Rose, and other family members, have been helpful in this extensive process and continue to be to this very day. I am very close to my mom and talk to her and try to see her on a daily basis. Of course, my mom and loved ones were very shocked and in disbelief to learn of my diagnosis. But they, like myself and wife, were finally relieved to receive not only answers but a definitive name at the root of my health history."

While 2020 was a difficult year for most because of the pandemic, Terry continued to persevere. He was not only appointed to the United States Adult Cystic Fibrosis Association (USACFA) Board of Directors but Terry's dream also came true when his book, *Terry's Journey to CF Land: Navigating the Adventures of Cystic Fibrosis* (a coloring book and children's story that can be found on Amazon), was published on November 4, 2020, coinciding with his and Michele's twentieth wedding anniversary. And acknowledgment for his contributions continued in 2021, as he was awarded the CF Star from the Arkansas Chapter of the Cystic Fibrosis Foundation and received an impact grant from the Cystic Fibrosis Foundation for his and Michele's organization.

Terry, who currently resides in North Little Rock, Arkansas, is a certified personal fitness trainer (CPFT) with more than three decades in various arenas of physical and mental coaching. "[My profession] has allowed me to effectively help meet the physical, health, nutrition, fitness, and well-being challenges often endured by CF sufferers," he says. Terry is also a certified master gardener and certified master naturalist, offering more than fifteen years of personal and professional experience in horticulture and herbology, which he believes has made him the positive person he is today. "I wholeheartedly utilize my deep-rooted passion for gardening, nature, agriculture, horticulture, fitness, nutrition, and health to help individuals from all walks of life achieve the best in health."

"I am so extremely proud of my husband, soul mate, and love of my life, Terry Wright," says Michele, "because I so admire his perseverance, respect his will to live, and value his spirit of love and determination to never give up! And not only is he a remarkable trailblazer and CF warrior, Terry is an inspiration to countless across the cystic fibrosis spectrum for not only today but for generations to come!"

Terry and Michele continue to spread amazing awareness, not only to those in the CF community but also those in the African American community about the lesser-known group of people with the disease so that people like Terry will not be misdiagnosed for years and can start working on getting stronger right away. "Now, I continue to reinvent history through the cofounding of the National Organization of African Americans with Cystic Fibrosis and my children's story and coloring book . . . If I can help make a difference and positively impact the life of just one cystic fibrosis patient, then my living, suffering, and CF journey will not have been in vain. At sixty years old, I am still going strong with a mission to bring awareness, education, and understanding to the potential lack of support, information, understanding, and diagnosis of CF in the African American community and beyond!"

DR. VICTOR ROGGLI

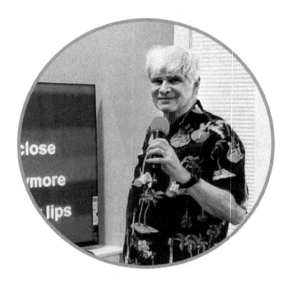

Age: 71
Resides: Durham, North Carolina
Age at diagnosis: 12

SHINING AT SEVENTY: THE MIRACLE OF TRIKAFTA

D r. Victor Roggli—who was born in Winchester, Tennessee, in 1951, and raised on a farm between Decherd (population two thousand) and Cowan (population three thousand), Tennessee—was doing pretty well until one July afternoon.

After a morning of hoeing weeds out of the corn, he returned home to find "these odd crystals on my shoulders and [I] was pale as a ghost," he says. "Over the next few weeks, I was diagnosed by the local doctors as having mumps, measles, and double pneumonia. From age seven to ten, I had a chronic cough and ate my parents out of house and home without gaining any weight. That is when my parents in desperation took me to a Chattanooga allergist, who found that I was allergic to a number of foods, including chocolate and ice cream." The allergist also suggested a sweat test, but it was filed and not acted upon. "So, from age ten to twelve, I had the same symptoms of chronic cough, enormous appetite, steatorrhea [the excretion of abnormal quantities of fat within the feces], and failure to gain weight," says Victor, "but now not enjoying chocolate or ice cream! So, in desperation at age twelve, my parents hauled me on the ninety-mile trek to Vanderbilt in Nashville, where I was finally diagnosed with cystic fibrosis."

Victor continues, "My family was more relieved than anything that they finally knew what was wrong with me. My younger brother and two older sisters, none of whom has cystic fibrosis, were particularly supportive, allowing me to be less concerned about the disease and more concerned with following my new CF protocol." Victor was treated with nebulizers and physical therapy with moderate results. With pancreatic enzyme supplementation, however, he doubled his weight from 70 to 140 pounds between 12 and 14 years of age.

Growing up, Victor played baseball, basketball, and some backyard football. He went to high school at a military academy because he and his family believed it would provide a better education than the public school system in his area. "But CF was an issue at the military academy," says Victor, "in that my doctors had me excused from drilling with my platoon. I was also excused from the overnight camp-outs. During the summer between my freshman and sophomore years of high school, my doctors at Vanderbilt noted an abnormality in my right upper lobe. They thought it might be histoplasmosis, a fungal infection which is endemic in Tennessee. Best treatment at that time was rest and decreased physical activity. Hence no sports activities at the academy." Victor believes his disease played a role in his time at the military academy outside of just sports. "I was never promoted to an officer in spite of my high academic performance," he says, "and I always expected that CF had something to do with that." Still, that academic success resulted in admission to prestigious Rice University in Houston, Texas.

It was in high school when he read that life expectancy for a CF patient was twenty-one. "Sure enough, it was when I was twenty-one, a junior in college at Rice University, that I was walking between classroom buildings on campus when I started coughing. What I spit up was pure blood, and I felt this bubbling feeling beneath my sternum. I went home and went to bed but continued to cough up blood. An ambulance carried me to the hospital where I was admitted for about a week of IV antibiotics. I had noticed in the past a little blood streaking in some sputum but never this amount of pure blood, and that was scary, especially not knowing what to expect next."

Victor would recover from this episode and not only graduate Rice but attend the equally esteemed Baylor College of Medicine in

Houston followed by a residency program in pathology with Baylor-affiliated hospitals.

Victor says, for the most part, he did well throughout his twenties. "I have always been extremely compliant with my prescribed treatments and have never hesitated about trying something new," he says. "My peak flow was over six hundred, which was better than even my doctor's!" In fact, Victor's latest CF medical team in Houston let Victor do whatever he wanted, as opposed to the restrictions put on him during his military days while seeing doctors at Vanderbilt. Victor began playing new sports like intramural basketball, water skiing, and tennis.

"When I got to college in Houston," says Victor, "my doctor was Gunyon Harrison at the Texas Institute for Rehabilitation and Research. His philosophy was that CF patients should be able to do any physical activity they wanted, as their own bodies would tell them when they had had enough. Besides, the physical activity accelerated the clearance of lung secretions."

Victor picked up another fun activity in his early twenties as he got his first guitar at the age of twenty-one. "I have been playing, singing, and recording ever since," says Victor.

He moved to Durham, North Carolina, in 1980 for his job with Duke University and Durham VA Medical Centers, and in addition to practicing lung pathology, he has been teaching first-year medical students every year since, with the exception of a one-year sabbatical.

Victor soon got involved with Duke's lung-transplant program, which included evaluation of the explanted CF lungs as well as tests for rejection of the newly transplanted normal lungs. Once the tissues have been fixed in formalin, there is no danger of bacterial cross-contamination.

"One of the great influences on my career was Dr. Don Greenberg, a world-renowned lung pathologist at Baylor College of Medicine," says Victor. "His enthusiasm was infectious, and, of course, the fact that I had a chronic lung disease myself had to be a factor at some level. When the lung transplant program took off at Duke, I was the senior thoracic pathologist and, along with our senior immunopathologist, we had to jump in and learn the ends and outs of transplant pathology."

Victor is currently a board-certified pathologist in Durham, North Carolina, who specializes in pulmonary pathology with an emphasis on dust-related diseases, especially asbestos. He has testified as an expert in courts in the US, UK, and Australia—"I won my first case as an expert witness sometime in the late 1990s or early 2000s against Big Tobacco," he says—and given lectures at international meetings in Europe, Asia, Australia, and North and South America. He has also written numerous articles, chapters in books, and texts on these subjects. He published the first edition of his book, *Pathology of Asbestos-Associated Diseases*, now in its third edition, in 1992 about diagnosing disease caused by asbestos and determining causation or attribution. He also published *Biomedical Applications of Microprobe Analysis*, now in its second edition, which is about using specialized analytical electron microscopic techniques in the practice of medicine, and especially for identification of foreign materials like asbestos. *So Far, So Good: Living and Coping with Cystic Fibrosis*, which details his life with CF and contains interviews from the perspective of both a patient and a physician, is, as yet, unpublished.

Also during that time, he met Linda, to whom he has been married for thirty years, and between them they have three children (Victor has a daughter from a previous marriage and Linda has two sons from a previous marriage).

"Linda and I got married shortly after I turned forty," says Victor. "My health was pretty good. We were able to do pretty much what we wanted. Linda had told me that even if we only had a few years together, that was what she wanted."

"I knew the risks involved with marrying someone with CF," says Linda, "I also knew that I wanted to have him in my life. *Is it worth it to spend the next ten to fifteen years with him or without him?* I decided even a short time together was worth the risk."

"A turning point in my health, though, was when I contracted pneumonia in my forties," says Victor. "After that, my lung function was never quite the same." Though Victor admits it wasn't all doom and gloom in his forties because he discovered one of his great passions—karaoke. "Karaoke cassettes have been available since about 1996," says Victor, "and I got into it around that time. CDs weren't far behind. I started going to karaoke bars around 1996 to 1997 and have won three local karaoke contests."

Things didn't get any easier for Victor as he got older. "In my fifties, I developed cardiac arrhythmia [atrial fibrillation], which curtailed many of my athletic activities, and then I developed pneumonia again in my sixties. My health was definitely in peril."

"I thought I was losing my husband," says Linda. "I was making funeral arrangements for Victor. He was dependent on oxygen night and day. The transplant team wanted to do extensive testing to make sure he was clearly eligible for a transplant and though he agreed, he told me privately he would never go through with it. He knew how to handle his CF after years of 'new normal' adjustments and changes in his daily treatment regimen. Dealing with transplanted lungs meant a complete change of strategy. He would be taking even more antirejection medication than his previous CF medication. Victor did not want to have a transplant. He simply did not think it was worth the risk; thus, he would prefer to continue fighting CF rather than fight a new enemy — rejecting foreign lungs in his body."

"Because of my strong immune system (extraordinary reaction to histoplasmosis, allergies to various foods) and my knowledge of rejection as a pulmonary pathologist," says Victor, "I was pretty sure that I would get into fatal difficulties with a lung transplant in terms of short- and long-term rejection. However, in 2015, I was desaturating significantly and in need of oxygen. I had had atrial fibrillation in the early 2000s with uncontrolled rates around 140, which had significantly weakened my heart. The work-up for transplantation at Duke cost around seventy thousand dollars. The actual transplant, around one million dollars. The transplant work-up included a cardiac catheterization, and I wanted to know how much my heart was contributing to my condition. So I went through with it. Turned out it was the lungs, not the heart, that was the problem. I was totally familiar with what it meant to live with CF, whereas I had no idea what was in store for me post-transplant.

"After 2015, my FEV1 had dropped to below thirty percent of predicted, and I was desaturating with exertion [moderate exercise, like walking] and at night [sleep apnea]. So I was dragging a portable oxygen concentrator behind me when I walked around the medical center and using oxygen with a BiPAP machine at night. Because of the guarded prognosis for an FEV1 that low, that is why my doctors had the palliative care referral. They [the doctors] sent us to end-of-life palliative care at Duke, thus my funeral home visit. I saw the palliative care specialist to humor my doctors."

Victor didn't stop fighting, though, and even admits he was still performing karaoke during this time. "I have a pretty nice system here at home with four microphones, wall-mounted speakers, a sixty-inch TV screen, and over three thousand songs on CD," says Victor. "One of my CF doctors believed singing was a key to my long survival, building a strong diaphragm (and hence, an efficient cough mechanism). After two years of seeing [my palliative care doctor] with little or no disease progression, he finally gave up and told me to call him when I needed it."

Beginning in 2015, Victor had been on O_2 at night prior to palliative care and with exertion which meant walking too fast, too far, upstairs, etc.

A few years later, Victor's life would change tremendously. "It was around November 2019 when Trikafta was first available in the CF clinic at Duke," he says. "I have always been gung ho about any new treatment modalities, so I jumped on the bandwagon. Within about a month, my sputum production became almost negligible. Within six months, I had discontinued using my vest (which I had been doing twice per day), hypertonic saline, and Pulmozyme. I went from albuterol inhalation three times per day to once in the morning (followed by a whiff of Trelegy). I no longer use (or need) my portable oxygenator. I still use my oxygen at night but that is mostly for the sleep apnea. The ejection fraction of my heart for a long time was thirty percent [normal greater than fifty percent], and my heart doctor was considering me having an ICD (implantable cardioverter defibrillator) implanted. However, [it] wasn't long until my ejection fraction went up to thirty-five percent (my heart really appreciated that my lungs were doing much better) and more recently, it was up to forty-three percent. I have also had a substantial improvement (about forty percent) in my FEV1. I cough up about one glob of thick sputum per week!"

"Victor was not so impressed with the first generation of 'genetic' medications," says Linda. "He could not tell much difference. But when the doctor switched him to Trikafta, things improved markedly. He was careful. He gradually withdrew support from some previously essential medications and treatments. And now he is taking only one treatment a day (imagine how much time this saves in his life!) versus seven."

Victor, who worked full time during all of his health complications, began traveling overseas again—"a miracle in itself," says Linda. "We always travel business class so he can plug in his machines for treatments in the air. But trust me, travel with oxygen is a huge hassle. He really needed it at night and when walking through the airports (those long treks were quite difficult, and he would have to stop and rest and catch his breath frequently). As he got worse, he needed it just to go to the cafeteria for lunch at Duke. He hated being on oxygen. To him, that felt like the end was much closer. He made the best of it because he couldn't function or work without it, but he was never happy about it."

Things are quite different for Victor now . . . and for Linda too! "I have always felt that I lived on the end of a bull whip with Victor . . . he's fine, he's dying; he's better, he's in the hospital," says Linda. "It's like living in limbo all the time, never knowing when the next 'hurricane' will hit. The sicker he got, the higher my anxiety. I worried constantly about losing him, the financial implications of being alone, thinking ahead to selling the house, but mostly missing his optimistic look on life. It is contagious, and since I was already prone to depression, I was afraid without him life would be hardly worth living. He has been my cheerleader for so long (he believes in me even when I falter) [that] I started recording some of his encouraging moments so I could hear his voice after he was gone."

Linda continues, "It took months for me to believe that he was truly on the upswing. His mood often reflected his physical health, so it had been rough on both of us. He tried to stay upbeat during the bad times, but we had the conversation again and again about what the latest calamity meant in terms of his survival. He was not his usual upbeat self.

"Trikafta changed everything. When he stopped taking some treatments that had long been part of our life together, it surprised me. When he could walk up and down stairs without stopping, it was shocking. In a good way. And today, he offers to take things upstairs or downstairs (previously, he had to ask me to do it). Rather than dragging a portable O_2 machine everywhere and stopping every few yards to catch his breath, Victor resumed walks with our four dogs and me—short ones, yes, but we loved it!

"After a year or so, I began to relax a bit," Linda says. "I realized that my own life had been on hold for years. My business had suffered because I was diverting attention from work to Victor. Now, for the first time, I was actually moving into profitability. I don't think I understood how much his illness had occupied my life until it was lighter and more under control."

Linda wants people to understand that it's not perfect. "When we walk the dogs," she says, "we stop halfway up a hill for him to rest. After all, his lungs are permanently scarred from previous infections. But the fact is that we take walks—that is huge.

"So, yes, going from funeral arrangements to travel (although COVID slowed us down)—it's like being normal! What a difference! Joy? You bet. Faded worry? Yes. Always cognizant of potential downswings again? Yes. But life is good. We are supportive of each other in ways that are tender and precious."

Travel is something else that has changed for Victor and Linda. "Victor told me early in our relationship that he had never wanted to be rich," says Linda, "but he wanted to see the world. With medical conferences, we were able to do that. It was always a hassle bringing along treatment equipment and meds, some of which needed refrigeration. As he declined, he couldn't even take walks on the beach with me when we visited Aruba. So it was lonely for me—I went out alone. He stayed in the room watching TV and taking treatments and resting.

"We thought our foreign travel days were over, but two summers ago, we visited Croatia and Victor walked the cobblestone streets without oxygen, pausing only a few times to catch his breath in the sweltering heat. Next April (2022) is my seventieth and Victor is finally able to travel with me (versus me traveling with him). Yay! I booked a Viking cruise down the Nile for sixteen days—our longest trip ever. We are both excited about it, and it would never have happened without Trikafta. Not only is it making Victor's life better; it is making my dreams come true!"

Victor, who says he missed a week or two while going through his transplant evaluation around 2015, is back to working every day as a practicing lung physician in North Carolina and is affiliated with Duke University Hospital and Duke Regional Hospital, though he has mostly worked from home since April 1, 2020, due to the pandemic. Now that he has had both doses of the COVID vaccine as well as the COVID booster, he has started going back to work one day a week. As a pathologist, he rarely works with patients. He believes that being in the medical profession has helped his CF. "I have always had a touch of obsessive compulsive disorder," says Victor, "which made it easy for me to take my medicines and treatments. Having medical training so I better understand what each does, what its side-effects are, and the consequences of missing a dose has certainly been helpful."

Victor celebrated his seventieth birthday in April 2021 doing what else but singing karaoke while enjoying a Zoom celebration fundraiser for the Cystic Fibrosis Foundation. He donates to the foundation every year, has worked with the Boomer Esiason Foundation, and has contributed three blogs to the CF Roundtable newsletter. "It feels pretty amazing to have made it to seventy," says Victor. "When I was diagnosed at age twelve, the CF brochures said that most patients don't make it past twenty-one. Then I got to twenty-one and was still doing okay. I went to medical school, where the textbooks said most patients don't make it past thirty. I got to thirty and was still doing pretty good. I began to realize two things: one, nobody had a clue as to how long I might make it; and two, I was dragging the average age upward as I got older and older. When I turned fifty, I considered that everything beyond that was gravy, which allowed me to enjoy every day, month, and year to the fullest."

"Never in my wildest of wild dreams did I expect to celebrate our thirtieth wedding anniversary as we did in [April] 2021," says Linda. "Back in the 'bad old days,' he teasingly said he would outlive me; we would wink at each other knowing it was quite unlikely. Today, that statement might prove to be true, even given my own good health!"

Even at seventy, Victor is still active at Duke. "I love teaching," says Victor, "because it is rewarding to provide information to young, eager minds that will help them in caring for their patients in the years to come. I turned seventy this year but have never thought about retiring. As Dr. Harrison explained, my body will tell me when I have had enough. I have taught first-year medical students every year except one since 1980—although in 2020 and 2021, much of our teaching has been by Zoom. [I] will be delighted when we once again have in-person classroom interactions!

"I have pretty much accomplished everything I set out to do in life," says Victor. "My dream is to climb to the mountaintop by showing [other people with CF] the way to a long and fulfilled life . . . and perhaps return to karaoke bars (when the pandemic is over) to win another contest or two."

4

FIGHTING FOR MY CHILD: STORIES FROM CF MOMS

JAIME PARSONS

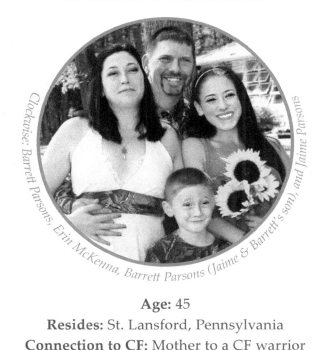

Clockwise: Barrett Parsons, Erin McKenna, Barrett Parsons (Jaime & Barrett's son), and Jaime Parsons

Age: 45
Resides: St. Lansford, Pennsylvania
Connection to CF: Mother to a CF warrior

#ERINSTRONG: A MOTHER'S QUEST TO GIVE BACK

"**E**rin was vivacious from the moment she was born," says Jaime Parsons about her daughter, Erin Lyn McKenna. "She knew what she wanted and who she wanted to be. I always say Erin was like a butterfly—breathtakingly beautiful and free, an old soul that could never be caged. She was outspoken, outgoing, and her smile lit up any room she entered."

Back in 1994, they did not do the newborn screening. Jaime was just a young mom (sixteen years old) at the time. Erin was sick on and off with what doctors thought were either allergies, pneumonia, or respiratory infections. Then one night, things got dramatically worse. "That night we ended up in the ER yet again," says Jaime. "She was feeling just awful. She was lethargic. They had said a few days prior that she had an upper respiratory infection, but things took a turn for the worse, and I rushed her to the emergency room.

She was not diagnosed there. They had no idea what was wrong with her, and this guy came into the room, and he was dressed all in white, and he said he worked at the hospital and could he look at Erin's hands and feet. As soon as he did, he said, 'You need to get her out of here now and to Children's Hospital of Philadelphia (CHOP). Have you ever heard of cystic fibrosis?' I said, 'No.' He said, 'It's a genetic terminal disease, and if you don't get her help, she will die' and then he left. No one at the hospital ever heard of him or knew who he was when I described him. We all believe he was an angel."

Erin was finally diagnosed with cystic fibrosis on May 17, 2003, just two weeks before her ninth birthday, at CHOP. "Our lives changed in ways that we could have never fathomed in a million years. We finally had answers after talking to twenty-nine different doctors and over one hundred trips to the emergency room."

While Jaime says the diagnosis changed things, it didn't prevent Erin from living her life. "Erin was scared at first when we found out she had CF," says Jaime, "but she just went with it. She took it like a true warrior. Our new life started, and her CF diagnosis never ever stopped her. Erin never allowed her CF to define who she was. She never backed down from anything.

"Erin was adventurous," says Jaime. "She loved the snow, and was the first one out and the last one in. She loved four-wheeling and being with her friends. She took pictures all the time and loved pulling pranks on people. We would go camping in the Poconos and a few miles from where we would camp, there was a hundred-plus-foot waterfall that we would go [to] and the kids would play in the water, hike, and explore. One day, Erin and her best friend Brianna climbed all the way to the top of the waterfall wearing flipflops, completely fearless. Nothing scared her. She wanted to experience everything she could. She was always pushing the limits and loving her life. I raised Erin to love life and to be fearless. And that she did and was. We both love animals and the outdoors, so Erin was raised with lots of pets and enjoying all that we could. Raising Erin was an adventure to say the least. She kept me on my toes."

Jaime says that Erin fought CF courageously. "No matter how bad things were, she kept pushing forward," says Jaime. "Living ten lifetimes in her short twenty-five years. The last year and a half of her beautiful life, she fought with so much strength, courage, and dignity."

Jaime was a single mom until Barrett Parsons came into her and Erin's lives three months after Erin was diagnosed with CF. "Barrett and I met at a friend's house," says Jaime. "We work very well, and he balances me out very well. We are best friends. And he raised [Erin] as if she was his daughter. He was at every doctor's appointment."

"It is an honor and privilege to have been Erin's dad," says Barrett. "To be in her life and to raise her and to be there when God took her home."

"Her brother, Barrett [Barrett and Jaime's son who was born ten years after Erin], was her love," says Jaime, who notes that Erin's passing has been extremely difficult for the younger Barrett, now seventeen years old. "They were two peas in a pod and did everything together. She was so excited to be a big sister."

Erin also had a few other special people in her life including her great-aunt Linny (Jaime's aunt). "She is the glue of our family," says Jaime. "Erin and Linny had an unbreakable bond from the time Erin was born. She was a second mother to Erin and even took her and her friend Carla on a week-long trip to Disney World when Erin was twelve just so she could experience it."

Then there was Kyle. "Erin met Kyle in middle school," says Jaime. "They were close friends and then started dating in high school. CF was always there but Erin never allowed it to define her or her relationship with Kyle. She never allowed it to stop her, not even in the end—she was still fighting. Erin loved Kyle with every ounce of her being and he loved her.

"Erin and Kyle worked so hard from a very young age to build their beautiful life together—hard work, love, trying times, of course, and thousands of memories of the beautiful love story they had," says Jaime. "They loved going on trips and adventures just as much as relaxing with their puppies, Moose and Ruby, watching their favorite TV shows together at night. They were best friends and had a love most would be lucky to experience, a once-in-a-lifetime kind of love. Kyle knew from the beginning Erin was sick and he still loved her at such a young age. What the two of them faced truly showed their love and strength and perseverance for each other."

Erin and Jaime had several Great Strides teams, from the Monkeys to the Salty Beaches to Erin's Eagles, to raise funds for the Cystic Fibrosis Foundation. Some of their teams had as many as sixty to eighty people walking with them to support the foundation. They even created their own fundraising walk, which Jaime says was a huge success.

"Erin was also an organ donor," says Jaime, "and believed wholeheartedly that we should never take anything with us. She fought to educate for CF and organ donation. Erin was, without a doubt, someone you would want to have fighting for you."

Times grew tougher for Erin as her lungs had irreversible damage and a transplant seemed to be the only method to save her life. "I have a lot of antibiotic-resistant 'bugs' growing in my lungs," said Erin on her GoFundMe page in January 2020 as she advocated for her transplant. "I am on multiple strong antibiotics to hopefully help, but along with that comes major side effects. Nausea has become a constant battle, and I am losing a lot of weight. I need to be a certain BMI for the transplant to take place, and right now I am way below that. I am keeping the faith and doing everything I can to get strong enough to get listed!

Jaime tried to get Erin a lifesaving double-lung transplant until the very end. "The fight to get a transplant hospital to take Erin was because she had antibiotic-resistant infections that can cause a lot of issues during and after transplant," says Jaime. "Erin was on cocktails of different IV antibiotics to try to desperately get them under control along with experimental drugs that ravaged her body. She was even prepared to participate in phage therapies, which use viruses, instead of antibiotics, to attack bacteria, since some people with CF develop an immunity due to a lifetime of overuse."

Jaime says that due to the state of the bacterial issues in Erin's lungs, many clinics did not feel comfortable giving Erin new lungs. "Erin and I had doors shut on us," says Jaime, "and we were heading to Duke when [they] called and canceled our five-day evaluation [to see if Erin could be a viable candidate for transplant]. That very same night, I called Duke and begged them and pleaded with them to let us bring Erin out for the five days. Erin and I were both on the phone with her doctors at ten thirty at night. Then they asked her all these questions and said, 'Can you get here in the next few days?' The amount of O_2 Erin needed to stay alive was nearly unsustainable in order to simply travel from home to the hospital, so Kyle hooked Erin's oxygen concentrators up to a generator on the back of his pickup truck, running her oxygen tubes through the back window in order to get her to the hospital."

Jaime continues, "The last year of Erin's life, she fought with such strength and dignity. She pushed through such awful things. I watched my baby go through things no one should ever have to go through, and she always fought to break through to the other side." In the last year of her life, Erin wanted to make a difference for the CF community and participated in antibiotic trials that further destroyed her body.

Erin wanted to marry Kyle, but due to her health, sadly, the two never had an opportunity to wed. "Erin never made it to transplant," says Jaime. "She passed before she was listed. My love for Erin has no bounds. I would have gone to the ends of the earth to save her. I would have given my life for hers. I have never fought harder for anything in my life than I did trying to save my baby. I was ready to travel the country to any hospital that would have taken Erin and so was she. We were a powerhouse together. We all were so thankful to be at Duke, to be given the chance at a lifesaving double-lung transplant. They knew how difficult Erin's surgery would be and they were on board to do it. But things took a turn for the worse, and we never made it. So close but yet so far. Erin was always, and will forever be, my hero."

Jaime says that despite Erin's strength and positivity, she knew deep down that every passing day, she was a day closer to losing the love of her life. "I was gutted," says Jaime. "I had no way to save her, and from the moment she was diagnosed, I was terrified of losing her, knowing that someday I would. Every birthday was literally a blessing. Birthdays were a Godsend, but then, I always felt we were getting a little bit closer and, deep down inside, I was scared every day. I can't imagine how she felt, but she never let it show. Erin was a light in darkness—a lover of all things. She did her best to live her best life no matter what. If people could live like Erin for just one day, they would know what it was like to truly live.

"When the doctors came into the room and told us there was nothing more they could do, we were gutted," says Jaime. "Those next few days, we loved, laughed, watched movies, listened to music, and just loved her so much. Erin always wanted to be in Kyle's arms, but that weekend was their last, so it meant everything to the two of them. He never left her side but to go to the bathroom."

Erin passed away on February 11, 2020, at the young age of twenty-five, in Kyle's arms "exactly where she wanted to be," says Jaime. "When she passed, a part of me went with her. I felt it as she took her last breath—a part of me died at the very moment. Only those that have walked this path can understand what it feels like. I literally felt a part of my heart and soul leave with Erin."

Jaime says that she wanted to give her daughter the legacy she deserved. During the last year of Erin's life, Jaime started reaching out on social media asking for cards. "That took off," says Jaime, "and she not only got mail but little gifts as well!" Remembering how much those gifts brightened their lives, Jaime started the #erinstrongbackpackprogram to "bring sunshine" to other CF patients and their families. She assembled a crew that included her husband, Barrett, and three CF warriors to help send #erinstrongbackpacks to those who are inpatient, battling CF like her daughter was for so many years. "We make them to fit the child or young adult's needs and interests," says Jaime. One of the program's staff members was Heather

McCoy, who resides in Myrtle Beach, South Carolina, and was the executive director of the program for a brief time.

"I saw Erin at rehab while I was finishing my session for the day and noticed her sitting alone with the RT," says Heather, who also has cystic fibrosis and had two double-lung transplants, one in 2012 and the other in 2020. "She was new and having been in that position before, I decided I'd introduce myself and offer that, if she needed anything, to ask me. To kind of give her that comfort that she wasn't the only one there—that despite seeing older patients, that there were quite a bit of CF patients. I sat my distance about two chairs in between, and as I introduced myself, Erin began to feel comfortable. The RT allowed us more time since the RT had known me for so many years; she knew I could be of help to Erin. It was about ten minutes total but I gave her my number so she could text or call me."

Erin texted Heather that same evening, and they began talking daily through text. "I'd see her a few times coming in for her sessions," says Heather. "We had different time slots. She actually was in the hospital and stopped by the floor to give her lung ornament [Erin painted several of these ornaments in different colors and made them out of pieces of wood, which depicted a set of flowery lungs, to sell as a fundraiser for her transplant fund but gave this one in particular to Heather as a gift] to my family as I was in surgery. After my complications, I wasn't able to communicate directly with Erin, but my sister would make sure Erin had updates on how I was doing. I was in the hospital when Erin passed but then I began talking to her mom more as the days passed."

Jaime spent so many days and nights in her lifetime decorating Erin's hospital rooms that she now uses much of that same energy to curate #erinstrongbackpacks to send to those CF warriors who are struggling with a hospitalization. "Inside the #erinstrongbackpacks are some of Erin's favorite books," says Jaime. "Erin loved to color, both as a child and as an adult, so we have adult and kids coloring books. She also loved *Girl, Wash Your Face* and *Didn't See That Coming* both by Rachel Hollis because the author never felt sorry for herself, and she never wanted anyone to feel sorry for her. [Erin] was a voracious reader." Other items depending on the child or young adult's age may include toys, crayons, and/or hand sanitizers.

Eventually, new items were added, including the #erinstrongCF-superherocape; the #huginabox, which includes huggable toys like stuffed animals; the #birthdaycardprogram, a card with stickers or something small sent in for the kids' birthdays just so they know they are being thought of; the #ultimatesnackbox, a box filled with all kinds of goodies for long hospital stays; #thelittleflowerlungornament, something similar to what Erin made for Heather as it carries a very powerful message of love and hope; #thelittleworrystoneheart, an amethyst stone shaped as a heart for the kids to have as a worry stone to keep in their pockets when times are tough; and coming soon, #storybookbuddies, a book with a matching stuffed animal.

"While the responses inspired us to continue our mission," says Jaime, "the brightening of one of those recipients, eight-year-old CF warrior Declan, was particularly impactful."

"He has been admitted over fifty times to Texas Children's Hospital (TCH) in Houston," says Declan's mom, Kayla. "When [someone is] inpatient that much, it can get really rough. When COVID hit, and he was there, that was worse for him. No visitors, no more fun activities, and nothing but sitting in your room, especially the children who can get sick more easily. That's when I found Jaime. She was exactly what Declan needed during those times. She sent him his first #erinstrongbackpack, and it was truly amazing watching his face light up. There was so much in it: toys, books, sensory fidgets, hand sanitizer, bathroom essentials, a stuffy [stuffed animal], and things to just make you feel better. Since then, she has been there for all his hospital stays, never missing a beat and making sure he is being taken care of. From sending him a snack box with everything his heart could desire and want to eat while inpatient to being one of her recipients of the #erinstrongCFsuperherocapes for being super and strong. She made sure his Halloween was awesome, too, while at TCH and sent décor for the room and Halloween fun. When Christmas came, she sent him an Elf on the Shelf, a Spider-Man Santa hat, and all the little goodies. She truly learned all his favorites. Everything has been personal. Jaime and the #erinstrongbackpackprogram was the biggest blessing to Declan and our family during a time when we needed it most."

"The backpack program is all my love for Erin," says Jaime. "I want to share it with our CF community. We have done about thirty-plus backpacks along with our #erinstrongCFsuperherocapes and #birthdaycardprogram."

Another one of those recipients is thirteen-year-old William. "The smile on William's face says it all when he receives #erinstrong gifts from Jaime while in the hospital," says his mom, Vickie. "[Jaime] sure knows how to brighten a child's day even when they are having a bad day."

Then there is four-year-old Marley. "[Jaime] is always surprising her with goodies from the #erinstrongbackpackprogram," says her mom, Brooklin, "and the only thing [Jaime] wants in return is to raise awareness for cystic fibrosis."

Feeling the impact #erinstrongbackpacks are having on CF patients like Declan, William and Marley, Jaime is primed to, in the near future, establish the Erin's Light Foundation, an idea Jaime and Erin thought up to be able to someday financially assist families to have anything, from day trips to events in their area.

"The reason behind wanting to do fun things for CF families," says Jaime, "is because we know firsthand what it meant for us. Whether it was a Flyers (Philadelphia's NHL team) game, the [Jersey] Shore, the lake house, camping in the middle of nowhere, we did it. We always had adventures. Making lifelong memories, memories that will live on forever. So I would like to someday be able to give that gift to other CF families. Memories that will forever be locked into time to hold on to."

Jaime says her children are the greatest gifts she has ever been blessed to receive. Losing Erin continues to be a struggle for the entire family; however, they have turned a lot of that heart-wrenching pain into philanthropic work by helping young people who are bravely fighting cystic fibrosis the same way Erin did.

Jaime now uses several hashtags on social media to reveal the character and heart that her daughter displayed so that those who never met Erin McKenna can understand what an incredible person she was. "To #livelikeErin is to wake up every day in the face of adversity and seize the day, making the most out of every moment, passionately moving forward without fear, regret, or apprehension. To #lovelikeErin is to love everyone and everything around you unabashedly in the moment. To be #erinstrong is to dig deep inside yourself to find strength to face anything and everything with grace, dignity, and a beautiful smile."

Jaime says that Erin gave her swift instructions about how to live her life before she passed away: "Don't wait around to live your life. Don't [waste time] and lose precious times and memories you could make with family and friends. Be grateful for every moment. Stop waiting for Fridays and enjoy the week. Stop waiting for summer and enjoy winter. Stop rushing your vacation you have plans for in a year and plan mini ones in between. Splurge and buy the appetizer or dessert. Don't live for the future; live for now."

MELISSA YEAGER

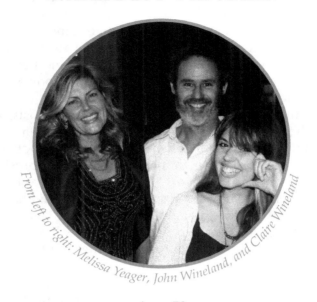

From left to right: Melissa Yeager, John Wineland, and Claire Wineland

Age: 52
Resides: Garden Grove, California
Connection to CF: Mother to a CF warrior

MELISSA'S STORY: KEEPING CLAIRE'S LEGACY ALIVE

Melissa Yeager's daughter Claire Wineland lived just twenty-one years, but her legacy will live on forever in the cystic fibrosis community. Claire's list of accomplishments is incredible: She was one of eight teens recognized at the Fox Teen Choice Awards 2015, named one of *Seventeen* magazine's "17 Power Teens" of 2016, and honored as *Glamour* magazine's 2018 "College Women of the Year" grand prize winner. She was also the recipient of the Global Genes' RARE Champion of Hope Award, World of Children Youth Award, the Gloria Barron Prize for Young Heroes, and winner of *Los Angeles Business Journal*'s "Small Nonprofit of the Year." She was featured on *The Dr. Oz Show*, CNN, the *Huffington Post*, ABC News, *Cosmopolitan*, *People*, *Ladies' Home Journal*, and many more. Claire was bigger than life, a public face of CF, whom many of us still quote today, but to Melissa, Claire was first and foremost, "an amazing daughter."

Melissa and Claire's father, John Wineland, found out something "wasn't right" at Melissa's last ultrasound appointment. "She was two weeks overdue," says Melissa. "The doctors came rushing into the room to look at the ultrasound screen and determined that I needed to head straight to the hospital and deliver her right away. I was terrified. She was born on April 10, 1997, in Austin, Texas, and they found that she suffered from meconium ileus, had a ruptured bowel, and a one-pound cyst in her abdominal cavity.

"They said these were the telltale signs of cystic fibrosis, something I had never heard of before but soon found out was a progressive, genetic, terminal illness and that her father and I were both gene carriers. At that time, the prognosis for people with cystic fibrosis was very grim. I felt the weight of the world on my shoulders at that moment and couldn't even hear the rest of what the doctor said because I was already far off in the future, imagining this beautiful baby and what a terrible life she had been sentenced to. I did as much research as I possibly could. The information I found scared me, and for a while I was very depressed and lived in the distant future of 'what if.'"

Melissa lost Claire to cystic fibrosis in 2018 when Claire was only twenty-one years old. Claire received a double-lung transplant on August 26, and one day later, suffered a massive, ischemic stroke caused by a blood clot in her carotid artery. "We made the decision to remove life support on September 2, 2018," says Melissa, "after taking into account the tremendous damage the stroke caused to her brain and her body and Claire's personal wishes of not wanting to be kept alive if she didn't have any quality of life."

In the twenty-one years in between, Melissa says her life was nothing like she feared the day Claire was diagnosed with CF. "Raising a child with an illness like CF is not easy," she says. "However, hearing the diagnosis and those first few days of reading about what the disease was, what it meant to live with it, life expectancy, pain and suffering, etc. left out all of the beautiful gifts that it brought to me and to my family. The lessons I learned about living in the moment and the spiritual practice of acceptance changed me, and I didn't expect that. I also didn't expect to be so entirely and wholeheartedly in love with her. I worried I would pity her. We were unusually close. I think that might be something many parents with a terminally ill child feel.

"Every milestone was special because it may be their last; every accomplishment was celebrated in an over-the-top sort of way. The people Claire attracted into our lives were exceptional, movers and shakers, celebrities, people bent over backward to help her, to make her life incredible. She had this light about her, even before her CF was so apparent with her oxygen cannula [a device used to deliver supplemental oxygen or increased airflow to a patient or person in need of respiratory help], people were drawn to her like a moth to a flame, and I felt so fortunate and so proud that she was my daughter.

"Her illness gave her a simple and beautiful outlook on life, a gratitude that most people don't naturally come by, a loving and kind spirit . . . I saw the world through her eyes, and there was so much magic in it. She truly was a blessing in countless ways . . . these are the things I could not see in those first few days. It was anything but the doom and gloom I read about—it really was quite a different and more beautiful world with her in it."

Melissa continues, "Raising Claire was a blessing in disguise and showed me how resilient human beings are. There were many times over the years where things would feel hopeless, usually during an extended hospital stay, but I saw miracles happen. Raising a child with a terminal illness is a unique experience for parents. We have to find that balance between being realistic [and] staying positive. Something I have learned is that we provide the basis of how our child will deal with the ups and downs of this disease—we must remind them and ourselves that life is a struggle for most people, not only people living with an illness. It's part of what makes us human and provides an amazing opportunity to relate to others on a deep level. Living life with death on your heels creates a feeling of living in the moment and of extreme gratitude for everything: the good, the bad, and the beautiful.

"Claire was a magical soul, so intelligent, full of life and love and joy! Cystic fibrosis did not define her. She used to say, 'My life is amazing, not in spite of CF but because of it,' and I just could not understand what she meant by that. Later, she would explain that CF was her greatest teacher . . . it taught her how to look at things with a profound sense of gratitude for the good things in her life, how it gave her a platform to share her story of perseverance and help others, how she enjoyed her times in the hospital because it was like her own little world. I had to learn how to accept this for exactly what it was. It was an opportunity to live a life like very few others did. To understand how incredibly precious each and every day is and to get past the 'feeling sorry' for her and for us as her parents."

Claire went on to become a public speaker, an author, a YouTube starlet, an actress, and the founder of Claire's Place Foundation, though Melissa admits that while the world grieved the loss of Claire, it's the family that suffers the most. "As it often is," says Melissa. "As her mother, though, losing her has been devastating for me, her father, John, and her sister, Ellie. I have days and weeks where I am in a rage—cursing the words 'cystic fibrosis'—but then I remember what she taught me, and the next week I am full of gratitude for the blessing that she was and for the privilege of being her mother. It's not easy having a child with this disease. I would not want anyone to believe that that is what I am saying. It was the most difficult experience of my life, but I feel like the lessons it taught me can be applied to any circumstance. I am not sure I would have experienced so much personal and spiritual growth if not for this role. I continue to work with the cystic fibrosis community and share my experience with other moms and that feels wonderful. I think being able to speak with another parent going through a similar experience is where the magic and the healing happens."

Melissa, Cofounder and Executive Director of Claire's Place Foundation, never stopped fighting cystic fibrosis after Claire's death. "I cofounded the foundation with my daughter Claire when she was just thirteen and coming out of a coma," says Melissa. Claire's Place Foundation, Inc., a 501(c)(3) nonprofit organization, provides heartfelt support to the families of children and to individuals diagnosed with CF. The foundation works to heighten awareness and provide education, skills, and financial and emotional support. "Until there's a cure, there's Claire's Place," she says. "As the executive director and board member, I work diligently with the board of directors. I am responsible for the organization's consistent achievement of upholding its mission and financial objectives. However, the most rewarding function of my job is reaching out and making a difference in the lives of families and children living with CF. I work each and every day to ensure no parent should have to decide between work and being by their child's side during hospital stays. No parent should have to endure the stress of possibly losing their family's home while their child lies in the hospital." Claire's Place has impacted more than 3,000 people worldwide, has given more than $630,000 in extended hospital-stay grants, and provided 380 COVID-support grants during the pandemic.

Though Melissa admits, her personal experience with the disease doesn't make her efforts any easier. "I do know that Claire wanted her foundation to live on. It was something that gave her life so much meaning and made her feel very proud of the impact she made, so I trudge on," she says, "but honestly, I struggle with this almost daily. I don't know how to put it without being offensive to anyone but hearing from a mother whose child got a transplant and is doing great or taking Trikafta and going to climb mountains makes me very bitter sometimes. Of course, I am happy for them, but the pain is always with me. Why Claire? Why not Claire? Nothing makes sense in the universe some days. Some days are easier than others, and I would say I am healing in many ways but still, there's the feeling of never wanting to hear the words cystic fibrosis again! That's just me being as honest as I can be."

Still, Melissa is driven by her daughter's spiritual legacy. "Claire committed her life to traveling the world and speaking about her experience, from the beautiful and humorous to the painful parts of her life," says Melissa. "She inspired all who followed her journey and broke down barriers for those who live every day with a chronic illness. As painful as it is to lose my dear Claire, I get up every day to fulfill the needs of other families living with cystic fibrosis."

Melissa has helped mainstream awareness to CF through her involvement with two films. "*Five Feet Apart* was inspired by Claire, and her undying passion for living a life to be proud of," says Melissa. "It was directed by her dear friend Justin Baldoni, whom Claire met while filming CW's *Our Last Days*, a docuseries profiling folks living with chronic illness. The story is not her life story, but it is the first major motion picture to cast a spotlight on people living with CF." Claire, unfortunately, was never able to see the final film. "We know she would be proud of raising awareness about truly living life fully," says Melissa, "regardless of whether you are lucky enough to be born healthy, and especially if you are faced with CF or other chronic illnesses."

And in September 2019, on the one-year anniversary of Claire's passing, the documentary *Claire*, directed by Oscar-winning filmmaker Nick Reed and Ryan Azevedo, was released exclusively on YouTube. The film tells the story of Claire through interviews and footage, spotlighting her unique outlook that inspires millions to find purpose and to live proudly. "Nick and Ryan masterfully use their film to allow Claire's message to resonate with the audience," says Melissa. "Claire turned down many filmmakers before accepting the opportunity with Nick and Ryan. The difference was they were willing to do it the way Claire wanted. I was by Claire's side through the filming of the documentary. Although the filming was met with Claire's unexpected passing, I am so grateful to have this beautiful film to carry on Claire's work and legacy."

And despite Melissa's great, purpose-driven responsibility vis-à-vis the foundation, her devotion to her family remains her first priority. There's her husband, Brett Yeager, whom she married back in March 2017 and her younger daughter Ellie, who she knows had a lot of pressure to live up to her big sister. "Growing up in Claire's shadow must have been very difficult for her, and it shows in parts of her personality today," says Melissa. "She is strong but silent. Independent and a bit distant. Incredibly smart but sometimes falls prey to being an overachiever and a perfectionist. Due to the unpredictable nature of Claire's CF, there were many missed holidays, missed events, canceled vacations, and many times that she was the last kid picked up at aftercare by a neighbor or a friend of mine because I was stuck at the hospital with Claire, again, for the hundredth time. I remember telling her how grateful I was that she was so healthy, strong, intelligent, and flexible because for many years I was a single mom and taking care of Claire and all her medical needs, which sometimes left Ellie feeling like she didn't want to 'bother' me with her own issues.

"She learned to be very self-sufficient, but as time goes on, especially now that Claire is gone, we have had many talks about this and how difficult it was for her some days. Of course, she adored and loved Claire with all her heart, but the resentment was there, directly or indirectly, and I understand that completely." This self-sufficiency has served Ellie well in some ways. For example, she taught herself how to play the guitar and how to cheerlead by watching YouTube videos and practicing for hours. "She plays guitar beautifully now," says Melissa, "and made the high school cheer team the first time she ever tried out for the sport!" Ellie has expressed a desire to study abroad at Oxford University after graduating from high school next year and maybe study environmental science or biology.

Ellie participated in Claire's Place fundraisers, she went to the flash mob as a young child, has done every Glow Ride, and attended the Claire's Place Foundation's first Clairity Ball. Since Claire passed, though, Melissa says that Ellie has not participated in anything else. "Not sure if it's because it's too painful for her or if it's just not interesting, especially now that her sister died from the disease. Maybe as she gets older, she will take an interest; I don't push her.

"The day that Claire got the call for lungs was Ellie's first day of high school," says Melissa. "Claire took an Uber over to our house at six a.m. so that I could drive her down to UCSD [University of California San Diego], and we were all crying happy tears, hugging and taking pictures. Ellie had a moment where she got a panicked look on her face and said, 'Sissy, shouldn't I come with you in case anything happens?' Claire said 'No, no, munchkin, you should go to school . . . I promise, everything will be fine and then you can come see me tomorrow or the next day when I wake up with new lungs and you can tell me all about your first day!' This, of course, has become a source of such pain and regret for Ellie as Claire never woke from the original sedation due to the stroke. She is very private with her feelings and her emotions, but this one thing makes her break down every time she thinks of it."

Melissa and Brett are also loving foster parents to Aurora, for whom they began caring a year after Claire's death. Aurora was a friend of Ellie's who had dealt with abuse, neglect, trauma, group homes, and several foster homes over a two-year period. "One thing I have learned in this life is that being of service to others is the best medicine for self-pity or a broken heart," says Melissa. "This has been true with Aurora."

Melissa continues, "Claire found a beautiful way to make something of her experience, to share what it was like living with chronic illness, but she was not a Pollyanna [someone who is excessively or blindly optimistic]. She admitted that it was indeed very tough at times but that she was determined to make something of her suffering, something to give back to the world and to find empathy for others who might be suffering with their own issues, be it health, mental health, financial fears, all of it. I know for me personally, when I am having a tough time dealing with the constant grief of losing her, I find a way to be of service to someone else and that seems to take a bit of the edge off."

In 2021, Melissa and the rest of her team celebrated the tenth anniversary of Claire's Place Foundation. "When Claire dreamed up the mission of the foundation from her hospital bed at the age of thirteen, I could have never imagined that we would still have the privilege of helping CF families ten years later!

"I am so proud of Claire and the impactful life she lived," says Melissa, "and my own goal is to likewise, 'Live a life you are proud of.'"

MARGARETE CASSALINA

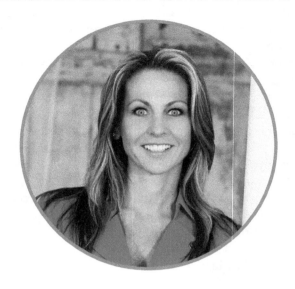

Age: 53
Resides: Milton, New York
Connection to CF: Mother to two CF warriors

INSPIRED BY JENA: MOM REVEALS HOW TO BREATHE BRAVELY

"**M**y dream since the diagnosis of my son, Eric, in 1991," says Margarete Cassalina, "was to one day tell my grandchildren what their daddy used to have."

Margarete became a member of the CF world when she and her husband, Marc, welcomed their first child, Eric, in 1991. Born with meconium ileus, Eric was flown immediately to Westchester Medical Center to have the surgery to unblock the intestine. "They ran tests for two days, trying to figure out what was wrong with my baby boy," says Margarete.

Three days after his birth, a sweat test confirmed what Margarete had feared. "The tests are positive," she says the doctor told her. "Your child has cystic fibrosis. Cystic fibrosis is a fatal genetic disease." Marc looked at Margarete and then at the solemn expressions on the other doctors' faces. Margarete says that over the next three hours, seven doctors would explain all the things that Margarete and Marc never wanted to know about the disease. Eric's life expectancy at the time was nineteen. Margarete was twenty-two. "Your world stops. And you think 'What do I have to do to save him? Breathe,' I told myself (ironically), 'Breathe.'"

Margarete quit her job working at Marist College in the Office of Student Accounts as a financial aid assistant immediately after Eric's diagnosis. She also stopped going to school full time at Marist, studying political science, became a full-time stay-at-home mom, and became an advocate for the cystic fibrosis community, "doing all I can to save my child's life.

"I've been involved with CF Foundation since 1991," says Margarete, "the year my son Eric was diagnosed. I began at a local level raising funds and awareness through CFF events like Great Strides. I began to chair multiple events in both the Greater New York Chapter and in the Northeastern New York Chapter where I sat on the board."

Meanwhile, Eric was doing well his first eleven months. "No damage to his lungs," says Margarete. "No complications at all. In fact, we wanted to try again."

"I wanted a girl," Marc admits. "We realized that there was a twenty-five percent chance the next child would have cystic fibrosis, but our attitude was that the odds would be in our favor."

In 1993, two years after Eric's birth, Margarete and Marc welcomed a daughter, Jena, whose failure to thrive resulted in the dreaded sweat test that confirmed a diagnosis of cystic fibrosis. Now, Margarete and Marc, who have been together since 1989, were raising two children with an incurable disease. Margarete was doing physical chest therapy on both children two to three times a day—which she jokingly admits was like a workout for her arms—and while Eric had few CF-related medical complications throughout his childhood, Jena's case was considerably more severe.

Margarete and Marc continued their hard work to make a difference in the CF community. "Marc and I attended the National Medical Updates in the late 1990s," says Margarete. "The Medical Updates eventually became the Leadership Council Conference which then turned into the Volunteer Leadership Initiative, which has now become the National Volunteer Leadership Conference. Marc and I were involved with all stages of those programs. We were involved with [Public] Advocacy since its inception in 2004."

Unfortunately, despite all of the hard work put in by the Cassalinas,

Jena's CF was only getting worse. In her first thirteen years, Jena had to be hospitalized twenty-two times. Then, on December 4, 2006, days after being listed for a double-lung transplant, Jena's lungs collapsed. "Monday, December 4, 2006, at 9:57 a.m. was the exact moment I knew how horrible cystic fibrosis can be," says Margarete. "It was the moment my daughter, Jena, took her last breath . . . I will never be the same. The death of a child is the worst crisis of all because nothing prepares you for it. The first breath I took after my daughter, Jena, took her last made it painfully clear that I didn't want to breathe; I never wanted to breathe again." Margarete still remembers her young son, Eric, whispering to her soon after Jena's passing, "Isn't it ironic how we have to suffer because Jena's not, and we have to be sad because Jena's happy?"

Still, Margarete knew that the best way to honor her beautiful daughter was to remember her fondly and make a difference. She turned her heartache and passion toward helping others, whether speaking to groups or sharing her heart in her writing, which, along with supporting the CF Foundation and its community, are her favorite hobbies. "Pain is not a valid reason for stopping," says Margarete, conjuring a quote she took from Jena—the same words that Margarete hears when it seems too tough to move forward.

Margarete, who is, today, widely known as a motivational speaker, award-winning author, and national advocate for the Cystic Fibrosis Foundation, continues to move forward, incentivized by Jena's words and by a mission to help her beloved CF community. "I will not stop until all one hundred percent of those with cystic fibrosis have a cure. And I won't stop. Knowing how hard my children fought to live a happy and healthy life, that was all the influence I needed to do all I could with what I had to make their lives, and all those with cystic fibrosis, better."

So Margarete and Marc continued the fight. "We were the Advocacy chairs from 2008 to 2010," says Margarete. "Yes, we were advocating for both kids while we were caring for both kids; in truth we were advocating, raising funds and awareness, for all those with cystic fibrosis and still do to this day. Our involvement was inspired by supporting the CFF mission: to cure and control CF for all those with CF. We will continue to do what we can from where we are to support the continued mission of the Cystic Fibrosis Foundation."

Margarete is a frequent speaker at CF fundraisers and events across the country including the annual presentation of the Rose in the Garden of Life Award, which became known in 2011 as the Jena Award and goes to the person who has made a big contribution to the CF community but has no direct DNA connection.

Margarete memorializes her daughter with a 65 Roses rose garden in her own yard, but perhaps the most notable relics are the pennies. "It started with the one I found on the floor of the funeral home after Jena's funeral," says Margarete. "There on the floor, under a table, was a penny, and it was in the center of a perfect heart-shaped spill of wine. You could not have drawn a more perfect heart if you tried. Jena and I used to tell each other, 'Heart to heart, that's what we are,' and there on the floor was my answer. I knew Jena left that message for me that day, to remind me—because I had obviously forgotten—that she and I are 'heart to heart.'" Margarete now has a special rose box with all the "pennies from heaven" that she and Marc find. They also have a Facebook page called "Jena Penny" dedicated to all the pennies found in Jena's memory.

Margarete is the author of *Beyond Breathing*, a memoir that was written after Jena "moved up to heaven"; *See You at Sunset*, in which Margarete introduces readers to a group of memorable, fictional characters who quickly become near and dear despite "or maybe because of" their idiosyncrasies and shortcomings; and most recently, *Embracing the Beauty in the Broken*, a motivational non-fiction tale inspired by Margarete's own story. Through it all, Margarete adheres to her passion of bringing awareness and a human-face to cystic fibrosis.

She is passionately involved with the Cystic Fibrosis Foundation having served as National Public Advocacy cochair, National Volunteer Leadership cochair, and National Leadership council member and has sat as a board member in New York because she is committed to creating awareness and raising funds for scientific research, "which includes going to Capitol Hill and pleading lawmakers to help those with cystic fibrosis to live better lives." Margarete and Marc were also named 2021 honorees at the 2021 Breath of Life Gala for all they have done for the Cystic Fibrosis Foundation, which, due to COVID concerns, the event was pushed out to November 17, 2022.

While Margarete and Marc think about their children every day, they are now basking in new roles as grandparents to Easton, who was born to Eric and his wife, Kourtney, on April 22, 2020. "I have lived a life full of hope, dreams, and optimism in the future," says Marc, "but living through the incredible pain and reality of watching

Jena fight and lose her battle to CF shook my beliefs. Even through that pain, I still carried the dream of one day being a grandpa. Seeing Eric thrive on Trikafta and becoming a dad, has realized that dream, and renewed my optimism in our future."

"While I do not have cystic fibrosis myself," says Margarete, "I have learned a lot from parenting my children. Eric and Jena taught me more about life than I ever taught them. I want to be that person to help other people. I have dedicated my life to finding the ultimate cure so that one day CF will stand for 'Cure Found.'"

Margarete thinks back to the dream she has had since the diagnosis of her son, Eric, in 1991, to tell her grandchildren what their daddy *used to* have. "Easton will one day hear that story," says Margarete, flashing a smile.[1]

---

[1] Some of the responses above are taken directly from Margarete's first book, *Beyond Breathing*, and her third book, *Embracing the Beauty in the Broken*, the use of which the author was granted permission by Margarete Cassalina.

BETH VANSTONE

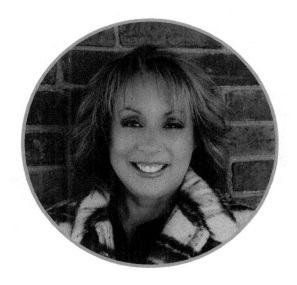

Age: 59
Resides: Beeton, Ontario, Canada
Connection to CF: Mother to a CF warrior

MOTIVATED BY MADI: THE ENDLESS FIGHT FOR LIFESAVING MEDS

Beth Vanstone knew little about cystic fibrosis until her second child was diagnosed. "My daughter Madi had been a very sick baby and was hospitalized for the first time at eight months with pneumonia when her weight dropped from sixteen pounds to twelve pounds," says Beth. Her diagnosis came soon after. After spending a day at SickKids in Toronto with the CF team, Beth, her husband, Glenn, and Madi returned home with two large bags of medications, a nebulizer, and fear of what her future held.

Beth remembers Googling cystic fibrosis and how devastating the disease appeared. Yet like many CF moms and dads, giving up was not an option for Beth. "I immediately rolled up my sleeves to battle for Madi's life," says Beth. "We decided that we would do everything in our power to keep her healthy until there was a cure. We then started doing whatever we could to get to that cure, including participating in research studies and lots of fundraising. Madi was enrolled in studies while she was still a baby. I made the decisions while she was very young, and she became more involved as she became older. She agreed to each and every study in an effort to make things better for others. She still participates in research studies."

"Madi had a tough time, and despite our best efforts, keeping her healthy was tough," says Beth. "She was very congested within weeks of being born. I would watch her breathe and see her chest concave as she inhaled. She had digestive issues and had a very swollen, hard abdomen. I ended up resigning from my job only a month back to work after maternity leave."

Madi and Beth spent at least two weeks in the hospital every spring and fall as she fought constant infections, and when she was five or six years old, Madi's lung function dropped into the fifties. "It was terrifying," says Beth.

When Madi was about five, she asked Beth why she had CF and her friends and family did not. "It caught me off guard," says Beth, "but I quickly responded, 'Because God knew you could do this, and you have a family who will always be with you to fight this.'" Beth didn't realize it then, but those words made a big difference. "It seemed to make her feel better, and years later after a speaking engagement, Madi was asked the same question by someone in the audience. It surprised me when she recited what I had told her all those years ago."

"It's a very delicate balancing act," says Beth, "never wanting Madi to be defined by her disease, but I also didn't want her to be ashamed of it. As a family we chose to fight this disease with all we had. Like many, we fundraised every year, Madi participated in research studies, and we used our voices to raise awareness."

Beth began fundraising within months of Madi being diagnosed in 2002. "Our family began participating in the annual CF Canada Walk," says Beth. "Both of my daughters formed their own teams, Jesse's Jammers and Madi's Maniacs, allowing their friends to participate and help raise money for CF Canada. I was soon holding my own fundraisers for the cause. We held a local five-kilometer run, and aerobathon [rhythmic exercises performed to music] for a couple of years. We [also] did paint nights and raffles."

While Beth continued to work to raise money and keep her youngest daughter healthy, Madi, who had probably participated in nearly twenty research studies, was asked to participate in another study at the age of eleven in 2012, a blind study for a CFTR modulator called Kalydeco. What transpired next shocked Beth, Madi, and their family. "It was life changing," says Beth. "Her lung function shot up in thirty days, her headaches and stomachaches were resolved, and her energy soared."

And yet the drug was very expensive and not covered by insurance or public plans. "So we took up the battle to have this amazing drug covered for eligible CF patients," says Beth. "Madi and I went to our local member of Parliament Jim Wilson and explained our situation and the desperate need for Madi to gain access to Kalydeco. We made several trips to Queens Park with our MPP [member of Provincial Parliament] where he repeatedly asked when Kalydeco would be funded in Ontario. We were writing letters to our health minister, our premiere, and collecting signatures for a petition. With our many trips to Queens Park, the media picked up the story. We did countless news interviews, shared our story on many news shows, and the story was followed in all of the major and local newspapers. The story took on a life of its own.

"After two years of meetings with politicians, a trip to Queens Park in Toronto, and countless television interviews to share our story, the drug was covered!"

Madi has thrived along with other CF patients who were able to access Kalydeco, but not all CF patients benefit from Kalydeco, and though new modulators have come to market for those patients, it is so difficult to get these drugs into their country. "Our government has made it extremely difficult for patients to access these lifesaving drugs," says Beth. "Although Madi is doing well, we continue to meet with politicians both federally and provincially to advocate for patients. We have spent a decade advocating for these drugs and patients."

Madi and Beth speak across Ontario spreading their story. Beth was also a director of a grassroots advocacy group CF Get Loud (which she retired from in September 2021), a group that works tirelessly educating, empowering, and elevating the nearly four thousand advocates from across Canada who are working for access to these lifesaving modulators. A CF Canada fundraising highlight for Madi and Beth is traveling to China in September 2019 and spending five full days trekking the Great Wall. "But I wish this wasn't a fight we needed to have," says Beth, "and I will not stop until each patient has what they need to live their best life. It shouldn't be this hard."

"My mom is my angel," says Madi. "Because she fought for me, I'm here today. When I was diagnosed with cystic fibrosis, she put her entire life aside to care for me when I was sick, and for that I will forever be grateful. She is the reason I am who I am today. She's not just my hero; she's a hero to the CF community."

Beth, Madi, and the Vanstone family have raised over $200,000 over the years for CF Canada while advocating for those who do not have a voice. They distribute ballcaps all over the USA and Canada with an image featuring the words on Madi's only tattoo: "Just breathe."

Madi's older sister, Jessie, (shortened from "Jessica") and Jessie's friends have raised funds on walks for Cystic Fibrosis Canada with their Jesses Jammers team (Madi, herself, created Madi's Maniacs). "I'm happy that Jessie is taking an active role in fighting cystic fibrosis," says Beth, who worked for years to get Trikafta approved in Canada—a drug she believes will benefit Madi and so many others—before finally having success in September 2021, "but it's not easy to have a 'sick' sibling. And yet if you are fortunate enough to have people who support you, let them. They want to help and be there for you. As a CF mom, I want to see both my girls achieve all of their dreams. One thing we often think of is the 'shadow siblings' who live in the shadows of the sick child. My daughter Jessie did this. She has made me proud every day as she has worked toward her goals.

"I think the first thing every parent wishes for their child is for them to be healthy and happy," says Beth. "When Madi was diagnosed with cystic fibrosis at eight months of age, we needed to redefine what we wanted for our daughter. Happy remained on top of our list. Having a child with any health challenge quickly reprioritizes what you want for them. I am not saying that you can't have the same hopes and dreams you would have for every other child, however, you do need to recognize that they may require a little more of themselves to reach their goals.

"My goal for Madi remains for her to be happy and to keep chasing her dreams."

Beth continues, "Whether having a difficult procedure done at [the] hospital or being the center of a scrum at Parliament, I always wanted Madi to know she could do it. I tried to lead by example often masking my own fear in an effort to show her an example of strength. I truly feel this helped her immensely as she was generally looking to me as an example. Madi has used her voice to speak for herself and others in the battle for modulators in Canada. She continues to use her voice both publicly and privately within the CF community to support patients.

"I am so proud of both my daughters," says Beth. "Jessica who is completing teacher's college and Madi who is studying social media. Despite the challenges, both of my daughters are compassionate and strong women who are choosing to live with gratitude for what they have and determination to achieve their individual goals and, of course, joy celebrating each day. As a mom, that is all I can ask for them."

LAURA BONNELL

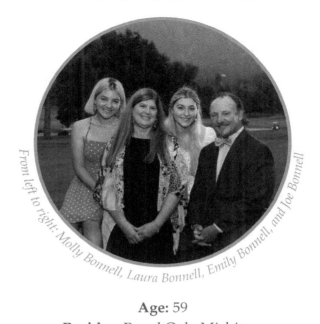

From left to right: Molly Bonnell, Laura Bonnell, Emily Bonnell, and Joe Bonnell

Age: 59
Resides: Royal Oak, Michigan
Connection to CF: Mother to two CF warriors

TV REPORTER TURNED CF ADVOCATE: THE CREATION OF THE BONNELL FOUNDATION

Michigan-native Laura Bonnell knew she wanted to be a news reporter from when she was twelve years old.

"My dad was an attorney and involved in local politics," says Laura. "Reading the newspaper was mandatory. We were always expected to know and be invested in what was going on in our community. I loved watching anchors and reporters on TV. I loved the news so much I became a papergirl. I was told I was the first female papergirl for the Observer and Eccentric newspapers. I was born to report the news, to tell other people's stories. I thoroughly enjoyed my television and radio career. I felt I was making a difference in people's lives. I went jogging with candidate (President) Clinton at Michigan State University (until my nylons ran and Clinton left me in the dust). I have met politicians (then Attorney General Janet

Reno, US senators, and representatives), rock stars (Kid Rock, Ted Nugent, Joe Perry), activists like Jesse Jackson and civil rights icon Rosa Parks, along with ABC News anchor Peter Jennings. The list goes on, but truly the best stories I did were about people trying to make a difference in the world. Then suddenly, I had a story to tell."

In 1989, when Laura was twenty-eight, a year after she met her husband, Joe—"who I'd met at a café right after my father died; I believed he brought the two of us together"—she took a year off from reporting the news and went to work for the United Way of Washtenaw County (UWWC). "I had no idea at the time how, during that one year, my life would change forever," says Laura. "At the UWWC, I was putting together a promotional piece on its agencies."

In 1989, Dr. Francis S. Collins, who would later become the director of the National Institutes of Health, announced the discovery of the gene that causes cystic fibrosis. "I was there, to witness the press conference on behalf of the UWWC," says Laura. "It was an exciting, exhilarating day to be at [the University of Michigan]. All the Detroit media gathered for a news conference to interview Dr. Collins. I had no idea, at the time, my future was on a CF path."

In December 1994, when Laura was a reporter at WWJ in Detroit, an all-news station, she and Joe had a baby girl named Molly. "I noticed she had greasy bowel movements, she had gas a lot, her stomach was distended, and she tasted salty when I kissed her," says Laura. "The dog licked her all the time. I thought back to a TV commercial where a local news anchor was talking about kissing your baby, if they tasted salty, they might have cystic fibrosis." Laura and Joe did not know they were even carriers. Joe had seven siblings and Laura had two and none of them had CF or had any children with the disease. "I started reading about CF and was certain she had it," says Laura. "Molly's pediatrician said I was a first-time mom and should go back to work. I ignored what I knew was true for about two weeks. And then I demanded Molly get tested. I was on my way to a breaking news story and the doctor called. She told me to pull over, but I knew. Molly had CF. She confirmed it. My journey had begun."

Laura was in radio/TV because it was her passion, but her passion had quickly changed. "The day Molly was diagnosed with cystic fibrosis, Joe and I sat on our front porch, drinking a beer, crying," says Laura. "Our lives as parents flashed before our eyes. We planned on a healthy child that would live a long life. Cystic fibrosis was not part of the plan. We were devastated. We planned to have between four to six kids, but our dream was crushed with the diagnosis. CF is a rollercoaster, then and now. Within an hour, we decided that we would just educate ourselves and give Molly a normal life. And we also decided we were going to have one more child.

"It was also within that first hour, as so many things flashed through my mind, that I became obsessed with documenting every part of our life. I took photographs, constantly, and still do. We started talking to other families about their paths and gathered information that helped us. Molly didn't have any hospitalizations early on, and that made moving forward easier for us. I was still scared and still wondered how long she would live. Just shortly after Molly was diagnosed, the CF Foundation [Michigan chapter] asked me to speak at their Tennis Auction Ball event. I said yes. I was a news reporter at WWJ. I was well known (a million people listen to WWJ on average). I was at the podium, I spoke and then started crying, and couldn't stop. When I composed myself, I did talk about our newly diagnosed experience. I felt free, like I got a big secret out. I was starting to heal from the diagnosis that blew up my idyllic dreams of motherhood. Then I re-alized—this was my journey, my purpose in life. And then I couldn't be stopped as I decided to one day start my own foundation, raising awareness and funds. My foundation turned into my much-needed therapy. I can never do enough to help the CF community, or to raise awareness. They're my people."

Emily would follow Molly two and a half years later. Although there is only a 25 percent chance another child would have CF, the results were the same. "The day Molly was diagnosed we realized how scary it was, and many times after that," says Laura. "We decid-ed to have a second child because we wanted Molly to have a sibling. We knew there was a one-in-four chance she could have cystic fi-brosis but naïvely we thought, 'How could it happen twice?'" Emily was officially diagnosed with cystic fibrosis through a sweat test at six weeks old and battled pneumonia several months later. "When Emily was eight months old and had pneumonia," says Laura, "that scared me as much as the day that Molly was diagnosed." Still, Laura says the day of Molly's diagnosis was the day they knew they were going to fight.

"This is when I asked for and got help from my peers in radio, tele-vision, and the print media," says Laura. "Public service announce-ments aired on TV and radio stations. Newsworthy stories about CF were written in the print media and aired on TV and radio stations. A celebrity baseball game began, media versus law enforcement."

Laura also asked the Detroit Tigers Major League baseball team if they would help her start the first Celebrity Softball Game. The Tigers agreed. Their wives played and the players watched. "It was amazing," says Laura. "All these people came to raise awareness because I asked them." Laura also noticed that the Cystic Fibrosis Foundation featured a calendar with different roses representing each month. Laura took it a step further. "The Portraits of CF calendars came about, featuring people with CF showing their strength in spite of the disease.

"Everyone has something," says Laura, "we have CF. I always told my girls they were never going to use CF as an excuse to get out of a test, a track meet, etc., and honestly, they never considered it. They actually worked harder to be normal because of the disease. But the girls must also be realistic—if they were sick, we had to deal with it straight on. We also tried to empower them at all ages and stages of their disease. From the beginning, we wanted them to be in charge of their disease, age appropriate, but they need to have a voice."

Laura remembers one example specifically. "Emily was terrified to get her blood drawn after several nurses poked her too much and didn't listen to her fears," says Laura. "It traumatized her. So, we decided the only way to conquer this fear was [for her] to have a say, even as just a five-year-old. One very large nurse came into the room and was bossing Emily around about getting her blood drawn and minimizing her fear as irrational. So Emily looked at me and I gave the look of approval, and in her little voice, she told the nurse she wanted someone else. And that was that. Emily had rules for blood draws: You had to wait until she calmed herself down. You had to acknowledge she was more than just an arm and you had to count down to the poke. It helped her slowly turn a corner."

As adults, Molly and Emily deal with the pharmacy and insurance challenges but call Laura in for backup when they need her help. "Nothing is ever easy when it comes to either of those," says Laura. "The insurance company denies coverage incorrectly. The pharmacy doesn't recognize the secondary insurance. It's a part-time job getting everything straightened out." Laura admits, though, she is not just the teacher with regard to her children. "My girls, now twenty-three and twenty-six, have taught me a lot," she says. "They have outlived the life expectancy of seventeen years old. That makes me so happy. The biggest accomplishment is that they are in charge of their disease, and they know their bodies."

As a news reporter, Laura was always trying to raise awareness about the disease, and she felt if the family was open about it from the start, then it wouldn't be awkward for them to talk about CF. "Everyone knew about their CF," says Laura, "and kids just asked questions and the girls answered. The girls have raised awareness about the disease their entire lives. From the classroom to speaking engagements, to videos or COVID-19 when they were part of a social distance squad campaign. In college, they didn't hide it but fewer people knew about it. I could not be prouder of both of my girls."

Molly, a graduate of Parsons in New York and Central Saint Martin in London, England, has incorporated design and research into her life and developed an undergraduate project about CF (featured in the New York Times) and in graduate school as well. Her undergraduate project was the development of hospital gowns for chronically-ill people and clothing that accommodates IV lines and PICC lines. Molly currently works for HospitalRooms.com in England and is a curator bringing artwork into hospital mental health departments.

Emily graduated from Michigan State University majoring in marketing and Spanish and currently works for a social media influencer. She has a deep understanding of her disease and sometimes a desire to be a spokesperson for CF. She spoke before a crowd of scientists to tell her CF story and inspire them to continue their CF work.

For years, Laura and Joe contributed to the CF Foundation Great Strides walk and the University of Michigan CF clinic, "and then we realized it was time for us to start our own foundation," says Laura. "We started a 501(c)(3) called the Bonnell Foundation, whose mission is 'to give emotional and/or financial support to parents who have a loved one with cystic fibrosis.' The foundation's hope is that one day no CF parent will experience the pain of losing a child to the disease." Since its inception in 2010, the Bonnell Foundation, whose tagline is, "Live, Breathe, and Inspire," has raised $500,000, which they have given out in college scholarships, financial assistance, and lung transplant grants.

"Watching my mom create this amazing foundation that's grown so beautifully into a community of assistance and healing has been incredible," says Emily. "I always say she's a superwoman because she truly is. She eats, sleeps, and breathes the efforts of her foundation and makes sure she can help as many people as possible."

"I left radio two years ago to give all my energy to the [Bonnell] Foundation," says Laura. "I do podcasts that have shed light on CF in Egypt and stories here in the US that people can relate to. I use all my radio and TV skills to document, photograph, write, and record our life with CF. My passion is my foundation—raising funds to help other CF families."

In July 2022, Laura went to Egypt to meet other CF families and bring them two pediatric CF vests that her daughters outgrew. "It's like stepping back in time," says Laura. "The CF care is so far behind the United States."

Dr. Samya Nasr, Molly and Emily's pediatric CF physician, did a study in 2004 to see if there were CF patients in her native country of Egypt. She diagnosed sixty-two patients with cystic fibrosis. After Dr. Nasr's study was published in the Journal of Cystic Fibrosis in 2007, Dr. Maggie Naguib sweat-tested more patients and another 538 patients were diagnosed.

"Thousands more are expected to be diagnosed," says Laura. "The parents are desperate for information and medications we have in the United States. When they met me and saw the photos of my twenty-seven- and twenty-five-year-old daughters, they had big smiles of hope and tears in their eyes. This was the first time they had talked to an American CF mom in person. We bonded instantly. The language barrier didn't matter. We hugged for a long time. We couldn't let go. We cried. I cried because it took me back to my diagnosis day. I remembered how scared I was and there was so much unknown. But at least we had the proper medications. They do not in Egypt. So the challenge is to get the Ministry of Health to understand. They're willing but they're just not completely informed. Doctors are trying to connect with them to get a distributor to ship meds to Egypt."

Laura is doing her part too as she received a positive response from MVW Nutritionals, a privately held company out of Huntsville, Alabama, after requesting much needed vitamins for the country's CF population. The organization's mission is to provide nutritional supplements and vitamins for persons who have CF and other gastrointestinal disorders. The company has confirmed that they will be sending vitamins to Egypt to help CF patients there.

"Going to Egypt was life-changing for me," says Laura. "It didn't matter that we could not speak the same language. We are the CF community and we are here for each other. Where you live shouldn't determine if you live."

"There've been too many nights where my mom's up all night putting all of us before herself and brainstorming how she can problem-solve issues, provide assistance, and be there for those who need it," says Emily. "I'm so incredibly proud of her for the way she's so selfless and such a force in her efforts. It's been incredible watching her do it."

DIANE SHADER SMITH

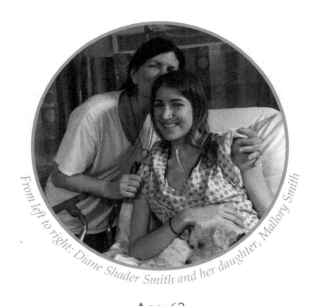

From left to right: Diane Shader Smith and her daughter, Mallory Smith

Age: 62
Resides: Los Angeles, California
Connection to CF: Mother to a CF warrior

MEMORIALIZING MALLORY: SALT IN A MOTHER'S SOUL

World-renowned speaker, writer, and publicist, Diane Shader Smith has built an impressive résumé. She was on the writing staff of the hit ABC-TV series *General Hospital*, ran public-relations and marketing campaigns for corporations and celebrities at Rogers and Cowan, and has authored four books. But her most important work, and the work she will be best known for, is her current work . . . as a cystic fibrosis advocate using her daughter Mallory's posthumously published memoir, *Salt in My Soul* (Random House, 2019) as her platform.

It all began in 1995 when Diane and her husband, Mark, were trying to figure out what was wrong with their daughter, Mallory, the younger of their two children (their son, Micah, is two years older). "Mallory displayed a lot of symptoms—a persistent cough, a chronic runny nose, and severe GI problems," Diane says. At age three, Mallory was finally diagnosed with cystic fibrosis. "We were devastated," Diane continues. "The doctor seemed hopeful when he said that the lifespan for children with CF had increased from five (when the disease was first discovered in the late 1930s up until the 1950s) to twenty-five and that he expected it to get even longer, but all Mark and I heard was that our child had an expiration date. I was bawling my eyes out and so I asked the doctor how he dealt with hysterical parents and very sick children. He said he had treated kids who had been beaten, burned, or abandoned. He saw the love we had for Mallory and the smile on her face . . . and promised us she would have a happy life, which she did."

Early on, Diane knew that it was important not to keep Mallory's disease a secret. "I was desperate for a way to explain the disease to Mallory and her brother, Micah," she says, "but there was no children's book about CF back then—so I wrote *Mallory's 65 Roses*. [The term,] 65 Roses is what kids hear when adults say, 'cystic fibrosis.'" Diane and Mark read the book, which has sold more than thirty thousand copies, to Mallory's class at the start of every school year and gave copies to her friends. They wanted those around Mallory to treat her like everyone else, not to be intimidated by the disease.

"That first year, Mallory hated doing treatments," Diane explains. "Every day when it was time to start, she would hide . . . in the closet, under the bed, anywhere she thought we wouldn't find her. To make it less traumatic for her, Mark made up a game he called 'Astronaut and Pat Pat.' *Astronaut* for the mask that delivered her inhaled medicines, and *Pat Pat* for the chest percussion therapy. For the first year we did manual percussion, then at the age of five Mallory got The Vest (a mechanical airway-clearance system). She followed standard protocols—Vest, nebulizer, bronchodilator, Pulmozyme, TOBI, rotating antibiotics (twice a day when she was healthy, four times a day when she was sick)."

One year, when she came home from sleepaway camp, Mallory had lost ten pounds and ten percent of her lung function, which led to her first hospitalization. Her lungs had been colonized by Burkholderia cenocepacia, a strain of the bacteria B. cepacia. Mallory and her family understood the severity of the diagnosis. This bacterium can spread throughout the body, causing cepacia syndrome, which can kill a person within a few weeks. But even if you are able to live with it, it eventually turns into a superbug, developing more and more antibiotic resistance over time. "Mallory would often say, 'The doctors are only focused on my lungs because that's what will kill me, but the GI problems are what ruin my life,'" says Diane.

As Mallory got older, Diane steered her into sports. "I knew physical activity would slow the progression of the disease, and I couldn't stand the thought of her sitting inside on a sunny day, playing piano," says Diane. Mallory was named team captain for her high school's varsity water polo, volleyball, and swim teams. "Mallory identified as an athlete and thrived on competition," says Diane. "Athletics made her feel a part of a community and generated deeply bonded friend-ships. She was a quiet leader and people flocked to her. Mallory was an incredible athlete and a very respected captain. The physical mo-tion helped her bring up mucus. I was a working mom but was fortu-nate to have a job that allowed me to sit courtside for every volleyball match and poolside for every swim meet and water polo game; these were my happy places."

"Mallory was memorable for a lot of reasons," says her high school water polo coach Rob Bowie. "Not only was she this statuesque, phys-ically gifted athlete but she was one of the kindest, most thoughtful, and quiet yet intensely competitive kids I ever coached. She never made any excuses, never wanted to be treated differently because of her CF. I think sports let her feel like just an ordinary kid, the gym and pool were her refuge from disease, allowing her to get lost in fun, camaraderie, and competition. I remember her yelling at her mom for making her miss morning practices so she could squeeze in treatments before school. She hated feeling like she was getting a pass that her teammates didn't.

"I was in constant awe that she could even make it through a water polo game. Anyone who's ever played the sport knows how demand-ing it is on your lungs and here was a girl grinding it out, having to breathe through what she once described to me as a 'snorkel full of glue.' She laughed when she told me that, like it didn't faze her. It was just her reality, and she rolled with it. She was always upbeat and laughing and good natured. It was almost as if she was putting her fears and discomfort on hold just to make everyone else around her feel like everything was going to be okay. That is extremely powerful and selfless. That is being a true warrior."

Mallory's high school volleyball coach Marla Weiss remembers one incident when Mallory proved her warrior skills. "We had a CIF [California Interscholastic Federation] playoff game, at home," says Marla. "Mallory was in the hospital fighting for her life . . . we did not expect her to be at the match as we knew she had been hospi-talized. We were all motivated to win for many reasons, but also so Mallory would be able to join us in the next round. A bit before the match began, in walks Mallory. She had checked herself out of the hospital . . . against medical advice . . . to be able to compete for the team. Dedication, desire—wow!"

Marla says that became the norm for Mallory. "Mallory's leadership abilities were through actions, more than words," says Marla. "But in a tight match, when things were tough, Mallory's words meant more than anything. When she did speak, to advise or motivate or strategize, everyone listened. Mallory rarely missed practices or any team event or activity. She did not want CF to hinder her high school experience or her sports season. If she wasn't feeling well, I wouldn't have known. If she coughed strongly, I always asked, 'Are you okay? Do you need time, or do you need to stop for now?' Mallory's answer was always no. And she got right back into the drills. Coaches often talk about the 'Four Ds' in athletics: desire, determination, discipline, and dedication. Often our athletes possess one or two, maybe three, but Mallory lived all four. She modeled all four. She was that good and that remarkable of a person."

As a senior waiting to attend Stanford, Mallory's lungs continued to get worse, and she started to need supplemental oxygen, yet despite being hospitalized for much of that year, she was named prom queen by her high school class.

"Mallory was kind, loving, brilliant, lovely, athletic, and fun," says Diane, "and the best daughter and friend you could ask for. She modeled patience and perseverance . . . she was the single most inspiring person I've ever known. She did not sweat the small stuff and taught everyone around her that you have to live every day in the moment because you're not guaranteed a tomorrow."

Mallory eventually went on to Stanford and despite dealing with many hospitalizations and various surgeries, she graduated Phi Beta Kappa, majoring in human biology with a concentration in environmental anthropology. Mallory put her environmental skills to work during and after college as a senior producer at *Green Grid Radio*, an environmental podcast, and as a freelance writer for the National Wildlife Federation.

Following her graduation from Stanford, Mallory met Jack Goodwin at a New Year's Eve party. Jack was working on his masters at Stanford. The two began dating in spring of 2016. "Mallory was special in a million ways," says Jack, "but what most impressed me was the delicate balance she maintained, between patience for my shortcomings and encouragement to become a better partner."

Still, Mallory's health was worsening. She and her doctors knew she would need a lung transplant soon, but she was rejected by transplant centers around the country, because the antibiotic-resistant B. cepacia bacteria lodged in her lungs could reinfect new lungs after transplant. Finally, the University of Pittsburgh Medical Center accepted Mallory for evaluation.

While Mallory was hopeful, she also knew the reality of her prognosis.

So did Diane: "I adopted a mantra—'No Pity Party'—and taught Mallory from a young age to prioritize love and friendship . . . to enjoy the small things, both of which she did. Mallory went on to adopt her own mantra: 'Live Happy.' She suffered a lot—with extreme physical pain, constant nausea and vomiting, bone-crushing fatigue, and anxiety about her future. But she never complained."

Jack also realized Mallory's prognosis was bleak. "After Mallory's doctor told us she wouldn't live more than one year without a double-lung transplant," says Jack, "I was terrified and needed to take a few days to process the reality of the situation. She was patient, giving me space to process that news on my own and to figure out the right questions to ask. I asked a lot of wrong questions, but the right one ended up revolving around identity: 'What kind of man do I want to be? Do I want to be the kind of man that loves someone only when it's easy, or also when it's hard? Not just also when it's hard, but *especially* when it's hard?' After a lot of reflection, I came back to Mal, told her I loved her for the first time, and that I wanted to be the type of man who stayed."

Diane says, "As Mallory's life narrowed, she fought hard to reinvent herself without giving up on her dream of working in environmental education. Instead of doing field work, she got hired to write a book—*The Gottlieb Native Garden: A California Love Story*, about the importance of using native plants and gardening for wildlife. The publication of this book enabled Mallory to realize that she could still make a difference, despite her limitations."

Mallory was always writing. Some of the time for publication, some of the time privately. She kept her journal strictly private. But in the end, she gave Diane the password. "Mallory had a lot of insights to share with anyone living with, or loving someone with, cystic fibrosis," says Diane. "She wanted her words to be published after her death since much of what she wrote was too personal to share during her lifetime. After Mallory had her transplant, she signed with a New York agent and was going to have her memoir published."

Unfortunately, Mallory didn't get to see that happen. She survived the nine-hour transplant surgery, but the antibiotic-resistant B. cepacia bacteria in her upper airways recolonized her new lungs and led to her death just two months after.

"I didn't open Mallory's journal until after she died. Then, I started reading it, hoping to find something to say at her memorial service . . . maybe something in her own words," Diane says. "It was immediately clear that the two thousand and five hundred pages Mallory had written was more than enough material for a posthumously published memoir. My sister came up with the title, *Salt in My*

Soul: An Unfinished Life. Random House published it, calling Mallory's writing life changing."

Diane decided to speak on Mallory's behalf—to share her words with the world since Mallory wasn't here to speak for herself. She's given more than two hundred talks about Mallory's life and legacy to hospitals, medical schools, high schools, ladies' luncheons, and many other venues. The consensus is that Mallory has important insights to share. The book has sold more than thirty-five thousand copies.

Fundraising is another way Mallory's family is honoring her memory. During Mallory's lifetime, they raised $5 million through their annual fundraiser, An Evening in Mallory's Garden, and through an online viral campaign, Lunges4Lungs. Mallory started Lunges4Lungs with two friends after learning that their transplant rejection research was woefully underfunded, and the *Today Show* did a short piece on the campaign.

After Mallory passed away, her family established Mallory's Legacy Fund at the California Community Foundation to support phage therapy. One hundred percent of the profits from *Salt in My Soul: An Unfinished Life* (the book) and *Salt in My Soul* (the documentary film) will be donated to research. The documentary was released by 3 Arts Entertainment in January of 2022 and has been used to raise money and awareness for antimicrobial resistance and phage therapy. The documentary, directed by Will Battersby, has received rave reviews which can be found at www.saltinmysouldoc.com from various publications including the *New York Times*, the *Los Angeles Times*, and the *Boston Globe*. Shortly after the film aired, a panel discussing the making of the film hosted by *The Office* star Rainn Wilson discussed how Mallory's journals led to a best-selling book and acclaimed documentary and the future of phage therapy which featured experts in the field.

Mark, Mallory's father, had heard about an experimental treatment called phage therapy and pushed hard to get it. Many doctors said no, either because they hadn't heard about it or because they didn't believe in its potential. But Dr. Joe Pilewski at UPMC (University of Pittsburgh Medical Center) listened to Mark and agreed there was no downside since Mallory was out of options. Mallory made history on November 14, 2017, becoming the first patient with CF to receive phage therapy. Her autopsy showed the phages had started to work— she just didn't get them in time to save her. Distraught that he couldn't save Mallory, Mark was determined to save others with cystic fibrosis. Mark convened a meeting with Dr. Mike Boyle and the Cystic Fibrosis Foundation where Mark introduced his vision of treating kids with CF with phage therapy before infection ravaged their lungs. The foundation is now funding several studies.

Mallory's case set the stage for others to receive phage therapy, so this is part of her legacy. Mark and Diane are supporting both the clinical trial at IPATH (the Center for Innovative Phage Applications and Therapeutics at UCSD) and compassionate use cases at Yale. They have also donated money to EVLP research (*ex vivo lung perfusion,* which is a technique to keep lungs viable during the time before a lung transplant) to help make more donor lungs viable for transplantation.

Scientist Ella Balasa is one CF patient who has benefited from phage therapy. "Diane Shader Smith is a devoted mom and an incredibly strong and determined advocate for the use of phage therapy to treat antibiotic-resistant infections," says Ella. "I am honored to know Diane—meeting her after I received phage therapy to treat a devastating lung infection. Her tireless work to help other patients struggling with the same infections that took her daughter does not go unnoticed in the CF community. She pushes for new research advancements and funding in Mallory's honor. I admire her tenacity and spirit. Mallory would be so proud of you, Diane."

"Diane and her husband, Mark, arranged to make the inaugural gift to IPATH, based on donations they'd received for Mallory's Legacy Fund," says Dr. Steffanie Strathdee, award-winning author of *The Perfect Predator* and codirector of IPATH. "It was deeply personal since my colleague Dr. Robert (Chip) Schooley and I had worked so hard to obtain phages to save Mallory's life. Their gift is an inspiration to us, and it also allowed us to hire a coordinator to field the many requests for phage therapy that we receive on a daily basis. Apart from their financial support, Diane has given literally hundreds of talks which have raised awareness about the need for the CF community to tackle superbugs and how phage therapy can be part of that solution."

Dr. Strathdee says they have a lot more to accomplish. "We'd like to ensure that phage therapy is evaluated in rigorous clinical trials so that the FDA can consider approving it as a therapeutic alongside antibiotics. IPATH is already involved in two clinical trials, and several others are on the horizon. We're also working to develop a phage library that is large enough that phage can be matched to superbug isolates within a day or two. Because when someone is fighting a superbug infection, and there are no antibiotic options left, every minute counts."

Dr. Strathdee still remembers how she was introduced to the Smith family. "Mark reached out to me after Mallory's B. cepacia started attacking her new lungs, and she was very ill," says Dr. Strathdee. "I talked to Mark and Diane on the phone, and I could hear the desperation in their voices. I immediately reached out to Chip, and we enlisted the help of the same scientists who found phages to save my husband's life. These were phage researchers at Texas A&M, the navy's Medical Research Unit in Maryland, and Jon Dennis in Canada. It was a race against time. I even used Twitter to crowdsource phage for Mallory, and the response was overwhelming. My tweet was retweeted 432 times! I was so optimistic that we could save her, but we were just a little too late. Diane, Mark, and I are now extended family, bound through our stories. Diane and I have also presented together at book events, and the response has been outstanding."

IPATH's Burkholderia Patient Registry, initiated in 2020, is now compiling a library of phages including lung specimens from Mallory, which are still in the process of being researched. The Cystic Fibrosis Foundation is now invested in a study, thanks to Diane and Mark, to evaluate inhaled phage therapy, and biotech companies are also looking to get involved.

"The work of Diane and Mark in promoting Phage Therapy has been nothing short of incredible," says Jack. "The Smiths are well aware they are fighting a battle against an opponent much larger and better resourced than themselves (i.e., the pharmaceutical industry, medical regulatory landscape, and insurance lobbyists), but that hasn't stopped them from continuing to give everything they have in a bid to drive change. It's not hard to see that being a CF parent comes with an abnormal set of life challenges, but also an inner strength and perspective that lends power to every decision they make."

Diane says one of the best descriptions she's ever heard of her daughter is from one of Mallory's best friends, Talia Stone, which Diane included in *Salt in My Soul*. "Mallory was always the tallest, smartest, most athletic girl in the grade—even at five years old," says Talia. "We'd chase boys around the playground, and she'd run faster than all of them. They all had crushes on her. Mal was every teacher's favorite student, and every kid wanted to be her friend. She was the friend whose advice everyone wanted: she coached you when to text or not text the boy you liked, how to say the right things to convince your parents to let you go to that party, and gave you the best hug when you needed it most. Mal was the girl who missed forty days of the school semester and still got the highest grade in the class. She was the girl who laughed so hard she snorted, which made her laugh even harder. She was the prom queen—and would hate that I [told you] that."

Jack has his own description of the woman he fell in love with. "Mallory had the highest maturity-to-age ratio I've ever seen," says Jack. "That's probably no surprise to those in the CF community, but her calm under pressure, kindness to others, and all-around positive spirit filled every room she entered with a beautiful brightness. She was also really beautiful, which at first made it challenging to listen to and learn from all she had to share while not staring too much. I miss the fact that she could be all of these amazing things and still be goofy and playful. I miss our deep chats about life and purpose. I miss the camaraderie we shared in taking on CF together. And though at first I had to keep myself from staring at her too long, I miss being able to stare endlessly into her eyes, especially when she was doing treatment or on a ventilator, and know what she was thinking without having to speak."

"Through her writing, Mallory is the young woman who shows us the power of personal story," says Diane when speaking about her daughter's legacy. "The patient who teaches healthcare professionals that if you're really going to deliver patient-centered care, you have to listen to the patient. The environmentalist who wanted to heal the planet in some small way through her words and her work. The girl who prioritized love about all else. The daughter we lost too soon."

5

ALL IN THE FAMILY:
CF AFFECTS "EVERYONE"
IN THE FAMILY

MARTHA GARVEY

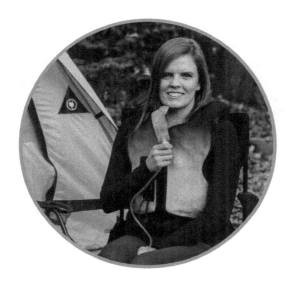

Age: 28
Resides: St. Paul, Minnesota
Age at diagnosis: Birth

RAY OF HOPE: THE SUPPORT OF A CF SIBLING

Martha Garvey was born in 1993 to Rusty, a policeman, and Darla, an elementary school teacher. Her older brother, Ray, born in 1988, had CF so her parents knew she could have it too. "Ray was a beautiful, happy, healthy-looking baby, but for all that he ate, he was slow to grow," says Darla. "Everything seemed to go straight through him, and we were changing diapers left and right. I kept telling his pediatrician that something was wrong. It just didn't seem normal to me. Not until Ray was nearly a year and a half and had dropped down to the fifth percentile on the growth chart did his doctor order a sweat test."

Two weeks later, Ray was diagnosed with CF. "He was hospitalized for baseline testing while we learned how to do bronchial drainage (BD) treatments by hand," says Darla. "We developed a routine, but CF care on a good day is still a lot to manage. So you can imagine my fear when I found out I was pregnant with our second child. I couldn't imagine how my husband and I would care for two CF children if our second child was diagnosed, as well."

Sure enough, a couple weeks after she was born, Martha was diagnosed with CF. "We were devastated," says Darla. "I felt responsible. I kept asking myself, 'What have we done?' It took more time than I'd like to admit, for us to come to terms with the fact that both of our children had a life-threatening disease."

"Ray immediately embraced his little sister," says Darla. "He couldn't wait for Martha to wake up from her naps so he could hold her. He liked to feed her a bottle and was amazed that she could already swallow an enzyme . . . as a baby. Ray had spent nearly five years protesting each and every respiratory treatment, but I think knowing that he was no longer alone in doing treatments led to better compliance without the fuss. CF was a common denominator, bringing a brother and sister especially close. They were in this fight together.

"The bond that Ray and Martha shared, and the relationship they formed, was so special and remarkable, that we felt blessed to be a part of it. We took their lead and embraced the life we were given, no matter its challenges. We put our fear of the future aside, for the most part, and focused on the present. We engaged in everything we could. As you well know, CF is pretty much the epitome of a life interrupted. Interrupted by pulmonary exacerbations and other CF complications. So the time between setbacks becomes almost golden."

Before the technology advancements of the airway clearance machine, a. k. a. The Vest, Darla had to do both her children's treatments by hand. "For a half hour on each kid, twice a day," says Martha. "She washed and made our neb cups every day, she made sure we took all our medication no matter how much we hated it. My mom made home-cooked meals most nights to ensure we had the high-calorie diet we needed. She learned how to administer feeding tubes, IV antibiotics, and, eventually, insulin pumps. My parents advocated for us and our education when we would miss large amounts of school. On top of all the medical hoopla, my parents gave us a sense of normalcy. We were always encouraged to participate in sports, school activities, church events, and neighborhood gatherings. With my parents' positive attitude, I never felt like I was missing out or not capable of doing something. They have this great balance of caring for me but not babying me."

Every three months, Ray and Martha had to go to the CF clinic at the University of Minnesota for pulmonary function testing, but that didn't make their lives any less fun. "For the first seven years of my life I had the best brother ever who let me tag along on every neighborhood adventure. My childhood consisted of tree forts, street hockey, ding-dong ditching the neighbors [ringing a neighbor's doorbell and running away before the neighbor knows who rang the doorbell], and running around with our dad's police dogs. I didn't think of my brother or myself as sick kids when we were younger. We played outside twenty-four-seven, went to school, participated in every sport possible."

Darla says Ray took the big brother role very seriously and he played a huge role in her toughness. "I wish I could say that it was all our doing—that Rusty and I are these two amazing parents who taught Martha to fight through the tough times and embrace the good times," says Darla, "but in reality, she had the best role model in her brother. Ray was a vivacious, humorous boy with a huge smile. In spite of having CF, he was a very positive person."

Ray also provided answers to Martha's CF questions that Rusty and Darla couldn't provide with the same depth or understanding. "For example, one day when Martha was three or four years old, she burst into tears when we had to leave the playground to go home to do vest treatments," says Darla. "She screamed, 'Why do we have to have CF?' Before I could muster up a lame answer, Ray put his arm around his sister and said, 'Because God doesn't give CF to weak people. He only gives it to tough people, and we're tough, Martha!' I marveled at his quick response."

Unfortunately, Ray and Martha's beautiful relationship ended unexpectedly. "My brother died in 2001 at the young age of twelve from a heart condition that was unrelated to CF," says Martha. "It would be another fourteen years before I talked to or met another person with CF. I was now fighting the disease by myself."

"To be honest, I'm not sure I did right by Martha for quite some time after Ray died," says Darla. "I felt so destroyed myself. I fell short in providing Martha with all the comfort she needed and deserved. Fortunately, we live close to my parents who were a huge emotional support to their granddaughter. Martha also had wonderful friends and teachers who stepped up to the plate.

"One thing that broke my heart each day was watching Martha do her vest treatments alone. She and Ray always did their treatments together while watching movies or playing board games. She always looked forlorn and lonesome after Ray died but having to forge on with CF care alone was especially difficult."

Three years after Ray passed, Martha had her first CF-related scary moment without her brother. "I remember a medical intern, who was not my usual doctor, came into my room and started talking about how lung function decreases in people with CF and that CF is a terminal disease and I most likely wouldn't make it to my twentieth birthday," says Martha. "I didn't know people could die from CF! I was terrified. I kept it to myself and didn't even tell my parents because it was so scary to me at the time. I remember feeling like I was going to throw up right then and there. Whenever I got scared about something with CF, though, I just thought of Ray and everything he had to endure and that he went through everything first so I could do it too. I told myself I was fighting this disease for not just me but for both of us now. Nothing motivates me more than my brother to this day."

In 2006, five years after losing Ray, Martha was diagnosed with CF-related diabetes. "Then I lost both my grandparents to cancer shortly after, only to then watch both my parents fight their own battles with cancer," says Martha. "In 2007, my mom fought breast cancer and was finally cancer-free after several surgeries and chemo. Four years later, my father was diagnosed with cancer but, fortunately, the cancer was removed with surgery, and he did not need any chemo." And still, Martha maintained this inspiring resolve.

"Life can be incredibly hard, and it can feel like the world is against you," she says, "but I am convinced it can still be great. If my parents have taught me one thing, it's to take your pain and make something good out of it. Find your reason and go." Martha's reason, during this hard time was Ray. "He was my CF role model and paved the way for me," says Martha. "We fought this disease together growing up. Ray's death was . . . life changing. I know I have a different perspective on things because of losing him. I don't take people or moments for granted. The everyday things in life have a greater meaning because I know they aren't always a given."

At fifteen years old, Martha was hospitalized (yet again) with a lung infection. While she was happy to be discharged before Christmas and didn't have to spend the holiday in the hospital, she felt bad for all the other children who weren't as lucky. That year, she was hired to work at a concession stand in a hockey rink (she had a PICC line at the interview). Remembering the children still hospitalized, she used the money from her first paycheck to buy Christmas gifts for them. "It has been our tradition ever since and has grown into a huge gift drop," says Darla. "In 2020, she threw a Christmas party and asked guests to donate a gift. We delivered over 250 gifts to three different children's hospitals in the Twin Cities."

Martha believes a turning point in her life came when, at eighteen, she left Minnesota to attend college at Colorado Mountain College in Steamboat Springs. "I wanted to prove to myself that I could do anything I wanted," she says. "I was living in the mountains on my own. It was the first time in my life that I didn't have my parents to help with my daily care. I didn't have my Minnesota CF team of doctors with me. I learned to rely on myself one hundred percent. I moved into my single dorm room with a baby bottle washer for cleaning my neb cups, a giant suitcase filled with medications, and the determination to make it work. I didn't have a car, so I had to bike down the mountain to my CF appointments, the grocery store, or post office to get my medications. It wasn't always easy, but it was the best experience of my life."

Martha ended up transferring to Minnesota State University, Mankato to finish her bachelors degree in recreation, parks, and leisure services, which was not available at Colorado Mountain College, with a concentration in resource management. This college experience proved to Martha that she was more than capable of handling this disease.

"Graduating college in four years was a big accomplishment for me because of yearly hospitalizations and a very ugly attendance record because of CF-related complications," says Martha. "I was usually admitted for lung infections that required PICC lines for IV antibiotics. My PICC lines always caused blood clots which then led to blood thinner shots throughout the hospital stay. It was a lot of stress to balance being a full-time college student, working part time at a recreation center for individuals with intellectual disabilities, coaching Special Olympics, and trying to stay on top of my CF and CFRD. I often had to take summer classes to make up for lost credits throughout the semester due to illness. I was able to intern out in Steamboat Springs, Colorado, as a teacher my junior year of college. I never wanted CF to stop me from accomplishing my goals."

After graduating college, Martha was hired as the program coordinator for LEEP (Leisure Education for Exceptional People), a nonprofit organization that offers recreation programs that enhance the quality of life for people with disabilities. Currently, she is a college instructor at MICC (Minnesota Independence College and Community) where she plans social engagement activities for students who are on the autism spectrum. "She has a special knack for knowing just what her students need," says Darla. "She even brings her dog, Charlie, to campus to provide comfort and support to her students which has been especially helpful to calm their worries during the pandemic."

Martha put her voice to use when she discovered cystic fibrosis was not on the priority list for the COVID vaccine in Minnesota. She was furious that people with CF were told to shelter in place because they were at high risk of not surviving if they contracted COVID, yet they were suddenly not high risk enough to be on the priority list for the vaccine. She called on her Instagram followers to put pressure on the Minnesota Department of Health. Within a short time, CF was added to the list.

In the middle of the 2020 COVID pandemic, Martha and Darla started their own business and developed the first of its kind: Sunny Rays Neb Cup Holders, a product that helps store and organize nebulizer cups, medication vials, and syringes. "By a CF family, for CF families," says Darla proudly. The product launched in January 2022, and one of their main objectives is to get it into hospitals to aid respiratory therapists in setting up patients' meds. They've named their company Sunny Rays in honor of their inspiration. In October 2021, Darla also published her memoir *Muddy Thursday* which discusses the family's battle with cystic fibrosis and Ray's abbreviated life.

While the launch of her new business comprises much of her current focus, Martha finds time to enjoy kayaking, snowboarding, hiking, and playing with Charlie. "They're simple hobbies but they keep me happy and healthy," says Martha, who is involved with the Cystic Fibrosis Lifestyle Foundation, for which she is a regular blogger in addition to being their 2021 Winter STROLO ("Stronger Longer") Star. In June 2022, Martha, who fundraises for the CF Foundation through the Minnesota/Dakotas chapter (her team's name is Ray of Hope for Martha), accepted a position with the chapter as an event support specialist. "My hope is that with today's remote way of work, and with the medical advancements in the CF community," says Martha, "that maybe the foundation can start to employ more people with cystic fibrosis."

Martha knows her life has not been easy compared to most people her age but the difficult times have helped her develop a unique perspective compared to most individuals in their late twenties. "I don't see a point in complaining about small things like homework, bad weather, or any other minor inconvenience. Ray didn't get to attend high school, didn't get his driver's license, or graduate college. He was robbed of many experiences. Ray didn't get to benefit from the new advancements in medicine like I do. I get to try the newest insulin pumps on the market. I get the new CF medication coming down the pipeline. I get to . . . keep going. Out of respect for Ray, the only thing I am after in life is happiness."

MELISSA KANDEL

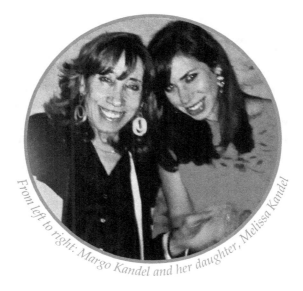

From left to right: Margo Kandel and her daughter, Melissa Kandel

Age: 34
Resides: Newport Beach, California
Connection to CF: Daughter to a CF warrior

MY MOM, MARGO: GROWING UP WITH A CF PARENT

"**M**y mom, Margo, lived with the disease, persevered, and ultimately passed away on April 18, 2012, when she was sixty," says Melissa Kandel, who doesn't have CF but knows intimately what it's like to be part of the village that copes with the disease. "Nothing got in her way. She even graduated college and attended Woodstock!"

Melissa says that cystic fibrosis was "very much a main character in the narrative of my early years. From as far back as I can remember, a nebulizer followed our family on vacations, the hours between dinner and bedtime were for my mom to inhale her medicine while I sat with her and my dog, watching TV as she puffed on her medications, and I eventually fell asleep. When she got really sick, she'd have an at-home IV and I got used to seeing the pole frequently standing in the corner of her bedroom." Melissa says it was scary for her whenever she saw a PICC line in her mom's arm. "There was a shelf, I remember, in her room, right below a big window that looked out onto the yard. It was never empty—always filled with bright orangish-yellow prescription bottles, vitamins, and whatever else my mom needed to survive. It doesn't feel like *my* story but cystic fibrosis, through my mom, was always a big part of my life."

Melissa says Margo, who was born December 31, 1951, came from a very close family, was tall and skinny, and had "intensely blue eyes and a head of wild curls she could never quite tame." Margo had one sibling, an older brother named David Golub who was fifteen months her elder and who later became a physician.

"Our relationship was always quite close," says David, "and we spent a lot of time together in our household, which valued family. Margo was always a thin child who notably had 'spoon' nails and other minor health issues which we all noted, but in no way was she ostracized or made to feel set apart by our family. She received regular pediatric checkups and care, but no mention was ever made of the consideration of a diagnosis of CF. In 1951, I believe CF was considered an illness that had a much more dramatic and unfortunately severely life-shortening presentation than the one which Margo demonstrated. She had a good appetite. I would not describe Margo as a sickly child and, fortunately, her early course did not include episodes of serious respiratory infections. Although a skinny child, she developed well and, by the time she was a late teenager, had grown to her adult height and weight and was an attractive and well-proportioned young woman who had a good appetite but never seemed to 'put on an ounce.'"

Margo was not diagnosed with the disease until the age of eighteen after the doctors misdiagnosed her with tuberculosis. "While in college in Florida at the University of Miami," says David, "she developed an intimate relationship with a young man who cared for her greatly and, being a Florida native, was able to help her navigate the health care system there when she developed a chronic and somewhat debilitating cough. She was seen by a respiratory specialist who diagnosed her, based on a chest X-ray and sputum testing, with tuberculosis. She went on a lengthy course of antituberculosis drugs and improved remarkably, though she was left with a slight persisting cough. To the best of my recall, I believe she had further workup after she completed her course of tuberculosis there and was diagnosed with CF based on sweat testing.

"She graduated and returned to New York where I put her in touch with a pulmonary specialist I knew. This was in the mid-1970s and this physician, who was a general pulmonary specialist, essentially recommended she go on a daily dose of the antibiotic Keflex. She did this for a year or so and then became involved with the cystic fibrosis center at Long Island Jewish [Medical Center] under the care of a physician named Dr. Jack Gorvoy. He managed her more aggressively, utilizing bronchodilator therapy and nebulized Pulmozyme and continued antibiotics as well."

David says that his sister remained relatively asymptomatic. "Margo was always quite physically active and socially she always had friends and was an extremely kind and thoughtful person," he says. "Growing up, the undiagnosed CF really did not limit her in any manner. I would describe her as being mildly anxious for much of her life. The anxiety, albeit mild, always made sense to me in the context of the chronicity of the illness she had been diagnosed with and had lived with her entire life. The impact of having a progressive illness manifests in many ways emotionally, and in Margo's case, what I have described as mild anxiety was her particular response. However, it did not interfere with her ability to function. Margo loved playing tennis and actually was fairly good at it and was able to play quite actively without restriction into her early forties. For many years, she worked managing one of the Broadway theater concessions in New York City, which was part of [our] father's business. She thoroughly enjoyed musical theater and being in that atmosphere. Her husband (Melissa's dad) did as well, and he frequently joined her at the theater in the evenings after his optometry practice day was completed."

David says that his sister had one particular desire. "I would say that one of Margo's primary hopes and wishes was to have a child," he says, "which as you well know is often quite difficult, if not impossible for CF patients. She and her husband tried for several years to conceive yet were unsuccessful. At the time, I was working in a holistic health center as a nutritional counselor and physician and was utilizing the best of my knowledge to try to improve her chances. I encouraged her to follow a diet in an attempt to provide the most fertile ground for conception. Margo was the ideal patient in the respect of following my recommendations assiduously.

"As I see it, the major turning point was that a Chinese acupuncturist was also working at the center where I was working and Margo became her patient. Margo began to see her on a very regular basis and took this treatment with absolute serious intention, never missing an appointment or failing to follow instructions and treatments to the letter. She was taking herbs prescribed by the acupuncturist as well as receiving acupuncture treatments. It took about six months and with great joy Margo became pregnant. Actually, I was involved in obtaining a pregnancy test (which at the time was not available with the ease that it is today through over-the-counter kits). I learned of the positive test result and was the one who communicated this information to Margo. I recall her breaking down with tears of joy."

David continues, "The pregnancy generally went well. She was closely followed by a high-risk-pregnancy obstetrician. However, in the third trimester, as the compression of the enlarging womb pushed up on her diaphragm, causing increasing restriction of her breathing, she required hospitalization for supplemental oxygen and monitoring. I believe she was in the hospital for the last four to six weeks of the pregnancy."

Still, the final result was a successful one. Margo gave birth to Melissa when she was thirty-seven. "All went very well, and a healthy baby girl was born who became the supreme joy and focus of Margo's life," says David. "She dedicated herself to giving her child every opportunity to succeed in finding joy and develop into the fine young woman she is today. [Melissa] had many innate talents, and they were cultivated through her parents' encouragement and provision of opportunities to be under the guidance of skilled teachers in multiple fields such as music performance, dance, singing, songwriting, and sports. Melissa had outstanding success academically and was supported happily and proudly by her parents through her post-graduate education."

Beginning in her mid-forties, Margo started to periodically have more serious respiratory infections, which were often treated with lengthy courses of, at first, oral and then intravenous antibiotics. She also developed insulin-dependent diabetes. "I recall a few very short hospitalizations for intensive management," says David, "which at that time included intravenous antibiotics and supplemental oxygen. As time went on, the option of home infusions of antibiotics became available when these infections required this form of management. However, her approach to these complications of her illness was always one whereby she followed instructions of the physician implicitly and additionally followed a very strict diet to help control her diabetes. She showed tremendous fortitude and conscientiousness in managing these complications. At no time can I ever recall her complaining about her health as a difficulty nor bemoaning her clearly progressive condition.

"As time went on," says David, "the infections became more serious and more frequent, though she actually never had what would be formally diagnosed as pneumonia. She had ongoing severe progressive fibrosis and bronchiectasis in her lungs which led to a state of worsening breathing issues. She never stopped seeking solutions. At one point, a mechanical vest was prescribed which vibrated and was intended to loosen secretions. In keeping with her general approach, she utilized this somewhat cumbersome device regularly and without complaint."

Still, Melissa says it would be a misconception that her mom's illness precluded her from enjoying her daughter's childhood, entertaining her own fantasies, and, most meaningfully, having a present and loving mom. "She was very much giving me extra attention and care," says Melissa. "If anything, I grew up slower because she really wanted to protect me and make sure I had everything I ever needed. For instance, when I went to sleepaway camp, she organized every outfit I'd wear every day in Ziploc bags with dates on them, so I didn't have to pick out my outfits or try to figure out what to wear when.

"Mom was so selfless and grateful for everything," says Melissa. "And she absolutely loved me." From the age of six, letter-writing was a big part of Melissa and Margo's relationship, including Melissa asking Margo to write her own entry in Melissa's diary:

I love quiet moments in the evening and saying good-night to Melissa with a soft good-night kiss on her lovable, soft cheek. She tells me about the actions of her day, some good, some just fair, but by evening everything subsides and moving on looking forward to the next day and what it will bring. I feel fortunate on this night and nights to come to hear Melissa's tales and give her that reassuring peck on the cheek and she knows I love her.

"I went to sleepaway camp at eight years old," says Melissa, "and asked my mom to write me a letter every day for the two months I was gone. She did and continued that tradition each summer I went to sleepaway camp for about the next ten years. I remember some of my bunkmates were jealous because when the mail came around, there was always a letter for me from my mom (and sometimes presents too)."

Melissa and Margo shared a love of the written word. "My mom loved my writing," says Melissa, "and as a kid, I was *always* writing. She encouraged me to start doing the *New York Times* crossword puzzles in kindergarten. In first grade, I won a national writing contest for this short story I wrote called 'The Cherry Tree.' In third grade, my mom helped me type up and draw a book about witches and shoelaces (I still have it but it doesn't make much sense) for parent-teacher's day at school. We used wrapping paper for the cover and tied it together with string. The assignment was to write a few sentences and read them aloud to the class. Of course, I wrote an entire twenty-page book, and everyone had to sit through almost an hour of me reading my wrapping-paper book about witches. My mom loved it and listened to every word.

"My mom worked really hard throughout my childhood to keep things as normal as possible for me. In fact, I think I probably did more than the average kid. Growing up, I was very involved with singing and theater and wanted to be a singer-songwriter. She'd drive with my dad into the city for my voice lessons, drive me to the Manhattan School of Music pre-college program every Saturday morning, drive me to auditions and wait in the hallway of a dusty Manhattan walk-up as I auditioned for some commercial or show. In everything she did, she went above and beyond to make sure I was happy and had whatever I could ever possibly have wanted to live a fulfilled childhood."

Melissa continues, "Of course, there were moments between the 'normalcy' when things were far from normal. When we'd have to pull over while she was driving because her CF-induced diabetes, which she developed in her fifties, made her sugar drop way too low and her entire face was covered in sweat and she could barely speak. Sometimes we'd have to stay in the car a few minutes longer and wait for the chocolate bar to kick in before we could do anything. She was covered in sweat and couldn't speak; it was scary for me because I wasn't sure what to do except wait. Or times when she'd watch me play tennis and I'd hear her go into a coughing fit, so she'd leave the bleachers to find a cough drop and settle her lungs down. When I was twelve years old, there was one vacation to Costa Rica she couldn't go on because she had an at-home IV. Without hesitation, she told me to go with my dad, but I could tell she was disappointed that this disease, this thing beyond her control, was preventing her from spending time with the daughter she worked for almost a decade to bring into the world."

Because of how difficult it was for Margo to get pregnant and the difficulty in the latter stages of pregnancy, Melissa would be her only child. "Because of how hard it was for her to get pregnant and, I think, her sense that time was a precious commodity between us, she really spent as much time with me as possible," says Melissa. "In sleepaway camp, I was one of the only kids who got a letter from their mom every single day. She called, she wrote, she was just there. She was so connected, and in a way her cystic fibrosis made her hyperaware of how close she wanted to be to me, always."

Melissa says that CF wasn't something that was often talked about in her household. "CF was never something that had to be explained," says Melissa, "it just *was*. An irrevocable truth in my life and hers. I remember being very, very little and telling a friend, 'My mom has a lung disease.' CF was never explained to me, it just existed. This might not be the best analogy, but I'd imagine it's kind of like being born with four toes instead of five. You don't know what things would be like with five toes on your foot because you've only had four. To me, I never knew what life was like *without* my mom having CF, so it wasn't much of a question I ever thought to ask or that my mom felt compelled to answer. My mom did a great job of putting CF on the back burner, as much as possible, so it wasn't the main focus in our lives. Her medicine, her doctor's appointments, they fell into the normal routine of everyone's day-to-day. The tougher times were always when she needed at-home IVs. I can't remember her being in the hospital except in the last year, when she was sick a lot."

In her fifties, Margo's health deteriorated, and she ultimately had to undergo emergency surgery. "I had previously mentioned that Margo had an anxious element to her character," says David, "however, it seemed that as she met these ongoing complications, the anxiety actually lessened and was replaced by a determination to do whatever it took to combat and overcome what the world was throwing at her. Postoperatively she seemed to be doing quite well at first but then slowly developed increasing difficulty breathing. Despite aggressive testing, nothing other than her underlying CF seemed to be the cause of this. Within a few weeks, she was back in the hospital on a CPAP machine and was told that her condition was terminal. This was when Margo's deep character and inner strength had its ultimate manifestation.

"With close family regularly visiting and her condition progressing toward respiratory failure, she never once acted the victim. Rather, she showed incredible calm and acceptance. Shortly before she was unable to speak, she called me over and quietly looked into my eyes and asked me to always watch over Melissa. She had great faith in her husband's role as a father but, additionally, she fully trusted me to do what was right and necessary. It was an extremely strong emotional moment for me, but I managed to assure her that I would do as she wished. Margo was a gentle, kind person who was loved and trusted by many people. She gave much more than she took, and her presence was, and memory is, highly esteemed."

Melissa says losing her mom took her years to put into words. "I was twenty-five when I lost my mom," she says. "I wrote about it in a blog post for the Cystic Fibrosis Foundation, but it took me about four or five years after she passed to even think about the final few days. I definitely didn't handle things well, although I guess that's to be expected. It felt like suddenly where there was this warmth and sun and *mom* in my life, there was now a gaping hole that would never, ever be filled again. That's hard to recover from, at any age, and even though I think the sun has come out again, the hole never really goes away. I'd imagine nobody is ever ready for good-bye."

Melissa's grieving process ultimately led to not just an acceptance of what she had lost, but what she had uniquely gained from her mom in terms of her own lasting motivation. "Her unwavering will to breathe was once a cruel reminder of how small my own problems were," says Melissa, "but it put a lot of things in perspective for me in a positive sense. I miss her knowing what's happening in my life and I wonder sometimes if she'd be proud of the person I've become."

Melissa began volunteering for the Cystic Fibrosis Foundation in 2012 shortly after losing her mom. "I wanted to do something to sort of calm my mind by helping others who might be in a similar situation as I was," she says. "In Orange County, I serve on the board of several events. I also started a yearly bar crawl event in Newport Beach (on my birthday weekend) to raise money for the Cystic Fibrosis Foundation Orange County Chapter in memory of my mom. We raised about fifteen thousand dollars in four years of putting on the small event and got on the front page of the *LA Times Daily Pilot* in our third year."

Melissa's passion is also her profession. Two and a half years ago, she quit her nine-to-five job and started her own company called little word studio providing high-quality writing, content, and content marketing strategy to small-, medium-, and large-sized brands around the world. She says despite the pandemic, her business is thriving.

"The nine-to-five job was definitely a solid position and an amazing opportunity. I was the youngest director at an incredible company, sitting in an executive office working directly with the CEO, who is still an important mentor and client to this day. I came to that job after journalism grad school and after a year of working at a magazine with the intention that I'd become a professional writer. But to really follow my dreams, I knew I had to leave and pursue writing full time and start my own business. Around the time I was about to quit, I had a family wedding in Oakland, California (coincidentally, for a cousin who was very close to my mom growing up). I decided to drive up Highway 1, and somewhere along a curve of Big Sur coastline, I felt this overwhelming sense that I would do it. Maybe that was my mom, maybe that was her instilling her belief in me, which manifested years later in the determination to start a business."

Melissa believes she learned a lot from her mom. One of the things she noticed was that Margo's attitude was always positive, and she was incredibly kind to everyone she met. "I think it helped that her mindset remained strong even as her body grew weaker."

Melissa says she is working on a fictional novel these days based on her family's history. "Growing up, I'd always wanted to be a singer-songwriter," says Melissa, "so writing is an iteration of that dream. I still want to do something more with theater, which will probably come by way of the book I'm about to start writing that details the story of my grandpa (my mom's father) and his brothers starting their business on Broadway. I've completed some preliminary research and it's all very exciting to me, getting back into that sparkly world of glitz and glamour. I can't draw a direct line between my mom coping with CF and my writing/theater/singing because she did her best to make sure CF was in the background, and I was always center stage. That was perhaps her greatest gift, because it made me grow up with not only a very normal childhood in a not-so-normal situation but also and always surrounded by so much love."

KATE O'DONNELL

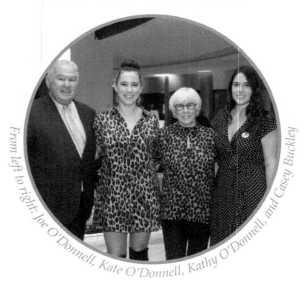

From left to right: Joe O'Donnell, Kate O'Donnell, Kathy O'Donnell, and Casey Buckley

Age: 35
Resides: Boston, Massachusetts
Connection to CF: Sibling to a CF warrior

KATE'S TURN: THE JOEY FUND GETS A NEW LOOK

On May 1, 1974, Joe and Kathy O'Donnell were blessed with the birth of their first child, a son they named Joey. Joey was born three weeks premature and weighed six pounds, three ounces. Kathy says she knew there was something wrong with her son, though, for weeks. She brought him to the pediatrician only to have him tell her that she was "overreacting." Five months later, on October 30, her worst fears were realized when Joey was diagnosed with cystic fibrosis.

Joe began getting involved in fundraisers shortly after to take action against the disease that his son was fighting. He developed connections through his once-small concessions operation that now sold candy to big theaters in the area and brought in millions annually. He eventually embarked on other business ventures making investments in restaurants, movie theaters, and amusement parks, and his now huge network brought him into contact with people in the cystic fibrosis community. People who could help him use his skills for the most meaningful mission of his life: helping his son and the community of which he now found himself a part. By the time Joey was two, Joe was elected to the board of the Massachusetts chapter of the Cystic Fibrosis Foundation and, for a short time, even served as a board member of the National CF Foundation. He and Kathy would make fundraising, awareness, and the search for a cure central to their lives.

The source of all this inspiration, of course, was young Joey, who Kathy says spent the first six years of his childhood like most kids. "He particularly loved playing baseball," says Kathy, "and Joe was his coach." Joey had daily postural drainage sessions; he took antibiotics for infections and enzymes to help with digestion; and, occasionally, he would be hospitalized when battling infections, "but it was far from the norm," says Kathy. After his sixth birthday, however, lung exacerbations and hospital tune-ups at Mass General became more frequent.

Joey lived only twelve years fighting the battle against cystic fibrosis, passing away November 23, 1986, just three months before his sister Kate Alexandra O'Donnell would arrive. "Joey read Frank Deford's *Alex: The Life of a Child*," says Kate. "Before [Alex] died, she helped her pregnant nurse choose the name Kate for her baby. After Alex passed away, her nurse chose Alexandra for her middle name, in honor of Alex. Joey liked the combination, and here we are!"

While Kate never met her late brother, she loves learning about him. "I love that [my parents have] always been so open about him," says Kate. "The stories have always made me feel some sort of connection. It's definitely interesting seeing your parents in an entirely different reality, but the movies and stories just bring that to life so much more vividly, and the love really shines through. It's amazing seeing how much life and love and fun they pumped into his twelve years."

Kate spent much of her childhood playing on the playground that donned his name—Joey's Park was built by the community three years after Joey passed with many of Joey's friends designing it and many of their parents contributing to the actual building of the structures, which included a zip line and plenty of good hiding places! But it was in the first grade that it hit Kate that someone who was a part of her family was gone forever. "I guess looking back," says Kate, "I was always very aware of being [at] the playground every day, and it was named after my brother, and I did get questions. I remember the whole idea of death, and the permanence, finally clicking one day and just completely melting down. I think my mom had to bring me home. It's such an intense idea for a little kid to wrap their head around. Knowing what my own reaction was, and remembering how that made me feel, when I didn't even know him—my heart completely breaks for kids who lose siblings they actually grew up with."

Kate's family history was never concealed from her or her younger sister, Casey. "I've always known what they went through with Joey," says Kate. "It wasn't a taboo topic in our house growing up at all. There are just as many photos of Joey as there are of my sister, Casey, and me, and my parents made sure that we knew exactly what happened. We celebrated his life and felt very welcome to ask questions about things that might be super uncomfortable, such as the topic of death."

Before each of their daughters was born, Joe and Kathy used a rather new test at the time called chorionic villus sampling, which would determine if the fetus had one or two copies of the CF gene. Fortunately, neither Kate nor Casey has cystic fibrosis, though they are both carriers.

"I know, as a result, genetics have always been really fascinating to both Casey and me," says Kate, "and don't scare us much. Having that background definitely helped in high school biology! I'm in the process of freezing my eggs and getting my own genetic test back was *fascinating* to me."

Following Joey's death, The Joey Fund was established in November 1986 to fund the science to treat, and hopefully someday cure, cystic fibrosis and to aid local New England families and CF clinics around the Massachusetts area. While approximately 5 percent of the money raised went to patients around Massachusetts, a great majority went to fund the work CF Foundation CEO Dr. Robert Beall was doing to invest in pharmaceutical companies to find drugs that could better treat the cause of cystic fibrosis.

Joe has been putting his fundraising talent to work since the turn of the century. From 2004 to 2011, he led the CF community in a capital campaign by raising an unprecedented $175 million in what the CF Foundation called Milestones for a Cure. He led a follow-up campaign called Milestones for a Cure II that raised another $75 million and will lead a third campaign called Milestones for a Cure III beginning in March 2022. Joe's work helped the Cystic Fibrosis Foundation invest in drug companies, particularly Vertex Pharmaceuticals which would eventually lead to the discovery of the CFTR breakthrough drug Trikafta which has helped tens of thousands of cystic fibrosis patients.

Kate says her parents preached to her and Casey the importance of giving back from a young age. But the two girls actively witnessed it while attending The Joey Fund fundraisers, beginning when Kate was six and Casey was three (Joey Fund events have been happening since before Joey died — it just wasn't called The Joey Fund until after his death. Kate attended her first event as a newborn in a stroller, and Casey began attending as an infant as well).

"When Casey and I turned thirteen, our parents told us that we could no longer get gifts from our friends at our birthday parties," says Kate, "and had to put 'in lieu of gifts, please bring a check to The Joey Fund, if you'd like.' Obviously, we weren't thrilled at the idea, but it was absolutely brilliant, looking back at it. Not only did we get excited about seeing how much we could raise every year, and if we could beat last year's amount, but something else happened that I don't think even our parents anticipated. Both of our groups of friends became used to fundraising at a very early age, and they were just as excited about it as we were. I think fundraising unfortunately has a negative connotation, and if it's not introduced early and young people aren't shown exactly how to do it and what it can accomplish, that connotation is really difficult to break through. Both of our groups of friends learned how to do that at a really early age, started bringing in their own friends, and are still incredibly involved. Many of them have started their own nonprofits."

"A huge part of our lives has been watching [our parents] start The Joey Fund from the ground up and make it into what it is today," says Casey. "The impact they've had on the CF community is something that must and will live on, not only through these patients and their families but through the work that we will continue to do."

The Joey Fund, for the most part, benefits the Cystic Fibrosis Foundation, but a small part of the funds also goes to helping CF families in the Massachusetts/Rhode Island area. Kate and Casey's contributions grew from just raising money at their birthday parties. "We started by walking in walkathons," says Kate. "We'd pull names out of a hat for raffles at events benefiting The Joey Fund and attending the Joey O'Donnell Film Premiere."

"So much of the groundwork has been laid by our parents and the CFF volunteers," says Casey, who is now a parent to two children herself. "We have this amazing platform and a leg-up just by association. We are so lucky that this community already exists, and our role is to keep the wheels turning. It's important to keep our feet on the ground and realize that the work is not done, and we won't be slowing down until it is."

Kate says there was never any pressure to partake in the family "business" of fighting cystic fibrosis. "I don't think there was any one thing in particular that made me want to get involved in CF," says Kate. "It wasn't even really an option (not in a bad way!). Casey and I were at the first Joey's Park built (I was two and a half and she was a baby). We both went to walks, and our family's film premiere started before we were even born. It was always made incredibly clear to both of us that we had a responsibility to help this community who had done so much for my parents and family through Joey's life and death."

"I'm obviously really lucky that I actually enjoy what I'm doing, no matter what it is," says Kate, "but the opportunity to work with the CF community is honestly such a blessing. The group is so motivated, and fun, and successful. The people I have met through this work are some of my absolute favorite humans and have taught me so much about this world and how to make a difference effectively."

Joe is known in the CF world as a master fundraiser for all of his work bringing better treatments to the CF community, but he is a dad first. Like Joey before them, Joe loved coaching both of his girls. "I played soccer, tennis, basketball, ice hockey, and other sports," says Kate. "My dad coached everything." Eventually, Kate became a stand-out rower. "I was a port [the left side of the boat], bow seat [the number-one seat or closest to the front of the boat] usually. My boat won the Head of the Charles [the largest two-day regatta in the world held on the Charles River between Boston and Cambridge, Massachusetts with more than 11,000 athletes, 1,900 boats, and 61 different events] twice in high school and finished fifth in nationals."

Kate attended Harvard as an English major after being recruited for her rowing (crew) reputation and her passion for her CF work. Kate injured her back the winter of her freshman year and was unable to continue rowing at Harvard, but still, that didn't put a damper on her time there. "I had an amazing experience, met my absolute best friends," she says, "and Casey also went there with me as a history of science major and graduated with honors after writing her thesis about the history of venture philanthropy and the Cystic Fibrosis Foundation!"

During her sophomore year, Kate spent a semester abroad in London and had her life in the CF world come full circle. "I had six flatmates," says Kate, "but only two of us were Americans. One night we were talking about health care, and I found out that Lauren has cystic fibrosis. We connected, as I didn't know many people my age with cystic fibrosis. We still keep in touch today." Kate also says that it was during her college experience that she began going to larger CF events and began becoming more immersed in the CF community. "I started meeting families," she says, "and that made a big difference."

In 2009, right after graduation, Kate started working primarily in advertising—Hill Holliday, then did creative advertising and locations for Sony Pictures and Happy Madison Productions. Kate had been a volunteer for the Cystic Fibrosis Foundation her entire life. Around 2011, she started taking more of an interest in The Joey Fund. "I was working for my dad at the time," she says, "and I was getting a ton of questions about our organization. We had an antiquated website, very few pictures, and not much of a social media presence. I wanted to contribute." So Kate spent the next three years working on the site and building up the social media presence. "I just wanted to get more eyeballs on it," she says. "When I hear about a nonprofit, I go straight to the website to learn about the organization's vibe."

She and Casey started hosting their own events. "We took on more responsibility," says Kate. "We both realized we really just enjoyed what we were doing. I also really just love working with people, non-profits, and event planning. Working on CF, especially in the last few years, you're able to see such a tangible difference, and it's so incredibly rewarding. This community is also *so* active online, due to not being able to hang out in person, which makes the online community so engaged. I'm able to get feedback so quickly, and change our own tactics based on what people want."

Around 2013, Kate and her family organized an extensive rebuild to a place she still often frequents—Joey's Park. "The whole town came together," says Kate. "Over two thousand people showed up over three weeks to rebuild this park from scratch." The park was built entirely out of wood. Kate was two and a half when it was originally built around 1989. "Things were breaking so there were safety concerns," she says. "No one got paid, everyone took off work, brought their own tools, and learned how to build a playground. All of Joey's friends showed up for the first build, but this time, they were bringing their own children to help, and watching them explain to their children what the park meant to them was so wild. Joey's teachers, coaches, family, even people who didn't know him, but who lived in Belmont—everyone was there. We had a lot of engagement online, so even people we grew up with, who couldn't go, donated online and sent old photos. It was a giant reunion, and truly showed me how much Joey meant to his community. As I've gotten older, lots of my friends will send me pictures of their children at the park. Seeing it become this deeply meaningful place for a whole new generation, and the ripple effect, is so touching."

Making changes to the organization's social media presence, and playing a big role rebuilding the park in her brother's memory, eventually led to Kate becoming president of The Joey Fund in 2013. She graduated from Harvard Business School (HBS) in 2016, after which she joined Snapchat in New York City as a creative strategist.

Then she decided she needed a change that would help her align her passions.

"New York City wasn't really for me," says Kate, "and I had just served as a cochair for my own one-year reunion at HBS. I loved that experience so much that I left my job and reached out to HBS to see if they had any openings. Coincidentally, they did—on the same team that runs the one-year reunion. I spent the next four years working there as the assistant director of student and young alumni engagement, which had so much overlap with my own nonprofit work."

Kate, who has been vice chair of Tomorrow's Leaders for the Massachusetts/Rhode Island Chapter of the Cystic Fibrosis Foundation since 2018, will be cochairing the Volunteer Leadership Conference in the near future. "I'm just starting to get more involved on the national level," she proclaims.

In July 2021, Kate left her job at HBS to focus on her role at The Joey Fund full time. "It was bittersweet [to leave HBS]," says Kate, "but I am moving on to more of a volunteer alumni presence, while increasing my own work with The Joey Fund, the CF Foundation, and our family office in Cambridge, Massachusetts. I was finding that a lot of my time was going into our events and fundraising, but I obviously had a nine-to-five job, so I'd have to fit it in during lunch, at night, or on the weekends. There's a lot I'd like to do but just didn't have the time to dedicate to it."

Kate's new role as *full-time* president has made her even more active with regard to the CF community. "As the president of The Joey Fund," says Kate, "I deal with a lot of the day-to-day things. I manage our social media and online presence, interact with people in the community, and answer questions. People order our Joey hats and wear them all over the world, so I post pictures of those as they come in. We get a bunch of emails every week ranging from people sending in stories about their loved ones with CF [to questions about] how to fundraise effectively, to requests for grants. The Joey Fund provides need-based grants to those in the Massachusetts and Rhode Island community, so a lot of time is spent on how much and where those go."

Kate also does a lot of work directly with the CFF in planning The Joey Fund annual events, like the Joey O'Donnell Film Premiere. "[During the pandemic], we had to move entirely online (like everyone else), and that was a huge challenge," says Kate. "We ended up working with a studio to secure three films, got personalized links to all of our attendees, and, based on their ticket price, sent out tiered gifts.

The CFF Massachusetts/Rhode Island team is incredible, and honestly makes my job even possible." The Joey Fund, which has raised over $1 million each of the last five to six years, raised a record-breaking $1.2 million to benefit those with cystic fibrosis in 2020, despite being completely virtual for the first time during the pandemic.

"I'm so lucky to have learned from the best fundraisers there are," says Kate referring to her parents. "I've learned so much just watching them in action and have realized how much of fundraising is about relationships."

And yet Kate holds in equal esteem the time Joe put into his daughters outside his copious work and fundraising responsibilities, coaching virtually every youth team Kate and Casey played on. "Having my dad as a coach was so much fun, and I have amazing memories of that," says Kate. "He's obviously a super busy person, and was home late a lot, but he never missed one practice or game, and that made a big difference. Of course, as soon as I hit high school, I started rowing and playing ice hockey, the only two sports he didn't play previously. But you can bet he learned everything he could and was just as involved as he had been with the other sports. The night I decided I was going to be an ice-hockey goalie, he strapped pillows to me, handed me a helmet and a racquet and spent the night pelting me with tennis balls." Kate now finds herself making time in her own busy schedule for cooking, traveling, and being a doting aunt to "the coolest niece and nephew, Blair and JD," while enjoying time with "the love of her life," her English bulldog, Chickie.

"My girls have always amazed me with their kindness and understanding of a side of life that might never have been a part of theirs," says Kathy. "At first, it was just a party where their parents' friends attended—they always begged to stay for the movie and free popcorn. But as the years went by, they asked more and more questions, became more confident, and became fully committed to CF and their brother's memory. Now even more so as they become strong independent women who honor their brother's memory. I know we are leaving our life's work in competent and loving hands. This is what fulfills them—they have involved their friends and friends' families."

"I truly believe that people inherently want to help, but they don't always know how," says Kate. "In telling your story, creating a relationship, and letting them know how they can help, you're giving them an outlet. And I also want to be clear: fundraising is not always about the money. Of course, we need to raise massive funds to find a cure for everyone with CF, but I believe that participation of any kind is outrageously important. Can people donate goods? Spaces for events? Donate their time to help you organize and run something? Serve on a panel to donate their own expertise in their field? All of these things count toward creating a community that can go ahead and make a difference."

And Kate will need lots of community support as her ambitions to support CF patients and their families have grown. "I'm looking to expand engagement with a younger professional group," she says. "Boston is such a melting pot of amazing nonprofits, and a lot of people in my age group are looking to get involved in something they're excited about. Now that the city is opening up a bit more, and I have more time to throw into this, fingers crossed we'll start to expand into this different demographic."

Kate's long-term goal is for 100 percent of people with CF to have a cure. "And once we're there," she says, "to continue to support that community."

KRISTEN BROCKMAN KNAUF

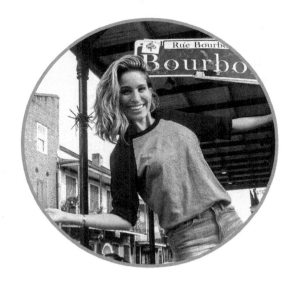

Age: 39
Resides: Manhattan Beach, California
Connection to CF: Sibling to a CF warrior

THE UN-BUCKET LIST: A SISTER'S UNDYING LOVE

"**I** remember very vividly when my mom got the call from the doctor to tell her Kelsi (at age two) had cystic fibrosis," says Kristen Brockman about her kid sister. "I was only about ten years old at the time and I was taking a bath, and my mom came in the bathroom with tears running down her face." At the time, Kelsi struggled with digestive issues. She developed lung issues as she got older.

Kristen and Kelsi grew up in the small town of Campbellsville, Kentucky. "When Kelsi was younger, I don't think I realized the severity of CF," says Kristen. "I was in fifth grade when Kelsi was diagnosed, and other than watching my parents sprinkle her enzymes in her yogurt and 'beat' her [chest percussions], she was relatively healthy. But when I was in junior high, my cheerleading squad competed in a cheer competition that was held in honor of a high school cheerleader who had passed away from CF. They let Kelsi come out onto the floor and do a little cheer pose, and I think at that moment the reality of CF started to set in with me."

Still, while Kristen eventually learned about the severity of cystic fibrosis, she says Kelsi was "pretty healthy for someone with CF, and I always thought she had a mild case and maybe she might be 'different.' Her health started to decline in her late teen years, and around that time, someone I went to grade school with who had CF, passed away at twenty-three years old. I think then it really hit me that this could be a reality for Kelsi."

Kristen says that she and Kelsi had a great relationship growing up. Kristen called her a "sassy, redheaded spitfire," while Kelsi called her big sister "Sissy."

"Since she was so much younger than me, we didn't have a lot of the sister issues that siblings close in age have," says Kristen. "She was kind of like my own little doll and I had a lot of fun with her, dressing her up in crazy costumes and making funny videos with her." Kristen jokes that they got in more fights when they got older. "And we could fight hard! I always said, 'She may be sick, but she's still my sister.'"

Kristen has such fond memories of her sister. "Kelsi was just one of a kind. The best thing about our relationship was that no one could make me laugh harder than her, and no one could make her laugh harder than me. It was the best! She was hilarious, artsy, talented, so fashionable, and even though she was my little sister, I looked up to her so much. She was the best gift-giver—anyone would tell you that! She gave the most thoughtful gifts to everyone she loved, complete with custom gift wrapping that she would draw, paint, design, create herself."

By the time Kelsi's symptoms worsened in her late teens, Kristen had graduated from the University of Kentucky and was now living in Los Angeles, where she had moved in 2005 to pursue a career in entertainment. Soon after, she began looking for a way to help her sister, even though she was so far away from her. So, in 2008, Kristen decided to get involved with the Cystic Fibrosis Foundation and discovered a passion for fundraising. She began volunteering for the Los Angeles CFF chapter and, in 2013, began chairing (and continues to chair) the Los Angeles 65 Roses Climb, a stair-climbing event now done annually at the world-famous Rose Bowl in Pasadena. Kristen's team, Kelsi's Klimbers, has raised $300,000 for the Cystic Fibrosis Foundation.

In August 2013, Kristen landed a gig cohosting a digital show called *Hollywood Today Live* covering topics such as entertainment, pop culture, and fashion. In 2014, *Hollywood Live Today* debuted to a national audience with Kristen still performing the cohosting duties while interviewing several big-name actors, including the likes of Vin Diesel, Reese Witherspoon, and Zendaya.

Still, being in Los Angeles, "I didn't get to experience the ugliness of CF as much as my mom and stepdad," says Kristen "When Kelsi was hospitalized, she would tell me not to come home to see her—but, of course, I still did sometimes—because she would rather me visit when she was feeling healthy, able to hang out and enjoy our time together elsewhere. There were times when Kelsi wasn't the best about taking her meds and doing her treatments. I know that's not what most teenagers and young adults want to be worrying about . . . so I definitely had a lot of tough-love conversations with her that usually ended up in tears for both of us.

"My fashionable and funny little sister Kelsi passed away from CF [on] September 4, 2016, at the age of twenty-six," reads Kristen's blog back in 2017. "I felt some sense of relief for Kelsi when she left this world," says Kristen, "no more pain, no more struggle to breathe, no more days and weeks in a hospital bed. Part of me was happy for her in a weird way. When you see someone you love go through so much, for so long, you get to a point when you know it has to be better on the other side."

Kelsi had told her family that, in the event of her death, she made requests for her funeral, among other wishes, and that Kristen would know how to locate them on her computer. "Unfortunately, shortly before Kelsi passed away, her computer had been wiped out from technical issues. Everything was gone: videos, pictures, etc." Kristen and her family frantically called the phone carrier who, after several nail-biting minutes, was able to help them retrieve the info from the cloud. "I'm so grateful for the cloud!" says Kristen. "Because not only did we know the dress she wanted to wear, the songs she wanted played, what she wanted inscribed on her gravestone, I came across something called the 'Un-Bucket List'—a list of things Kelsi wanted to do before she died but never thought she'd be able to do." Then and there, Kristen became determined to finish them for her sister. "It was almost like a puzzle I had to solve."

A few weeks later Kristen found herself at the legendary Biltmore Estate in Asheville, North Carolina, the enormous mansion built for George Washington Vanderbilt II between 1889 and 1895 and, at 178,926 square feet, the largest privately owned house in the United States. Why? "It was on her list," says Kristen, who, though she took a tour of the house by herself, could feel Kelsi's presence. "I saw so many sites that immediately made me think, 'Kelsi would love that!'"

Kristen posted a picture on social media wearing a shirt with a pink design of a pair of lungs in honor of Kelsi. "Some really wonderful people in our hometown made these shirts when Kelsi was struggling in the ICU before she passed away," says Kristen. "I wear this shirt whenever I check off an item from the list and I've also had them reproduced to sell and raise more money for my Un-Bucket List fundraiser."

When she posted that first photo, the response was incredible, with a number of people pleading with her to finish her sister's list. Kristen knew that this was not just an opportunity to explore the globe but rather a chance to raise awareness for cystic fibrosis and fundraise in memory of Kelsi. Her goal is to raise $100,000 along the way. As of February 2022, she has already raised more than $70,000! "I've crossed off visiting San Francisco and New Orleans (Kelsi had both New Orleans and the French Quarter on her list so that was a two-for-one so I went out that night on Bourbon Street). I've hugged a sloth and walked her dogs in Central Park," says Kristen. "And I went skydiving!" The items that remain are taking a cruise and visiting Punta Cana and Atlantis in the Bahamas. Kristen now blogs about the journey on her blog, *The Un-Bucket List.*

"My family also runs a nonprofit, the Kelsi Brown Foundation," says Kristen, "which helps cystic fibrosis patients and their families in Kentucky. Their main event is a golf tournament (and after-party) held every spring, and also a Halloween party. Kelsi *loved* Halloween!" Kristen's parents Jeanne and E. G. Brown pretty much run the show, "but I go home for the golf tournament every year to help out." Kristen also hosted the CFF Tomorrow's Leader's podcast *Breaking Through.* "It's my passion," says Kristen, "helping in the fight against cystic fibrosis."

Kristen is married to Jimmy, whom she met on a blind date. "Fortunately, Kelsi was able to meet him before she passed away," says Kristen. "There's a funny story I had the preacher tell at my wedding in 2018. A few weeks before Kelsi passed away, she was talking to a friend about her health and said she was worried she 'won't get to dance at my sister's wedding,' followed by 'who am I kidding, she'll probably never get married!' JimBob, as Kelsi called him, and I weren't even engaged yet, but I think she knew we'd end up together. She loved him. Unfortunately, I think she also knew her time on earth was almost up. Although she wasn't physically there on our big day, we all felt her spirit as my 'mer*maid* of honor.' Jimmy created the annual Kelsi Spirit Award for the 65 Roses Climb as my wedding gift."

Kristen often talks to her and Jimmy's now two-year-old son, Theo ("my greatest accomplishment," says Kristen) about his aunt Kelsi. "She would have been obsessed with Theo and spoiled him rotten," says Kristen, who even brought Kelsi's favorite stuffed animal (a sloth named Murphy) to the hospital when Theo was born so that Theo could keep it close to him as a reminder of his guardian-angel aunt. "My first year of motherhood in a pandemic has been challenging," says Kristen, "but one of the things that has encouraged me—that has given me a focus beyond the challenges—has been planning and completing Kelsi's Un-Bucket List and hitting my one-hundred-thousand-dollar fundraising goal for CF!"

MEGAN BARKER

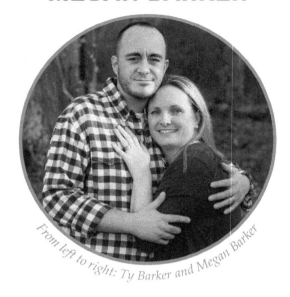

From left to right: Ty Barker and Megan Barker

Age: 40
Resides: Monroe, Georgia
Connection to CF: Spouse to a CF warrior

THE CF SPOUSE: A MISSION TO FIND SUPPORT

R espiratory therapist Megan Barker is a Georgia native who grew up in Conyers, about twenty-five miles east of Atlanta. The first time she heard about cystic fibrosis was as a teenager. "My mom's friend had ridden in a motorcycle ride for CF and brought me a T-shirt," says Megan. "I remember doing some research about CF after that because I wanted to know more. It's kind of crazy how that T-shirt sparked my curiosity about something that would become so meaningful to me later on. I had never met anyone with CF prior to working at Emory University in Atlanta."

Megan first started reading about respiratory therapy due to her grandfather dying from lung cancer when she was only three. Megan says she has some memories of him, "though they are not super clear. All my life, I've heard how much like him I was—mannerisms, temperament—and I think that created a supernatural bond between us. His cancer was the catalyst for me to become an RT."

Megan received her undergrad degree from Everest Institute in Atlanta and, in 2018, her graduate degree in respiratory therapy from Canisius College in Buffalo. Early in her career, she started working at Emory and one of her first patients was a gentleman named Ty Barker. "I went in to give him a breathing treatment, and he was watching poker, and we struck up a conversation," says Megan. "I knew immediately that Ty would be much more than a patient. He was my person. I have never thought twice about the conflicts associated with him being my patient. I feel like God puts people in our lives at certain times and, at that time, working a lot as a new therapist, God needed to put him where I could find him."

"It's hard to put into words just how helpful and important Megan has been in my life," says Ty. "Other than the obvious convenience of having my own personal respiratory therapist at home, she has been like a guardian angel to me. I thank God every day that he brought her into my life."

"I knew Ty had CF before I met him," says Megan, "so there was never that conversation about him being sick, which I'm sure was a relief to him. I am pretty certain that despite the nagging about treatments and stuff, he is pretty thankful that I understand CF and respiratory things like I do."

Megan worked with CF patients for about three months after she and Ty began dating when she changed jobs. "Thankfully, everyone where I worked was very understanding about exposing me to things that I could bring home," she says, "and I was typically assigned the non-cepacia CF patients."

Megan, who married Ty in 2008, wanted to help other spouses who do not have CF but would like to better understand how to be there for their spouse with CF. "I felt like I understood life with CF," says Megan, "but quickly found out that wasn't the case the first time my husband's lung function dropped into the teens. You kind of lull yourself into a routine with CF and know that tune-ups and treatments are just part of it. But when it's something new and something that is quite scary, it rocks you. I remember being quite freaked out and it took a while for me to find that comfort in our norm again. However, it's always in the back of my mind that the other shoe can drop at any time. It was during this worst of circumstances that I realized there were no resources for people like me who marry into the CF community, and after that episode, I wanted to ensure that no one had to use Google as their only guide for navigating life as a CF spouse/partner."

So, in 2016, with an impact grant from the Cystic Fibrosis Foundation, Megan founded Project CF Spouse, a nonprofit organization that provides spouses and partners access to resources similar to what someone parenting a child with CF would find. "It was such an unbelievable feeling," says Megan. "I had been working for several years to build a network of spouses and partners to support this part of the CF community and getting this grant allowed that work to continue to grow."

Megan had other reasons to start Project CF Spouse. "When I started dating Ty, I had only ever met patients or parents, not a partner or spouse. I stumbled across a blog one day written by a woman who was married to a man with CF. I sent her an email and it was an instant connection. We formed a friendship and leaned on each other for years. From hospitalizations to her husband's transplant to our IVF journey, we were there for each other. Our husbands even became good buddies and football [fanatic] rivals! She became a part of my family, and I am forever grateful for finding that blog! My friendship with her is what I hope to do with Project CF Spouse. A way of connecting to form those bonds because they are truly life changing."

And there is another complex issue in addition to that of health maintenance and, God forbid, emergencies. "Obviously, when Ty and I started talking about having kids, I knew that we would have to go through IVF," says Megan. "Ty and I had talked about infertility possibilities when we were dating, so when we decided it was time to start a family, we just assumed we would be in that boat. So, after consulting with an IVF doctor, we did testing and confirmed what we already knew. While it wasn't a huge shock to us, anytime you get news like that, it always brings a little unsettlement with it. I remember reading all these stories about crazy expenses and failed attempts. It was very overwhelming. Fortunately, at the time, IVF was partially covered by my insurance. I think we were both hoping for the best but preparing for the worst the whole way through our procedures."

Despite the anxiety, Megan says their IVF journey "was very smooth and successful" and the result was twin boys, Bryce and Ben, who just turned nine. Though neither has CF nor understands it fully, they both are an integral part of Ty's support team. "At nine, they don't really grasp all that CF is," says Megan. "They know that Ty has crappy lungs and that he has to do treatments and sometimes go to the hospital, but overall, I doubt that they truly understand. When we talk to them about it, we try to keep it at a level that they can understand so that it doesn't feel too overwhelming or scary for them. Honestly, they really handle his CF well. They remind him about doing treatments and ask lots of questions about his machines. So they want to know. The hardest part for them is when he is admitted. They don't understand why he can't just do his treatments at home and why they can't go see him. But even that has gotten better as they have gotten older."

In addition to running Project CF Spouse, Megan does a lot of CF fundraising for the CF Foundation through Great Strides. "I head a national team, and I run the Atlanta branch," says Megan who is also one of the Georgia Chapter's Peachtree Society alumni, a group of men and women in the state of Georgia, selected by the Georgia Chapter of the Cystic Fibrosis Foundation, who are committed to professional growth through a fundraising and awareness campaign.

But with all her CF advocacy, Megan still honors her calling. "Being married to a cystic fibrosis patient has helped me to be a better respiratory therapist," says Megan. "I get the bonus of having perspectives of both a family member and a clinician. This is something that has proven to be useful on many occasions! Obviously, I am looking at this from a spouse's perspective but for me, it's about building a support system. Having people to talk to who had been in similar situations or had similar experiences was a great source of comfort."

Megan says that while she wants to continue to make a difference in the CF community, she is focused on helping those with the disease survive the pandemic. "This has been the craziest thing that I have ever experienced," says Megan, who admits to being a life-long germaphobe and that meeting/marrying Ty has certainly heightened those concerns. "I never wanted to bring anything home to him. COVID has done nothing to calm that fear. I find myself becoming more and more OCD about things. I am constantly aware of what I touch and what touches me. I have never washed my hands so much in my life! It really is as emotionally and mentally exhausting as it is physically.

"From a healthcare worker's perspective, it has been a nightmare. I have seen more death in the past year than I have probably in my entire career. I have held the hands of people dying while their loved ones watched via FaceTime. I have cried with my coworkers when we've lost patients who had been hospitalized for long periods of time. I have seen families torn apart because one or more members succumb to the virus. I have seen doctors break down because they felt so defeated. I have seen a community go from hailing us as heroes to villainizing us. It's heartbreaking. I told my mom one day that working during this time is like being in the ocean with a really strong undertow. You never really can get your footing before the next wave hits and knocks you down."

Still, Megan sees the big picture and has goals to help the CF community. "I want to grow Project CF Spouse to a point that we have connected with all the spouses/partners in the world," says Megan. "I want these people to come into their walks with CF with resources that will guide them down all the paths they take, from transplant to infertility and even in loss. I just want to be able to continue to give back to this community that I love so much. To likewise help others find their people so they can truly lean on them in those hard times."

6

TRIUMPH AFTER TRANSPLANT: HEROIC STORIES OF DOUBLE-LUNG TRANSPLANT SURVIVORS

AMANDA VARNES

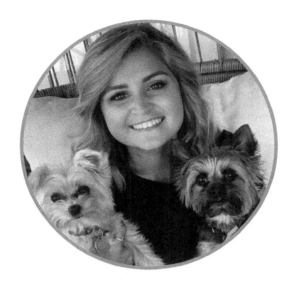

Age: 26
Resides: Lakeland, Florida
Age at Diagnosis: 1

TRIPLE THREAT: SURVIVING THREE LUNG TRANSPLANTS

Lee Varnes was the 94th Aircraft Maintenance Unit Chief of the United States Air Force and the proud maintenance chief for the F-22 Raptor Fighter Jet. Fighting, it turns out, is genetic in the Varnes family as evidenced by Lee's daughter, Amanda.

Third double-lung transplants are rarely performed given the risky nature of the procedure, but a year and a half after Amanda Varnes's second double-lung transplant—as she was celebrating what she and her family saw as a new lease on life—chronic rejection forced doctors to make the critical decision of whether or not her body could endure another.

Amanda was born at Tyndall Air Force Base just east of Panama City, Florida, in 1995 to Lee and his wife, Dina. "The first real symptoms my mom noticed were that I was pooping constantly and that she was breastfeeding me constantly," says Amanda. "Initially, I was 'failure to thrive' since I was not really getting any bigger. I didn't look like a sickly baby. I was just small. The doctors just assumed that I would be petite since the majority of my family is. I mean, in the end, they were right. I stand tall at four feet eleven. But mother's instinct kicked in, and my mom pushed for further testing, and a sweat test a year later, I got diagnosed with cystic fibrosis."

Amanda says she grew up feeling not much different from others her age. "I just assumed all kids used a vest and did breathing treatments," she says. She attributes that to her parents' attitude toward the disease. "They held me accountable like every other child," says Amanda, "but also gave me freedoms that others my age experienced. I respect them so much for that. I still do what I am supposed to, but I don't live my life in a bubble. I have my parents to thank for giving me that mindset and to always look for the positive and laugh when possible."

"Before she was conscious of it, I made a promise to Amanda and our family to raise her as normal, happy, and thriving as possible," says Dina, "and not let CF define her. Her very first CF doctor told us the difference between quality of life and quantity of life. We don't have control over the quantity, but we have control over the quality. And I latched onto that, and I let that guide me."

Amanda says being an "Air Force brat," she moved around a bit, from Florida to Texas to Virginia. "I was blessed with friends that just understood my CF," says Amanda. "My best friend from college, Ellen Fisher, is one of them. She would sit with me in my dorm room while I did breathing treatments. She would pick up food for me when I got a cold. She and I are still extremely close. She came and sat with my parents when I was in the operating room being transplanted. I feel so incredibly blessed to have her in my life."

Amanda says that growing up she found stability for her mind and body in physical activity. She played soccer in elementary school and a bit in high school, but it was dance that became her passion. "My mom put me in dance when I was three or four," says Amanda, "and from that moment I loved it. It became my escape. In that dance studio, my CF didn't matter. I performed like everyone else. It felt freeing in a way. I still dance around. In shopping aisles, around the kitchen when I'm cooking, when I feel happy, or a tad sad. I just dance it out.

"I stopped dancing when I went to college. I did stay active by going to the gym and walking everywhere but felt the big decline my sophomore year of college, which lead to my first transplant."

In third grade, Amanda contracted a rare fungal infection called Trichosporon which led to a hospitalization. "I don't know how my parents did it, but during my first hospitalization after my initial diagnosis of the fungus, I didn't feel scared," says Amanda. "We all just took things in stride. We, as a family, knew that in order for me to not succumb to this fungus, we had to be extremely aggressive and proactive in my CF care. I truly believe that I am here because my mom asked questions and also did a lot of legwork behind the scenes. I truly am an advocate for being proactive in your care."

Over the years, the fungal infection led to her pulmonary function results slowly declining and continued to manifest around the time Amanda was in the eighth grade. "Because the fungus was so rare, there weren't a lot of 'traditional' CF treatments, so I had to go in the hospital to receive some 'off label' antibiotics combos so they could monitor side effects, place a PICC line, and establish home health care," says Amanda.

"I will say that the majority of my CF exacerbations we were able to treat at home with home IVs. When I was in the hospital, a lot of my friends were able to come visit a few times and spend the day with me. My teachers worked with me to get me caught up and I also had a re- mote teacher who would come and work with me after school as well. I always knew I had CF, but it really wasn't until this hospital stay that I truly understood the depth and seriousness of it. I do remember having a couple of people in some of my classes treat me differently because of it. Some made back-handed comments such as 'Aren't you the girl that is going to pass away soon?' or 'the sick girl,' but I knew that I was so much more than that. CF doesn't have me; I have CF. For the most part, those comments didn't bother me. I truly didn't let my CF hinder my social life. My parents would do what they could to help me so that I could live as normal as possible."

In high school, Amanda continued to notice a decline in her health. "Lyrical was one of my favorite dance forms," says Amanda. "I could tap into my CF journey and dance with so much emotion. At dance practice, I would have to take a couple of breaks when I became short of breath. I didn't make a big deal of it. I would just step to the side, get some water, catch my breath, and join in when I could. My teachers were understanding when I would be out or miss class.

"When I was a junior in high school, I became very sick, and my doctor told me that I would need a lobectomy [specifically, the remov- al of a section of her lung]," says Amanda. "I had been in the hospital before for tune-ups and such, but it was different this time. I would be missing a lot of school, and I almost missed my junior prom. I had my true first 'why me' moment. I did everything correctly. I took my meds, did my treatments, and was very active. It made me realize that CF had a mind of its own.

"My PFT's would continue to decline each year," says Amanda.

"During my senior year, they stabilized in the mid to low twenties. I believe I got mono that year which led to another hospitalization. I was in the hospital, and the doctor told my mom and I (my dad was overseas) that we needed to get the Red Cross to get my dad back home. I was then able to go home and spend Easter with my family. I had a follow-up appointment soon after.

"Over the course of a decade, all antifungals became resistant, and the only next course of action was a lifesaving double-lung transplant. My doctor told me that because I had such a rare fungus, we needed to start looking for a high-risk center sooner rather than later. It was so sudden, and I got so sick so fast—close-to-death sick. I remember my heart dropping and an almost out-of-body experience [when the doctor told me I needed a transplant], but I buckled down and knew that now more than ever I had to tap into the strength my parents raised me with. My family and I were, of course, scared but knew the alternative was much worse. After graduation, I was accepted into Duke University Hospital's Lung Transplant Program. I wasn't in my transplant window yet, so I was able to go to college."

Still Amanda endured, completing her high school career and being admitted to Longwood University, a small school in Farmville, Virginia—two hours from her home—where she selected a major in communications and public relations. "Heading into college, we knew that when my lungs gave out, it would be fast," says Amanda. "So I took each day as a blessing and loved every second of it and still had a wonderful college experience."

The surgery took place on May 23, 2015, at Duke University Hospital. She would return to college at Longwood three months post-transplant, but not without serious post-surgical complications. "I was completely stripped of my independence and relied on my mom [her dad was deployed] for everything," says Amanda. "She needed to help me up and down the stairs, I needed her with me twenty-four-seven. It was in one of our many talks that she really just lit a fire within me to fight. I knew I wasn't ready to leave my parents yet. I had so much more life to live and things that I wanted to accomplish. CF had never defined me before, and it wasn't going to start then.

"After I finished cardiopulmonary rehab," says Amanda, "I felt amazing and, with the permission of my transplant team, returned to college." Her journey to recovery was then interrupted by a donor-specific virus as her body began to reject the new lungs. "When her doctor told us that Amanda would need another transplant to survive," says Dina, "we told Amanda that it was ultimately her decision, and we would respect her wishes."

On January 11, 2017, just a month shy of her twenty-second birthday,

Amanda was back at Duke University Hospital for the second emergency transplant. "The second transplant surgery took longer than the first because my old lungs were essentially glued to me," says Amanda. "But when I woke up, I felt amazing. I felt recharged and ready to see what these lungs and I could conquer. This recovery was one hundred times easier than my first. I felt like because I had an idea of what to expect it made it mentally easier for me. I am optimistic by nature. I definitely get that from my parents. We always look at the bright side of things. That things could always be worse. That's how I truly get through all that I've been through."

A new lease on life seemed possible. Amanda even completed the UNOS 5K in Richmond, Virginia, three months after her second transplant! However, chronic rejection came into play a year and a half later, and Amanda would have to fight for her life a third time. "This rejection was slow moving," says Amanda. "I was truly shocked when my results showed rejection.

"When I got the news that I had chronic rejection and needed a rare third transplant," says Amanda, "I felt a wave of fear I have never felt before, but that fear quickly turned to grit and fight. I started training for my third transplant. I started eating high fat-high calorie foods and exercising as much as my body would let me."

Amanda wasn't sure she'd be approved to get a third transplant, but that didn't stop her from putting in the work. "I was definitely shocked when Duke told me they wanted to evaluate me for a third," she admits. The news came on February 15, which just so happened to be her dad's birthday. "I got a call from my transplant coordinator, and she was setting up a rejection treatment and let me know that the transplant committee met and told me that they would do a third transplant. I remember my mom and aunt embracing me and we all just cried. I then called my dad and then we cried. I was so relieved and ready to conquer this head on."

Though Amanda's situation was urgent, the donor lungs were not as fast coming as the prior ones. "My first transplant, I was so unaware of my surroundings," says Amanda. "I didn't even know that I had gotten a transplant. But I did cry when my parents told me. For my second, I knew. I was scared that lungs wouldn't come in time. When my mom received the call, I was actually being transported to the ICU. I was so relieved but sad because someone was mourning their loved one. During my third, I spent the days waiting just praying for my donor. I prayed that they were spending time with the people they loved and doing what they loved. I was grateful for the gift they gave me."

Amanda says she has built a special rapport with the people who have saved her life. "I am extremely close with my transplant team.

My transplant surgeon and I are really close as well. He has done all three of my transplants and has been such an advocate for me and my success. My team has never given up on me, even in dire times." Amanda's team at Duke came up with a plan to add another antirejection medication and keep her very immunosuppressed this go around.

"When I received the call that this was a 'go,'" says Amanda, "I knew this time would be different."

Amanda received her third transplant on May 17, 2019, at the age of twenty-four, and it wasn't without serious complications. "A catastrophic spinal injury caused by a spinal hematoma crushed my spine and temporarily paralyzed me," says Amanda. "Doctors told me that it would be a medical miracle if I could walk again within six months." And yet, within forty-eight hours, she was standing. And within seventy-two, she walked. "In my mind, not succeeding just wasn't an option," says Amanda. "I set my eyes on what I wanted to accomplish outside of the hospital and kept that at the forefront of my mindset."

Amanda remained in the hospital for fifty-six days, and after a course of physical rehabilitation, she returned home. "Post-transplant life was an adjustment," says Amanda. "I traded CF for transplant basically. The medicine regimen is more extensive, but I don't have to do vest treatments anymore, but today I feel the best I have ever felt! I can play around with my dogs and not feel short of breath. I can bounce my nephew around with ease! I can walk around the mall without getting tired. I can sing in the car!"

Amanda considers herself a "Peloton junky" and rides a few times a week, but she says what's helped her most has been journaling, prayer, her dogs, Georgia and Jet, "and talking through my anxiety with my mom. She is strong like no other. She never wavered or broke down. She's truly my best friend. When I was little, a lot of kids wanted to be doctors or lawyers. I always told people I wanted to be a mom, just like my mom."

About being the third person at Duke and the eleventh person in the country to get a third transplant, Amanda says, "It's scary because it can mean my immune system keeps rejecting my new lungs." But it's afforded her an elite community of third double-lung transplant survivors. "They're some of my best friends," she says. "We have a bond like no other on a level that is indescribable. We understand the fear of repeat rejection. And what that could mean for us."

"She is my rock, she is my inspiration, and of course, my 'Duke' mentor," says Cassie Stanley of Oak Park, Illinois, who's thirty-six and another three-time double-lung transplant survivor with CF. "Positivity beams out of her like sunshine and I'm so grateful to have her by my side living our third transplant journeys together. There have been so many times when I went to her and she always knew how to turn my negative attitude right around. No one quite knows what we have gone through, and I feel, because of this, our bond will always be unbreakable. She is my forever third-lung sister."

Amanda, who, along with her family, has raised $100,000 for the CF Foundation since her diagnosis, says that all of these near-death experiences have given her a different outlook than most. "I am not afraid of dying," she says. "I have faced death before, but what I am afraid of is not living this life I've been given."

NICOLE KOHR

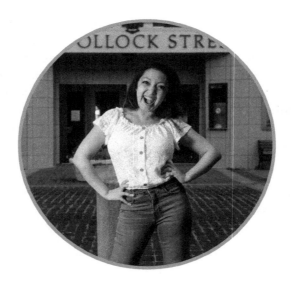

Age: 29
Resides: New Bern, North Carolina
Age at Diagnosis: 5

MY TWO CENTS: THE INSPIRING LIFE OF A FALL RISK

It takes an evolved mind and a unique talent to have the imagination and tool set to turn cystic fibrosis and a double-lung transplant into a musical comedy. And that is exactly the concept for which theatrical juggernaut Nicole Kohr has received two grants, en route to fulfilling her Broadway dreams.

Despite having symptoms from birth, it took until Nicole was five for her to be diagnosed with CF. "I had a failure to thrive, a never-ending respiratory infection, terrible GI issues—you name it," says Nicole. "I was finally diagnosed after years of my mother begging and searching for a doctor who would diagnose me with . . . something."

"As a first-time mother, I felt that something was seriously wrong," says Nicole's mom, Patty, "but I couldn't get anyone to believe me. Many said I was a paranoid first-time mother or ignored me and Nicole altogether. I found a few doctors who took note of her severe breathing issues—her chest would cave in when she breathed, she was constantly coughing and snotty, back-to-back respiratory symptoms."

Doctors diagnosed Nicole with asthma and a reactive airway and began treating her for those conditions. The nebulizers and antibiotics would help for a short time, but the moment the antibiotic ended, Nicole was ill immediately. "I had done my due diligence and my research on my own time," says Patty, "relying less and less on doctors. I pitched cystic fibrosis a few times, but none would give my diagnosis the time of day. One doctor told me that it was unlikely because Nicole is mixed race—White and Hispanic.

"I remember the day she was diagnosed like it was yesterday. Her antibiotic had just ended, so she was suddenly very ill. I made an appointment to see her doctor that day, and I made a fuss, so they squeezed us in. Her regular doctor wasn't there, so the receptionist asked if I was okay seeing another doctor. I agreed. The new doctor listened to me for about fifteen minutes, looked Nicole up and down, asked me to lick Nicole's head, and unofficially diagnosed her with cystic fibrosis. Later that day, Nicole received a sweat test, which turned out to be overwhelmingly positive. The next day, Nicole was admitted for her first tune-up."

"We praised that day that my doctor asked my mom to lick my head, confirm that it was salty, and send me for an immediate sweat test," says Nicole. "I was told, like many, that I would die around the age of ten."

Nicole, an only child whose parents divorced when she was only a few months old, says she was fortunate to be raised by her "strong, divorced mother" and her grandparents, with whom they lived until her grandparents' passing (her grandfather passing when she was eight and her grandmother passing when she was seventeen). "My mom is my best friend and the most supportive, nurturing person you'll ever know," she says. "But she also taught me that you have to 'suck it up, buttercup,' if you want to make all of your dreams come true."

Nicole says she was always a "bubbly, confident, ham of a child . . . but only around my family. In public, I was so shy, most doctors overlooked my respiratory symptoms and narrowed in on the fact that I was completely nonverbal in public. Some thought I was deaf. Mom signed me up for musical theater classes at the age of five, and she hit the nail on the head. I knew from that moment on that I would be on Broadway."

"Nicole was a very easy child to raise," says Patty. "She was happy, patient, and recovered quickly—emotionally and physically." Patty admits, however, that Nicole was a very anxious child. "It took years for me to learn that her disease and medication were likely the cause in addition to her type A personality," she says, "but she was smart, kind, and resilient. I didn't really have to discipline her. Therefore, up until this day, if there was something that she wanted to pursue, I was on her team."

From the ages of five to eighteen, Nicole was credited in over one hundred community theater and regional productions, working as an actor and choreographer in and for musicals as wide ranging as *Cinderella*, *The Wizard of Oz*, *Rent*, *Peter Pan*, and *Jungle Book Jr.* She is also a principal actor for an audience of special needs children called the My Name is Matthew Program, created by Tina Lee and inspired by her special needs child, Matthew, now grown up. Nicole even has television credits from that time, including *SpongeBob SquarePants* and a TV short called *MommyTime*. And this despite being hospitalized at least three times a year since her CF diagnosis due to frequent sinus/lung infections which dropped her pulmonary function, though Nicole admits that some of it was her own fault. "I would run myself into the ground, starring in several performances and classes at once and requiring a lengthy tune-up shortly thereafter," says Nicole. "It was always my goal to keep up with my competitive classmates, and I did, but it came with a price."

Nicole refused to let her disease hold her back. "I was a stubborn bull and refused to accept accommodations from anyone," says Nicole, who only told a handful of friends and teachers that she even had cystic fibrosis. "I did my meds, of course, but otherwise ignored my CF altogether. I did not identify as a CF patient and, therefore, it did not exist. Even during hospitalizations, I practiced choreography and wrote lyrics. It was a coping mechanism, as was my dark sense of humor."

At the age of eighteen, she came to the crossroads of deciding, "what I want to be when I grow up. I wanted to major in musical theater but also knew that I needed a 'proper' job to provide medical insurance for my CF needs. A stable nine-to-five position would be the more responsible choice.

"I was offered several scholarships based on my entrance essays, high school academics, and lengthy list of extracurriculars. Mom and I pursued every scholarship and school in New Jersey. We knew a smaller school would be more understanding should I fall ill. Kean University was *much* smaller and offered the most financial assistance. I'm very money and career driven; I knew that was the school for me!

"When it came to deciding my major, it was one of the many heart-wrenching decisions I would face. I once again had to choose between my 'potential decline in health' and 'my dream.' My mom was always supportive when it came to these moments. She would state her piece, reminding me that I may not be able to do eight performances a week. Then, she would say that she supported me no matter what I decided. It was difficult watching some of my closest friends pursue their theatrical career, but I knew a path toward a nine-to-five position was better for my health. Seeing all of my friends posting their stage pictures on social media during my college years was like a stab in the heart, but I was at least somewhat able to express my passions through a major in public relations, through which I could explore journalism, media, creative campaigns, and even some radio.

"Luckily, I enjoyed my time in the communications department, dipping my toes into every platform and field," says Nicole, "but my lack of a BFA [bachelor of fine arts] in musical theater is *still* brought to my attention. It's those conversations that drive me to prove I am indeed a theater professional."

During Nicole's junior year, things got more difficult. "I was in the middle of planning my extracurricular projects, per usual," says Nicole, "when Mom invited me to Applebee's near Kean. It's where we met weekly to see each other and chat. She was teary-eyed, so I knew something was wrong. She said my social worker from clinic called and broke the news that I am growing mycobacterium abscessus. I was surprised. I knew the name, and knew it was bad, but I didn't know how bad. I honestly didn't feel any worse than I usually did. I was so accustomed to running myself into the ground, I always felt ill. It was once again a conversation where I had to decide if I should abruptly stop what I was doing to tend to my health, or soldier on.

"Despite my clinic's suggestion to stop school temporarily or altogether, I maintained my same level of full-time classes. I simply added two to three self-administered IVs on top of that. I would meet with my visiting nurse once per week at the disability center to change my dressing and organize my medication deliveries. I did this for seven months. My lung function dropped from seventy percent to fifty percent. I was miserable. I made the difficult decision to keep my CF a secret throughout this process as well, making my resentment sky-high. It was one of the hardest times of my life."

Nicole had started dating her soon-to-be-husband, Jared, two months before being diagnosed with mycobacterium abscessus. "He was studying IT, and he was my soul mate," says Nicole. "Jared knew that I had CF, despite my hesitation to tell him, but he didn't know what CF really looked like until my IVs started. He just knew I was bubbly and had blue hair. Going from that to full-time IV use for seven months was . . . challenging. Luckily, his breath-of-fresh-air existence in my life is what drove me to get up and shower every Friday per my IV schedule. I stayed on my routine because I knew he'd be outside after class, ready to take me to dinner. He sees things very logically and compartmentalizes everything. As far as he was concerned, there was not an IV popping out of my port; I was just his 'hot girlfriend.' His words. While I was completely sleep deprived, and occasionally an emotional basket case, he and my mom are what got me through the experience."

"Meeting Nicole, you wouldn't even know she had CF," says Jared, "I didn't. I don't mean to say like 'ahh, she trapped me,' but she assumed I knew because we had the same friend circle. Our dynamic worked because she never made her condition a requirement of our relationship—I was not expected to suddenly become her caretaker, but we are both there for each other."

Still there were some who wanted Nicole to slow down. "I was advised by my care team to temporarily or even permanently drop out of college," she says. Instead, she self-administered four IVs simultaneously for seven months while continuing classes. Nicole not only graduated on time, but with honors—summa cum laude—with a BA in public relations and a minor in child psychology. She also received her certificate in the theory and practice of child life online from UCLA that same year.

Not long after graduating, Nicole landed a "practical" job working at Princeton Theological Seminary, a religious nonprofit in Princeton, New Jersey. It was the "typical nine-to-fiver" that gave her those medical benefits, but it also allowed her enough time to work on children's books at night. Nicole self-published her first book, *Two Cents*, which is based on her experiences with CF, in 2018.

"*Two Cents* was my way of reintroducing myself to the writing community," says Nicole. "I write about what's on my mind, and people were constantly giving me their two cents. Especially medical advice, mostly from self-proclaimed social media doctors. I was always a writer at heart. As much as I loved and craved performing, writing was relaxing and came naturally. I wrote plays when I was in elementary school; I would write custom lyrics for my friends; I had a journal on me at all times. Writing wasn't new. But as far as everyone knew, I was just working a nine-to-five job.

"I was fussy. I needed to be more creative than my job would allow, so I wrote a few articles on LinkedIn and shared them on Facebook. Social media went crazy, sending me messages like 'I didn't know you could write!' I had fifty-plus ideas for stories written on my notes app on my phone, so I picked one. Then I interviewed students within my nonprofit job and chose one who I thought would be a good illustrator. I did a lot of research and made some educated guesses about self-publishing. My first book put me on the map, allowing my second book, *My Pants* (a story which teaches ways to advocate and cope while dealing with everyday social interactions), and upcoming third book, *Water Your Human* (a book about empathy and caring for another), to keep me on the map.

"I started my nonprofit career in September of 2015, four months after graduating college," says Nicole. "I was a healthy ninety-five pounds. My FEV1 was still recovering from my mycobacterium abscessus but was stable around fifty-five percent. Princeton Theological Seminary was *not* where I thought I'd end up, but I had a blast working in the development role. It enabled financial stability but allowed for creative flexibility. Mom and I were very excited about my health benefits and pay. It confirmed for me that my PR major was the right choice.

"I was able to work for three months before being hospitalized in December 2015. I would have rather run away than tell my boss that I had to be hospitalized for 'only two weeks, I swear,' but a grown-up has got to do what a grown-up has got to do! My boss was *very* understanding—always putting my health first. I had to be hospitalized every six months or so after that point, which I maintained until 2018. I'd self-administer IVs as needed, but nothing out of the ordinary. In 2018, I started to decline rapidly. No matter what I did, my infections wouldn't clear, and I was losing weight. I brought a family serving of pasta for lunch every day, in addition to my ScandiShakes [high-calorie weight-gain drinks] and feeding tube, but nothing helped. The office knew me as the sunshine of the office, always looking on the bright side. They knew something was wrong when my energy dipped to near-nothing, constantly checking in to see how I was doing. I was now administering a secret IV under my desk at work as well as a feeding tube," says Nicole.

"I had dropped to a mere seventy-nine pounds, so I was pounding the pile of pasta I had on my desk. I also had a glass beaker that I was casually coughing blood into to measure how much was coming up. I paused and said to myself, 'Have I finally crossed the line between a healthy work-life balance?' That night, my mom, Jared, and I had a long talk. We decided it was time for me to go on short-term disability. This led to an immediate hospitalization, long-term disability, and, eventually, social security disability."

Nicole says that social security disability and her "stubborn-bull" personality didn't go well together. "I tend to get depressed when I'm sitting still or not succeeding," she says, "and boy was that the case. I would find random projects just to keep myself busy, but eventually my body wasn't responding either. I could barely walk to the bathroom, and my dependence on Jared and my mother grew and grew.

My New Jersey care team said it was time to talk transplant, and I made my way to Pennsylvania to be evaluated at the University of Pennsylvania."

The evaluation was March 2019. The problem was that Nicole and Jared had just gotten engaged the previous summer, and their wedding date was coming up. "I said, 'We're getting married on June 1,'" says Nicole, "'You can't put me on the transplant list right this second!' The woman on the phone was *definitely* not expecting that response."

Nicole found herself in this strange place where she was discussing a living will and the colors she wanted at her wedding. "This leads to a strange mindset," she says. "My team at UPenn wanted me to put off or cancel my wedding because my transplant was the priority. I tried to explain to them that canceling is not how my life goes—we simply make it work. So, with my New Jersey CF team's assistance, they pumped me full of steroids."

But Nicole was not ignorant of the implications of her condition. "As I came to terms with these life-and-death circumstances, I harbored a wish that I could be involved with just one more show. Not just as an actor or choreographer, but as the creator. That's when *Fall Risk* occurred to me," says Nicole. "Everybody's a fall risk. There is no 'one size fits all' when it comes to a disability. Do the best that you can to balance meds and living and create your own version of normalcy."

"I submitted a poem called 'Fall Risk' to the Abbvie Scholarship program," says Nicole. "I won a thousand-dollar scholarship from Abbvie and my poem was displayed at the Abbvie Conference! *Fall Risk* was just something that kept my mind busy during hospital stays. Whenever I was bored or emotional, I would write lyrics—ranging from sad to comical. Eventually, the lyrics developed a storyline. As I matured and gained more experiences, I would update lyrics and scenes. By the time of my transplant evaluation in 2019, I had an entire musical draft collecting dust on my computer with 'Fall Risk' being the original poem which helped me earn the Abbvie scholarship. I tried a few times to get people to read it, but no one took interest until I started writing children's books and/or had my transplant. When I told my mom it was time to be transparent and public about my CF, I knew it was the right time to tell my story and apply for a grant from the CF Foundation in March of 2019. That led to winning a ten-thousand-dollar impact grant on June 1, 2019, the day of my wedding!"

With this morale reprieve, she walked down the aisle with her oxygen tank in tow. She named it O2D2, as a nod to *Star Wars'* R2-D2, and dressed it like a flower girl.

"On the day of our wedding, I weighed eighty pounds," says Nicole. "I had a lung function of eleven percent. I was on twenty-four-seven oxygen, six liters, and I was completely resistant to all remaining antibiotics, ravaged by infection, and was on ventilation and was high-flow dependent."

"Watching Nicole decline in 2019 was the scariest, worst time of my life," says Jared. "Somehow, typical [Nicole], she managed to plan the best wedding I've ever been to while she was being evaluated for transplant. Watching her answer calls about napkin colors and a living will within five minutes was emotionally exhausting. I have a hard time celebrating anniversaries of 2019. Nicole's mom would vent to me about losing Nicole to CF almost every day. At the time, I didn't want to make assumptions about what could happen to Nicole because I couldn't bear the worst-case scenario."

Two weeks later, on June 14, 2019, Nicole received her much-needed double-lung transplant. "As I was put to sleep, about to get my surgery, I remember assuring myself, 'You'll be in pain, but when you wake up, at least you'll be able to breathe,'" she says. "I woke up fully intubated, in a lot of pain, and I *still* couldn't breathe. I was angry, very angry, and the pain didn't help. I couldn't eat. I couldn't drink. I couldn't move. My mother, who was staying at the Gift of Life House [a residence in Philadelphia for patients and families to stay during their transplant journeys, where volunteers help to make the journey more comfortable], was at the hospital from six a.m. until nine p.m. with me every day. My husband was with us for as long as possible but had just gotten a new job that required travel."

"Seeing my intubated wife and then having to get on a plane," says Jared, "was one of the worst things I've ever had to do. I had *just* transitioned to a new, remote IT job (my current job), and they required travel. I had to go to Vegas on a plane for the first time by myself the moment that Nicole woke up from her transplant. I had a missed call on my phone the moment I got on my plane. I spent the whole plane ride to Vegas trying to distract myself from the missed call—thinking the worst-case scenario. I was numb for the length of Nicole's decline. Luckily, Nicole is the nicest and funniest person I've ever met—opposite of me, a realist. She never makes her disease anyone else's problem. In the end, I know that my Nicole is very strong, so I do my best to support her in whatever way I can."

"But, of course, I was stubborn," says Nicole, "and moved things along as quickly as I could. The moment they said I could walk, I walked. I walked three days after my transplant. The moment they said I could eat, I ate!"

While double-lung transplant stories are full of drama, Nicole maintains a practical, even humorous, outlook. "It saved my life," she says of the procedure. "My sinuses are a still a mess, my GI is still all over the place, and my hair falls out in clumps . . . but then it grows back. There are a ton of rules related to transplant that keep life interesting, but overall, my two nonsense mutations always give me a great story to tell."

Post-transplant, Nicole no longer requires nebulizers or CPT. "I take two antirejection pills," she says, "as well as an antiviral, an antifungal, an antibiotic, prednisone, an allergy medication, several reflux medications, two pills for my osteoporosis, a pill for my high blood pressure, a pill to manage my liver levels, a pill for anxiety, and a ton of vitamins. And I have to wear a mask and gloves in all public settings *forever*."

Still, with her new capacity for breath—her FEV1 is currently at 131 percent!—Nicole wasted no time in recapturing some of the theatrical joys that buoyed her during her first tour of CF. She began taking dance classes and even started making YouTube Broadway choreography workouts. "It brings me back to my days as a performer," she says. But her main objective has been working on *Fall Risk*, to which she returned just a few days after she woke up from transplant.

Between March and June 2019, despite dealing with a double-lung transplant and a wedding, Nicole's wheels were already spinning with regard to *Fall Risk*. "I contacted my friend Ellie Marie who put me in contact with percussionist and CF and transplant patient Adam Brostowitz (now, one of my best friends)," says Nicole. "Adam signed on as my composer and music director, and he's been with me ever since. My friend since high school, Nicole Dvorin, was already on the project, assisting me with the impact grant submission in any way she could. I communicated with both of them throughout my transplant recovery. I had a lot of time to write and reach out to people during my evaluation, surgery, and recovery. It inspired and excited me. After being awarded the grant in June 2019, the three of us quickly built a team of musicians, and music and volunteers were coming in hot until December 2019. I lovingly call my high-ranking team members my board up until this day even though we weren't officially covered under a 501(c)(3) entity until June 2021. Now, as of June 2021, *Fall Risk* is under Colie Creations, my 501(c)(3) writing entity.

"Three weeks after my transplant, I was out of the hospital," Nicole says, "and within days of my return home, I gathered my board of directors and musicians."

Filled with enthusiasm, Nicole filled out an application for a second grant. "The second grant was much easier than the first," says Nicole. "My go-to person at the CF Foundation was Melody Zelenz, Community Partnerships Coordinator Senior. She's a dear friend of mine to this day. I kept her updated with the ongoings of *Fall Risk* throughout 2019 and 2020, submitting summary and expenditure reports as needed. She always showed her support, love, and encouragement for the show.

"We were told to reapply for a second year (the max time allowed for one project), submitting an abbreviated version of the first grant to the board. We were awarded another ten-thousand-dollar grant for 2020–2021 in August 2020. The first year's grant allowed us to give stipends to *many* composers who helped us write music early on. We also invested in music producer James Hawkins, a well-known CF advocate and music producer in the UK. The rest went to PR-related things such as marketing fees, merchandise, and virtual production expenses."

Nicole continues, "The second grant mostly went toward staff and workshop costs. In order to host a virtual workshop of a musical over Zoom, you need really good equipment. We ensured every cast member had the technology they needed, and that staff was better accommodated for their time. While the pandemic was a horrific time with many innocent lives lost, it allowed our production to thrive in a virtual, online environment. A local community-theater production may only attract local performers. We have auditions from domestic and abroad talent, swinging our doors to opportunities wide open! We could not have done that without the CF Foundation grant."

Nicole continues to seek grant opportunities related to sheet music, royalties, production, and studio costs, among other things. In the meantime, *Fall Risk* had its first virtual workshop production in August 2021 and plans to release music for the production in summer 2022 and have its first in-person workshop in fall/winter 2022 (which, of course, is COVID-dependent). "*Fall Risk* is already bigger than I ever dreamed," says Nicole.

Nicole, Jared, their dogs, and her mom now live in North Carolina. When asked about activities and résumé items, apart from her success with *Fall Risk*, she modestly mentions she's a WEGO Health Award finalist, a patient representative for the Robert Wood Johnson Adult Cystic Fibrosis Clinic, and a Regional Lung Transplant Conference patient representative and a public speaker. She supports and praises the work of CF Yogi, Beam, Breathe Bravely, the Frey Life, CF Adventurer, and Emily's Entourage, and loves to blog for CF programs.

"I love to collaborate with others in the CF community," says Nicole, who becomes excited discussing a TikTok video she made with a few other CF warriors. And she has a special place in her heart for the Cystic Fibrosis Foundation. "I've been doing the Great Strides walk with my friends and family since I was five," she says. "I also make sure a portion of all my profits from *Two Cents* goes directly toward the CFF. I'll do the same with *Fall Risk* as it becomes a success!" Nicole—lights up as she returns to her favorite subject. "We already have people telling us to go to Broadway!" she says. "Chronically ill and able-bodied patrons alike are in love with this comedy, and I'm honored to be the creator."

CALEIGH SARAH HABER-TAKAYAMA

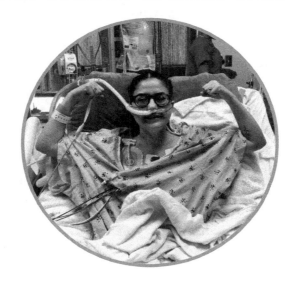

Age: 31
Resides: Los Angeles, California
Age at Diagnosis: Birth

FIGHT2BREATHE: TRANSPLANT SURVIVOR'S REMARKABLE JOURNEY

Fight2Breathe founder and CEO Caleigh Sarah Haber-Takayama's lung function was at 12 percent when she entered hospice at just twenty-two years of age. The goal was no longer to provide her with treatments to become stronger, but, as with other hospice patients, to maximize the quality of whatever life she had left. "When I was told I wasn't a candidate for the lifesaving transplant my body needed," she says, "I lost my passion to live."

Caleigh's (pronounced *kay-la*) "passion to live" started a couple of days after she was born, when she was taken into surgery for meconium ileus. A CF diagnosis followed, via a sweat test, which was performed two months after the surgery allowing her time to recover, and her fight had officially begun. "My parents had never heard of the disease," says Caleigh, "and had no idea of how it would be treated. Their immediate reaction was to ask how to fix it. They imagined that maybe another surgery or treatment would eliminate the disease. They were then educated on CF being a genetic disease which they hadn't known they were carriers. From that point on, they did everything possible to optimize my health.

"Being raised alongside two healthy children, my parents never treated me differently," says Caleigh, who likewise participated in sports, social activities, school, and camping. "This probably is one of the things for which I am most grateful to my parents, because it taught me to be confident with who I am. And who I am includes having cystic fibrosis."

Other than taking enzymes prior to eating, she was not unlike the average kid. "My favorite class was recess," Caleigh says, laughing. "The only difference between my siblings or peers and myself was that I had to be careful of getting infections. As a young toddler and child, my mom was very protective and attended my playdates. She wanted to be sure that I took my enzymes and any other medications I may have been on. She kept a close eye on my nutrition because I was petite and underweight."

Caleigh says that growing up her symptoms were mostly invisible to her and her family primarily because she did not have a heavy cough nor did she require a feeding tube or oxygen. She did notice a decline in health when she participated in sports. "I would notice my stamina and cardio being impacted the most," says Caleigh. "However, my day-to-day activities were not affected. Therefore, I didn't feel I needed nebulizers. Without sports, I might not have actually noticed drops in my lung function." These invisible symptoms lasted until she started having annual tune-ups in seventh grade due to depleting lung function. Still, her FEV1 was around the 80–90 percent range, approximately 10–20 percent from her baseline. And while she felt the drop in lung function somewhat, it was generally when she was feeling sick that she did her treatments.

"My mother enrolled me in as many extracurricular activities as possible, including Girl Scouts, National Charity League, the Make-A-Wish Foundation, volunteering at local hospitals, and numerous other local philanthropies," says Caleigh. Caleigh was also physically active growing up. "I lived in Southern California along the coastline," says Caleigh. "I grew up playing on the sandy beaches and swimming in the ocean. I was totally obsessed with my brother and sister and wanted to do everything they did; therefore, I participated in as many playdates and games as possible with them—including flag football, dancing, and jumping on trampolines." All her athletic adventures proved great for her health. In fact, one of the ways she loosened mucus from her lungs was jumping on the trampoline *before or after* gymnastics and cheer!

Once she entered high school, Caleigh joined the accomplished cheerleading team, and though weekday practices and weekend athletic events made membership a nearly full-time commitment, Caleigh found time to embrace her passion for charitable endeavors. She became a member of the Children's Hospital of Orange County club, and she founded the Cystic Fibrosis Club to help raise money for the Cystic Fibrosis Foundation by participating at events like Great Strides. She also founded the national program named Kids for Wish Kids.

"We raised enough money to fund two Make-A-Wish trips (each trip was approximately $4,500)," says Caleigh. "Our [Make-A-Wish] club did a send-off celebration for our first Make-A-Wish recipient. We threw a huge pep rally where I gave a speech to the entire school. I spoke about the impact of my New York City Wish trip on my family [when Caleigh was fourteen] and the importance of paying it forward."

Though she had become accustomed to annual tune-ups, Caleigh's sophomore year of high school was the first year she was hospitalized due to various infections associated with CF, including pseudomonas. Soon she was having complications from CFRD (later, she would deal with distal intestinal obstruction syndrome [DIOS], which is the obstruction of the small bowel).

"While in high school," says Caleigh, "I began to miss classes more and more due to my health and hospitalizations. I knew that I wasn't going to be able to keep up with college classes nor living alone due to [cystic fibrosis and the complications that came along with it]. I decided to shift my focus onto something I loved, which was food. Both my parents cooked in our household; however, my dad really enjoyed the process and included me often from a young age."

Caleigh got her first job in high school working in the food industry. "I was hired as a hostess at a local steakhouse," says Caleigh. "I loved the atmosphere of the culinary industry and often admired the chefs and cooks. Over time I was invited to export dishes and get closer to the kitchen. I felt a spark in me and became obsessed with the idea of cooking and the experiences cooking gave to others, even though I hadn't done it much previously."

Caleigh began researching culinary school programs during her senior year of high school. After graduating high school, Caleigh interned for a year and then spent the next couple of years in culinary school, as her passion was patisserie and baking.

"I decided to do something I loved that would also cooperate with my health schedule, which was culinary school," says Caleigh. "I did an internship for a year in Newport Beach which was required by the school before applying. I began interning in the culinary hot kitchen, but when the holidays came around, I was asked to help in the pastry kitchen. I knew it was the perfect place for me. It was more organized, and I found beauty in creating more detailed culinary experiences. I was able to learn many skills before going into school and confirmed it was my passion. I went to Le Cordon Bleu CCA (California Culinary Academy) in San Francisco from 2008 to 2010."

But in addition to the pressure of working side-by-side with the future great chefs of America, she had to navigate now-frequent hospital visits as she was hospitalized every few months, primarily for lung infections, and therefore had to take extended absences from working. "I was very upfront and honest about my disease with my academy chefs at the time," says Caleigh. Her health was not improving in culinary school. "While in school I did get sick often," says Caleigh. "I would usually pull out of classes then restart with the next graduating class. The school was designed to have training for separate courses six weeks at a time. This made it possible to get treatment at the hospital for a few weeks then return to classes after my health improved."

After graduating, Caleigh worked in some of the most well-known and successful kitchens in San Francisco, including Kara's Cupcakes, the Fairmont Hotel, and Restaurant Gary Danko, spending thirteen to sixteen hours a day working as a pastry cook.

She was spending more and more time in the hospital, two to three weeks at a time, and then returning a week after being released. "While working at Gary Danko, post–graduating the Le Cordon Bleu program in culinary school," says Caleigh, "I experienced a serious pneumonia that multiplied into other infections as well. I was hospitalized and immediately became oxygen dependent. Over the course of several months, my care team worked hard to recover my weight and lung function. After no success at either, I was forced to get a feeding tube."

Caleigh was sent home from the hospital to hospice care and, within a few weeks, was surrounded by her entire family. She was told that she needed a double-lung transplant to save her life. "When the doctor came in to first tell me that I needed a lung transplant," says Caleigh, "my mom was in the room with me. At that time, I was on high-flow oxygen and very weak. I wasn't even able to walk to the bathroom in the hospital room without the help of someone else and increasing my liter flow. My muscles had completely deteriorated, and I was about sixty-five pounds in a four-foot-eleven woman's body.

"The doctor came in early in the morning while doing rounds and told me that they'd be back to have a meeting with me. This is not the norm since usually they come in as a team and discuss the day's goals with any ongoing issues during rounds. When the doctor came back for our meeting, he came alone. He looked at my mom and I and told us I needed new lungs to survive. As I laid in bed, I felt it was true. I was dying quickly and everyone around me knew it. I had visits from extended family, which was very reaffirming that I was seriously ill (my family lives nine hours away from the hospital and had never visited before)."

Caleigh admits that she was not in a healthy state of mind at that point because of her body's deterioration and the impossible chance that she would return to the job she loved. "When my doctor told me I needed new lungs." says Caleigh, "he followed with the news that he wasn't going to recommend me due to being a noncompliant patient (putting my career and social desires over my health). I was then put on hospice and discharged from the hospital.

"Coming home from the hospital, I was still weak and completely dependent on oxygen and nutritional feeds through my G-J tube [a thin, long tube that enters through the abdominal surface, into the stomach, and down into the second part of the small intestine, which is also referred to as the jejunum]." Eventually, she decided to end her dream of working in the culinary world completely. "When my culinary career came to an end, I was crushed," says Caleigh, who then turned her focus to getting new lungs.

Hospice care included a unique regimen of Caleigh using a feeding tube to put on weight, supplemental oxygen to maintain her saturations, controlling her CFRD through insulin, continuing her oral medications, and pain meds to help her to manage. Her mom and brother relocated to San Francisco to help her prepare meals and live as "normal" a life as possible while also having a home nurse come to her apartment several times a week to do vitals, manage nutritional needs, and evaluate any other complications she was experiencing. "At first, the loss of independence was shocking," says Caleigh. "But I became closer with my mom and brother. We became a great team."

It was then time for Caleigh and her family to figure out how she could extend her life. "After much persuasion from my mother," says Caleigh, "my care team provided us with a list of my 'red flags,' or reasons why I wasn't a candidate for transplantation at this time and what it would take for me to be recommended to the transplant team. So, while the doctors diagnosed me as failing to thrive and needing end-of-life care, my family and I were fighting for new lungs. I had changed my mind and actions from depressed and not wanting a transplant to wanting to live and fighting for a transplant. I had a change of heart and mind to start working toward the list of requirements. The doctor agreed that if I succeeded at all, and *only* all, of the requirements on the list, they would indeed recommend me to the transplant team to be evaluated as a candidate for a double-lung transplant."

The requirements Caleigh had to achieve were lowering her A1C (which measures diabetes) from 13 percent down to 6 percent or less, gain weight to a normal BMI, attend clinic with her endocrinology team weekly, log her insulin and food, attend transplant clinic weekly and check in by phone once a week in between, do nebulizers and chest physiotherapy four times a day, and adhere to a specific medication regimen completely. Over the course of two years, Caleigh completed the list of requirements, completed a transplant evaluation, and was listed for a double-lung transplant.

Unable to put her energy into baking, Caleigh began blogging over social media about her life experiences. "I shared my failures and victories of living with a terminal disease and the decision to live through transplantation," she says. "People from all over the globe began following my journey." Caleigh then began posting videos about her personal life as well as her health regimen, often in the hospital, clinics, or at home. Oftentimes, she shot videos of herself setting up and doing nebulizer treatments, doing chest physiotherapy with her mom or brother, setting up her feeds, administering IV antibiotics at home, and organizing her meds. As her Instagram following topped eighty thousand after creating it in 2012, with the handle @Fight2Breathe, with many of her videos garnering tens of thousands of views, she realized within what might've been considered a tragic story was something special. Her followers were giving her hope and she was giving them hope right back.

Caleigh waited 565 days for new lungs when, at 1:40 a.m., on Friday, October 20, 2015, the lung and heart transplant team called her to accept donor lungs. "Within twenty minutes, we were out of our apartment," she says. "We picked up my brother at his place and made the traditional forty-five-minute drive to the Stanford University hospital. While driving, I texted all our friends and family that the day we had been waiting for had finally arrived. I thought of all the nights I stayed home crying because I couldn't go out with friends, and all the tough experiences my family went through because of me, and put absolute hope into a better future for all of us."

Caleigh says that despite the stakes, just prior to transplant, she felt "strangely calm and reassured. I kissed everyone good-bye and realized that if something went wrong, this would be the last time I saw them," she says. "I squeezed extra tight, told each person I loved them unconditionally, and was wheeled into the biggest operating room I had ever seen."

Within four hours of the procedure, Caleigh, with the aid of her new lungs, was breathing independently. After eleven days, she was discharged from the hospital. "Leaving the hospital," says Caleigh, "was the biggest piece of hope my family and I felt in years. We believed that it was the start of a new life for all of us."

And yet, while Caleigh's appetite never returned after her transplant, nor did her love for cooking, her passion for both living and for philanthropy did. "I was able to travel and attend more motivational-speaking and mentorship engagements," says Caleigh. "During speeches, I was able to speak on the miracle of transplantation and working hard toward a goal, despite someone [saying you] cannot achieve it. I was also able to get back into hiking and outdoor activities. Hiking felt like a freedom I hadn't had in a long time. It gave me the sense of health feeling the wind brush against my face and my lungs expand in my chest with every breath."

Her health was still full of ups and downs though. Three months post-transplant, Caleigh experienced an abscess full of pseudomonas. "Despite my doctors having seen a growing mass in my X-rays," says Caleigh, "they decided to do nothing because my lung function was still increasing. One morning, I woke up with pain in my left shoulder. I went to my pain management specialist who told me there was nothing wrong but that I was most likely experiencing pain from the surgery. His answer was to give me a cortisone shot to help the pain. When I returned home, my mom insisted that I get an MRI before treating me. Luckily, I had an MRI and received a call one day after from my actual transplant physician—on a Sunday—to come to the hospital immediately. I was hospitalized for over a month, having excruciatingly painful antibiotic flush treatments every four hours directly into the infected area through a chest tube. During the hospitalization, there was even talk of removing my entire left lung."

Her troubles culminated with a DIOS episode which became more frequent and more severe after her transplant. "I was on an eight-month, post-transplant celebratory vacation to Hawaii with my mom and brother. We spent a week in Maui. We swam, hiked, surfed, and lived like islanders. I didn't require any slowing down or rest and, for the first time, was able to participate in everything the island had to offer, even cliff diving.

"The second week, we flew to Oahu. When we arrived, everything was fine. I felt healthy and we spent the day by the beach and pool. The second day, my brother and I were in the sun all day on the beach without sufficient water supply. I became extremely dehydrated and backed up. That same night was my mom's birthday dinner. We all ate dinner, however, afterward, I excused myself back to the room to rest because my stomach wasn't feeling well. Not wanting my mom's birthday to be ruined, I told her to continue on to the lounge with my brother and not to worry about me. After a little while, my mom called and texted me but got no answer. After no reply, she decided to come back to check on me. She found me in severe stomach pain on the bed. She rushed me to the ER and things spiraled out of control from there."

Caleigh continues, "To be honest, I don't remember any of it. My brother and mom say I was in the worst pain of my life. I was receiving treatments via Stanford's orders, but nothing was working to resolve the blockage in my intestines. My stomach was filling with the fluids they were using to empty me out, resulting in my belly getting so big that it was pushing up on my lungs and cutting off my ability to breathe. I began to lose consciousness. I coded and was emergency intubated. I was then flown, via medical-jet air ambulance, back to Stanford to my care team."

Caleigh aspirated, spreading numerous infections within her lungs and stomach, and was placed in a medically induced coma for several weeks. "After weeks of being bedridden, I woke up still on the vent and ECMO machine," she says.

"When I woke up, I was confused and scared," says Caleigh. "At first, I had no memory of what had happened or even the fact that we had been on vacation. I didn't understand where I was until my dietitian came into the room and I recognized who she was. From that point, my mom slowly explained to me what was happening and why. She would repeat this every day. Once I understood those basics, we moved on to photos of the trip and photos of friends and family. The goal was to work my brain and memory of the people and places in my life. I was extremely anxious and scared the entire time. The doctors didn't have very optimistic tones in their voices as I was on five separate life-support devices. My family was there for me every moment of the day and night. They were what got me through such a difficult time. They also read me comments and messages from people in the Fight2Breathe community, which helped to motivate me and inspire me to keep fighting."

Once the life support was removed and she was able to maintain her saturations with only supplemental oxygen, Caleigh went through months of inpatient intensive therapy to learn to swallow, talk, hold her head up, sit, walk, use the restroom, and regain memories and knowledge. Caleigh says, "Going through such a traumatizing and life-threatening ordeal was evidence to me who and what is important in life. I learned a lot about myself and my strength in overcoming struggle—what skills I needed to develop and what skills I had in my toolbox to use when needed. Relearning the basics of life was very humbling and also rewarding. I knew that in order to eventually live the life of total independence I wanted, I had to accomplish the life skills I lost—at the very least. Each moment a goal was accomplished, I felt prouder of myself than ever before. The experience gave me confidence and respect in accepting myself for who I was on a new level."

When Caleigh arrived home from the hospital, she began working with an occupational therapist, a physical therapist, and a home nurse while regularly attending clinics at the hospital with her transplant and specialty teams. "The physical therapist worked with me at home to recover muscle loss and gain strength," says Caleigh. "When the woman first arrived, she instructed me to perform exercises while sitting in a chair in the living room. Over several weeks, we worked together with exercise bands, weights, and my own body weight with the goal of returning to daily activities and responsibilities. Every day, she left me with new exercises to do nightly while she wasn't with me. Eventually, the physical therapist helped me to gain the strength to walk without a walker in my apartment, then walk through the hall on a flat ground, then walk on the city sidewalk, and lastly walk the incline of a San Francisco hill.

"The occupational therapist worked with me on my ability to dress myself, to tie my shoes, to write my name, to understand the nerve sensations in my fingers for grabbing and touching to carry things around the house, to count money, and to accomplish other day-to-day responsibilities. My brother and my mom were really great [with] helping me relearn as well. They continued to use photographs to remind me of places and people. They took me to revisit friends to get reacclimated into society. They also took on the responsibilities of administering all of my medications and nutrition in order for me to regain the power needed to keep up with my appointments."

Caleigh's mom felt it was important for her daughter to find some sort of normalcy by attending events. "We made it a goal," says Caleigh, "to attend friends' weddings and huge life events. She came to all the events with me and helped me to feel beautiful and as much a part of the party as everybody else."

In October 2016, just four months after being on the ECMO machine and just one week after celebrating the one-year anniversary of her double-lung transplant, Caleigh and her mom made the last-minute decision to attend the wedding of Caleigh's childhood friend in Laguna Beach, California. They drove the long nine-hour car ride from her home in San Francisco with her mom behind the wheel and Caleigh sleeping in the passenger seat.

"Being surrounded by friends I had known since kindergarten was the paradisiacal space for me to get back into the groove of life again," says Caleigh. "I sat at the table with them sharing stories of our much younger years and catching up on current relationships, jobs, and goals. They all knew of my recent battle and were very understanding of helping me whenever needed. I laughed and ate and took breaks outside when the ambience became too loud or activity too heavy for me."

Eventually Caleigh walked up to the wedding bar where she was approached by a handsome gentleman named Bryan. "He had been attending the wedding on the groom's side," says Caleigh. "I hadn't seen Bryan previously but as I turned around, there he was clear as ever, standing, smiling back at me. I thought he was handsome and well-dressed and had a gorgeously groomed head of hair. We greeted each other and began conversing immediately. He wasn't focused on the normal questions a twenty-something-year-old often hears at a bar or social event—the 'what do you do for work?' or 'what school did you attend for your college degree?' Instead, he asked me, 'What makes you happy?' and 'What is your passion in life?' We did discuss where we lived and what we did for work in which I responded by showing him my social media, Fight2Breathe. I explained my scars, including my zipper sternotomy scar that was visible in my dress, all about CF and transplantation, and the basics of what my life consisted of."

Caleigh's recall in what immediately followed seems out of a Nora Ephron movie. She caught the bride's bouquet of flowers, the couple danced, and together, spontaneously planned an after-party. "Bryan asked me if I'd like to continue the night with him and his friends," says Caleigh. "I told him I already had plans for the night when he insisted by asking my friends along as well. My friends all chose to join, reassuring my mom they would look after me and reach out if needed. As we all walked along the Pacific Coast Highway together to a bar nearby, I walked slowly and carefully, which Bryan somewhat understood from my explaining to him my recent health challenges.

"Bryan felt like a forever friend as he listened and carried on easy conversation. I was able to be open, honest, and upfront about my disease and battles up to that point, I think mostly because I didn't feel the pressures of trying to impress him. At the time, I wasn't looking for a relationship, as I was just being reintroduced to society and still needed an extreme amount of help from my family day to day. However, Bryan had other plans."

Caleigh continues, "After a failed bar hunt, our group all sat together by the firepit at the close-by house [Bryan and his friends] had rented along the beach. It was a comfortable temperature, and I was enjoying feeling like I could function normally after so long. As the night came to an end, my girlfriends and I found ourselves desiring some alone time to chat and headed out to get some food. That is when

I discovered I had left the bouquet by the firepit. Wanting to get the bouquet back with the goal of drying out the flowers and returning it to the bride, I scrolled my Instagram for recent new followers—only problem was I had forgotten what Bryan's name was. I asked my girlfriends to help and, finally, we found him and DM'd him asking if he'd mind walking to return the flowers in exchange for some greasy french fries.

"When Bryan arrived, he handed me the flowers and spoke the phrase, 'This will be a story we tell all our friends at our wedding.'" Caleigh was charmed, but chalked it up to a night in which they were both caught in the moment. The day she arrived back home, she found a pot full of succulents. She knew the sender right away.

Over the next month Bryan, who was living in Ohio, traveled for work in Ireland, and Caleigh had a Nissen fundoplication surgery—an invasive procedure in which the upper part of the stomach is wrapped around the lower end of the esophagus and stitched in place, reinforcing the closing function of the lower esophageal sphincter to treat gastroesophageal reflux disease with various potential complications—to protect herself from a recurrence of aspiration. They frequently texted during their long-distance relationship in what became a deep dialogue about CF and the life she had built around it. "I told him I have always identified myself as more than my disease," she says, "as a 'regular' woman with passions equal to my peers. I believe from a place of total honesty, our love grew, with CF and transplant becoming a part of our lives, but never the center."

Bryan visited Caleigh in San Francisco in early December, a little over a month since they had first met. In early March 2016, after four months of a cross-country relationship, Bryan not only made the decision to move to San Francisco and move in with Caleigh, he worked hard to adapt to a life full of tough decisions and hospitalizations. He spent hours researching treatments, medications, complications, attending clinics at Caleigh's hospital, staying with Caleigh during hospitalizations, and learning from Caleigh and her family about how to prepare and administer medications. He was fully committed to helping Caleigh thrive as best as possible. And then, of course, there were the typical growth patterns of a romantic couple trying to explore each other's depths.

Unfortunately, the couple faced huge challenges almost immediately as Caleigh's health began to deteriorate. "I went through several surgeries, a bleb [a small collection of air between the lung and the outer surface of the lung which can rupture, potentially leading to a collapsed lung] in one of my lungs, respiratory failure, and, finally, I went into organ rejection," says Caleigh. "I worked endlessly to fight to get out of organ rejection. I spent weeks in the hospital again, worked out with a trainer to try and gain muscle mass, ate healthy, tried to gain weight with the assistance of my feeding tube, and attempted to control every factor we knew could be playing a part in my health decline.

"Gaining muscle was important at the time because I was weak from constantly being hospitalized and chronic hypoxia, which causes muscle wasting and weakness. Fighting infections and end-stage lung disease meant being couch-bound the majority of the time as well. The goal would be to gain muscle and therefore gain the ability to accomplish more daily tasks, plus exercise to gain lung function. I was using supplemental oxygen twenty-four-seven again and reliant on my feeding tube. Going through rejection was more emotionally and physically taxing than my first battle through end-stage lung disease. Eventually, I was told I needed a second double-lung transplant. I felt like I had failed to honor my first donor."

Caleigh immediately began treatment for organ rejection and worked tirelessly to overcome it. "I was fighting to stay alive until anyone would accept me into their transplant program," says Caleigh, "abiding by my medical regimen and forcing myself to do feeds to gain weight even when I didn't feel well. My family worked endlessly to support me during the moments I couldn't administer my medications myself." Despite Caleigh and her family's efforts, she was sent home and placed into hospice care once again. "We were told that unless my family couldn't manage my care themselves, we should not return to the hospital and that I would pass away very soon."

At this point, the couple made the decision to get married. With the help of others, they put on a wedding filled with 250 people in just six days.

Immediately following the wedding, Bryan went to work. "My husband searched tirelessly for a transplant center who would accept me as a redo candidate," says Caleigh. "I was life-flighted out of one hospital and into the next after ending up back in the ICU, requiring a BiPAP machine (a non-invasive life support) allowing me to breathe. I then persisted to fight a grueling and many times questionable 106 days in which I lived full time within my new hospital walls until my second lifesaving transplant."

On June 8, 2018, Caleigh received her new lungs. Immediately following, the surgeons deemed the procedure a success, but still, a fairy tale ending would have to wait. "I suffered from pericardial effusions from July to November, resulting in several emergent and lifesaving open-heart surgeries," says Caleigh, "the last being a pericardiectomy, the surgical removal of the membrane sac that surrounds the heart.

"I feel blessed that my incredible new transplant physician took a chance on saving my life when no one else would," says Caleigh. "My second transplant has allowed me to experience breathing in a way I have never felt before: without thought, concentration, or help. I am now one hundred percent independent and live a better quality of life than ever before."

With two diagnoses of hospice care behind her, Caleigh's resolve is to support others in the way she felt supported through her literal life-and-death experiences. "I was driven by hope and motivation to do more, see more, and help others," she says simply, though she admits she can't quite believe it herself that she's still here. Caleigh is expressing her passions in a variety of ways: as an ambassador for many foundations, including Rare Genes, Donate Life, One Legacy, and the Cystic Fibrosis Foundation; speaking at galas, hospitals, events, and conferences for everyone from medical professionals to pharmaceutical companies to supporters to families to individuals living with disease and/or transplant. She also returned to one of her passions in high school—the Make-A-Wish Foundation—by becoming a wish granter.

"Being a Make-A-Wish child provided my family with an escape from the financial, physical, and mental battles of cystic fibrosis," says Caleigh. "I'll never forget how I felt the first time the wish granters came to my house. It was an overwhelming feeling of admiration of their duties and role. When they asked me what my wish was, I thought about all that my family members have sacrificed to provide me with good health and made the decision to include them in a trip to New York City. The wish granters spent their time detailing out an itinerary for the trip to include everything on my New York bucket list. By the time I was on a plane headed to New York, I set a goal for granting children's wishes myself and paying it forward by being a wish granter for the Make-A-Wish Foundation in my future."

Caleigh is still passionate about her blogging exploits because it gives her the opportunity to more deeply discuss how she combats CF and deals with life after a double-lung transplant. "I hope that my blog shows others in the fight that their dreams are possible despite their struggles and encourages fighters to always pursue new passions, find worth within their new bodies, and to understand there are always positives in life, no matter what you are going through in the moment," she says.

Caleigh also makes time to mentor those in the cystic fibrosis community. "Parents, teens, peers, partners, anyone in need of support," she says.

And then, there is what might be called the linchpin for all her activities: Fight2Breathe. "Fight2Breathe.org aims to support the individuals and families of individuals living with disease by easing the burden they experience," says Caleigh. "We provide care packages to inpatients across the nation, help with financial concerns, and spread positivity. We are also working toward a 'little cysta/fibro, big cysta/fibro' mentorship program." As is evident from the tone of her story, Caleigh says her mission is to provide a fully transparent view into life with cystic fibrosis, chronic illness, genetic diseases, and organ transplantation. She also aspires to fund innovative research in the future.

"When I think about all I've gone through, my immediate thoughts are appreciation for the two selfless individuals who chose to be organ donors and save my life through giving me new lungs," says Caleigh, who has also returned to her culinary passions and is using her entrepreneurial know-how to grow a baking business out of her kitchen. "I think about their families and their friends and of the pain they must all be constantly going through. I don't take the responsibility of caring for their gifts lightly. These thoughts always end with sending them love and gratitude."

ERINN HOYT

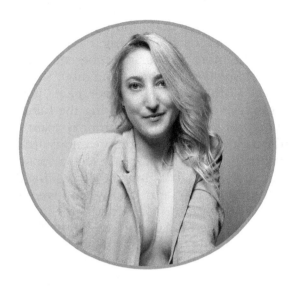

Age: 31
Resides: San Diego, California
Age at Diagnosis: Birth

BACK IN THE POOL: SWIMMER FINDS BEAUTY IN HER SCARS

"When I first woke up from my transplant," says Erinn Hoyt, "I awoke in a dark room. I remember trying to read the clock to see what time it was. The doctors had warned me that there is always a possibility of a 'dry run' when it comes to transplant. A 'dry run' is when lungs are believed to have been a match but upon closer examination they are not.

"The process truly begins when a seemingly healthy pair of lungs comes in from a deceased organ donor. The hospital sends out a team to assess and evaluate them in person so they can determine if the lungs are a good fit for you. All the while, you are still being prepped for surgery. I was told that if I see a surgeon, it means that the surgery will happen. However, I did not remember ever seeing a surgeon. So when I woke up, I was truly unsure if I had had the transplant or not. I also did not see my parents in the room. I assumed that if I had

had the surgery, they would be with me when I woke up. I signaled a nurse over and, with hand signals, asked if I could have a piece of paper to write on. I asked her if I had had the surgery and could she call my parents. She informed me that I did indeed have the surgery and my parents were in another room waiting. I still had a breathing tube down my throat. The more awake and coherent I became, the more uncomfortable I became with the breathing tube."

Erinn continues, "With my pen and paper, I kept begging her to call the team that was responsible for removing the tube. It seemed like eternity before my parents and the respiratory team arrived. At this point, I was fully awake and growing more and more uncomfortable. When the team finally pulled the tube, I was so consumed with that pain that I immediately started talking to them, asking them what took so long! It wasn't until half an hour later when I went to cough out of pure habit that I realized there was nothing there to cough out. It was a strange feeling and I tried to cough a few more times just to make sure there was truly nothing there. I had never felt mucus-free lungs."

Erinn was born in August 1990 at Stanford Hospital where she was diagnosed with cystic fibrosis at birth after a bout with meconium ileus. "When we were told that Erinn most likely had CF when she was just two days old," says Erinn's mom, Anne, "my initial reaction was fear for what her life would be like. I was familiar with CF because I grew up with a girl who had CF. I had gone all the way through school with her (from kindergarten through college). She was always very sick. I remember her almost always wearing a hospital bracelet since she spent so much time in the hospital, and she died when she was only twenty-one. I very quickly came to the realization that I wanted Erinn to live as normal a life as possible and do everything every other kid was doing."

Erinn's father, Scott, began running a charitable golf tournament for CFRI (which initially stood for Cystic Fibrosis Research Inc. but now is referred to as Cystic Fibrosis Research Institute) when she was just a year old and began volunteering at it when she was thirteen years old. The golf tournament, which has raised an average of $90,000 each year since its inception, has raised over $3 million in the last five years alone.

Growing up, Erinn describes herself as "very outgoing and overly talkative. I was the kid in class who always got in trouble for talking too much. I distinctively remember being forced to write lines in fifth grade that said, 'I will not talk to my friends during class.' I have always had a very outgoing personality. However, cystic fibrosis was not something I talked about with my friends. I do not remember ever saying out loud to anyone 'I have CF' until I got to college. I grew up in a small town, so I just assumed that it was something everybody already knew and there was nothing more to talk about. However, when I reflect back on that time, the truth is that I didn't want to be viewed as different. I never wanted to be treated differently or given any leniency in school or sports. I wanted to prove myself based on my own merit. One that did not include my disease."

Erinn admits developing insecurities from procedures done because of her CF. "Growing up, I was always insecure about my scars. I had meconium ileus when I was first born, leaving me with multiple scars on my stomach and belly button area. When it came time to put on a bikini, I was always self-conscious. I remember walking up to a make-up counter at the mall when I was twelve or thirteen and asking the employee if they sold anything that would cover my scars."

At five years old, Erinn's parents signed her up for a summer swimming league because they had heard that swimming could be good for her lungs, and by ten, she was ranked within the top ten fastest swimmers in her age group in all of Northern California. "I still, to this day, hold records for that age group that were set in 1999–2000," says Erinn. "I continually qualified for Far Westerns, an elite swim meet." She went on to qualify for the varsity team in high school as a freshman.

"Swimming was a blessing to me in the mental sense, in that it gave me an identity outside of my disease," says Erinn. "Swimming was my life. I was known as 'Erinn the swimmer' instead of 'Erinn the sick girl.' Swimming allowed me to find a passion, a hobby, and something to talk about that was outside of my disease. If I didn't have swimming, which also leads to having a love of competition and a love of sports, then what would normalize me? What would I relate to other kids about? The physical reward of swimming was an extra bonus. I got lucky that the sport I was good at just also happened to be the best thing for my lungs."

Erinn swam nearly every day. "Swimming was my treatment plan," says Erinn. "I have very few memories of myself doing nebulizer treatments as a child and prior to the age of seventeen. I swam six days a week for a minimum of two hours. If we had a meet that weekend, I swam seven days a week. I would sometimes do an extra nebulizer treatment here or there. However, my parents and the pulmonologist I saw at PAMF (Palo Alto Medical Foundation) agreed that I did not need any extra treatments outside of my swimming [though Erinn did take enzymes with food for digestion]."

Erinn admits that she was grateful for another thing. "The bathing suits I swam in for competitive swimming were always one pieces that covered [the scars from my meconium ileus].

"There were very few times I noticed the symptoms of my CF when I was swimming," says Erinn, "to the point of which when I began experiencing symptoms in the pool, I unsuccessfully identified them at first." That all started when Erinn was seventeen and a senior in high school, during her second semester. "I began to notice it when I started having a hard time walking from my last period of class to my car. I would get to my car and be extremely out of breath. I would have to sit for a decent amount of time in the car to catch my breath before starting it. It was then that the swim season at the high school started.

"The first few days of practice I assumed that I was severely out of shape. I had been so lucky with my health growing up that I failed to see the signs that my health was declining. I began to fall behind at swim practice," says Erinn, whose daily swim workouts proved to be harder and harder, leaving her increasingly out of breath.

"The first time I noticed my symptoms during practice was when we were required to do a drill in which we had to swim the entire length of the pool without breathing. We often did this up to sixteen to twenty-five times a practice. I have one specific memory in which I could not complete the drill. I could not go the full twenty-five yards of the pool without breathing; however, I was never given any sort of leniency due to my condition. My coach told me that I must complete at least one lap without breathing in order to stop the drill and move on to the next practice set. I think it took me a minimum of ten tries before I was able to complete it."

Erinn realizes outsiders may think that the coach was wrong to do this to Erinn, but she vehemently disagrees. "It is moments like this that made me who I am today. I never wanted a pity party or a pity pass. If that meant working harder than everybody else, then that's what I was going to do." Erinn says these issues had been going on for a few weeks. "I could not breathe at practice. This wasn't a 'I just had a hard workout and need to catch my breath sort of thing.' I was on the deck, doubled over, gasping for air and light-headed. I know now that my oxygen was low.

"I remember one of the first days of practice asking to be excused early. I went into the locker room and had to sit down for approximately thirty minutes and never could catch my breath. Here I was, a lifelong swimmer, used to swimming events back to back within minutes of each other. I had never needed thirty minutes to recover from anything. The next day, I asked to be excused early again. I felt like molasses moving through the pool. Again, I could not breathe or catch my breath. On the way home (the pool was only seven minutes away from my house), I had to pull over to rest. That night, I asked my mom to take me to urgent care.

Erinn continues, "When I got there, my oxygen was ninety-one. I was immediately put into an ambulance and taken to Stanford's Children Hospital. There, I was admitted to the hospital for my first time. I didn't know how to read my body in terms of CF. I knew how to read my body as a swimmer. If I had overstretched or underhydrated myself, I knew immediately the signs and symptoms. CF symptoms had never gotten in the way of my life in or outside of the pool. My life changed from then on out."

That night, Erinn was diagnosed with pneumonia. It was during these two weeks she spent in the hospital that her health continued to spiral. "When I was shown the MRIs and CAT scans of the irreversible damage done to my lungs, my first reaction was shock and then denial," says Erinn. "*Not me*, I thought, *I am the healthy one*. I had always been praised by doctors for my exceptional health growing up. The discussion of a hospitalization had never been touched upon. I was a successful athlete. Wouldn't I have known? How could I have performed for so many years with lungs that looked like that? I was naïve and truly never believed that I would one day be hospitalized. After the shock wore off and I had accepted what was happening, anger set in. I was now furious. I was furious with myself, for allowing myself to get this sick. And in return, I became angry with the doctors and hospital staff who were trying to transition me into my 'new normal.'"

Soon after seeing all of the images of her lungs, Erinn was introduced to The Vest along with many daily treatments that would become her new normal. "It felt that my identity was slowly transforming from Erinn the swimmer to Erinn the sick girl," says Erinn. When her friends would visit the hospital, Erinn tried to act as if nothing was wrong. "I figured if I could trick them into thinking it was a mistake then I would start to believe it myself. In reality, I felt horrible. I was exhausted, stressed, and most importantly, very sick." The worst outcome of this health episode: Erinn had to stop swimming.

"I was told I could never swim again," says Erinn. "I was frustrated that these doctors weren't listening to me, and I was devastated that this had a possibility of being my new normal. It later occurred to me that I had swum my last competitive swim race and had no idea it was my last. I didn't get to have the experience of being a senior and being able to step up to the block for that 'final swim.' I had been robbed of that."

Erinn eventually learned to adjust to her new normal during her senior year while doing IVs through a PICC line and using her new vest twice a day. "If there is one thing that can be said about me," says Erinn, "it is that I can adjust to pretty much any situation that I am in.

"Once I was released from the hospital, I felt the symptoms and there was no going back to life 'before.' I was tired, coughing more, and I had lost a significant amount of weight. While on home IVs, I would often attend the swim practices. It was a good way to see my friends and still receive the credit I needed to graduate. While in attendance of the practices, I understood why I could not swim anymore. Besides the obvious IV in my arm, my body was too weak. I had lost too much weight and my body was busy fighting against something much stronger at the moment. I could not have handled being in the pool. I was also looking forward to college. I had to allow my body to heal now. I understood that I never had any plans to be a collegiate athlete. The swimming at this point served no other purpose than to keep my body healthy. And I was still doing that — just now I had to learn to do it outside the pool."

Erinn graduated high school a few weeks later and attended San Diego State University (SDSU).

While Erinn was a sophomore at SDSU, Erinn's father revealed to her that her sister, Kristen, two and a half years Erinn's junior, was also diagnosed with the disease. Kristen was diagnosed at age seventeen after a chronic sinus infection and a persistent dry cough led to multiple tests which confirmed the diagnosis. Erinn still remembers her dad's emotions.

"He was angry and confused," says Erinn. "He was angry at himself and the doctors that she had been seeing for the past seventeen years. Kristen was born in 1993. In 1990, I had been diagnosed with CF. When Kristen was born in the hospital, the doctors quite literally just looked at her and told my parents she didn't have it. She was a chunky, healthy baby who passed her first stool. They performed absolutely zero follow-up tests for a baby who had an older sibling with CF. He was confused by this thought process of the doctors and angry at them for dropping the ball. He also questioned his own decision in not asking more questions. I told him absolutely not to blame himself. In my opinion, this was a total oversight by the doctors the day she was born and for the seventeen years after. If a doctor tells you that your baby is healthy then it is natural to believe them."

"I think that if I had been diagnosed at seventeen without any prior knowledge of the disease," Kristen says, "I would have been much more scared. I had grown up knowing that Erinn had CF. I had watched her live a very normal life and excel in her sports. It was a comfort to me to know that this diagnosis was not the end of the world."

Still, Kristen admits that dealing with CF has not been a piece of cake. "I had little to no emotion about it for the first few years because I was in denial and didn't fully believe the truth. I was mean to all of my doctors and didn't do almost any of my medicine. I wouldn't talk about it with family or friends. You can't tell someone after seventeen years of living a normal life, 'Just kidding, you have actually been living with a chronic lifelong disease and now it's time to change everything in your life.' You cannot just expect them to change their daily habits, mind-set, and way of life. When you almost expect them to go cold turkey on their previous life and jump into the world of being a CF patient, what you are actually doing is completely stripping them of their identity."

"I was surprised [by the diagnosis]," says Erinn, "because she had never even had a common cold. If I was considered 'healthy,' then she was iron woman. Honestly, my worries about her diagnosis were minimal. CF has such a broad spectrum of cases from mild to severe. If she had gone seventeen years without a doctor noticing that there is a possibility that a patient, with a sibling with CF, might actually have CF themselves, then I deemed her healthy. She had done all of this without swimming seven days a week or a single breathing treatment.

"I knew Kristen was struggling with the diagnosis. She understood that I had the disease. She had watched me live a full and normal life before my first health scare. I understood the damage it can do to someone's inner peace and identity to push something on them before they are ready. I love my sister and I intended on helping her with anything she needed help with in regard to the disease. However, the last thing I was going to do was scare her. I decided we would take it day by day."

Erinn continues, "When she was diagnosed, I was nineteen. I had been in college for almost two years by then. I had recovered better than intended from my hospitalization two years prior. My life had resumed as normal, and I wanted her to see that she could still lead a full life. Since my hospitalization, I had connected with more people with CF. I saw how a lot of them allowed it to consume them and make it their singular identity. I did not want that for myself or my sister.

"If I had to use one word to describe my college years," says Erinn, "it would be 'normal.' Of course, I had the new challenge of managing my health; however, I had a private dorm room so that was all done behind closed doors. Beyond those four walls, I was just like everyone else. Without swimming, I was finally able to successfully gain weight. I was at my highest and healthiest weight. With all of my newfound free time that normally I would spend in the pool, I was able to make new friendships and enjoy time that normally I would use training. I also used all of my free time to complete all of my vest and breathing treatments.

"I was in a new city, with new friends, and a whole new environment. I loved every second of it. I would 'vest' first thing when

I woke up and it was the last thing I did before I went to bed that night. Luckily, I was able to be placed on a disability list through the school, so I had first pick of my classes. This allowed me to schedule them around my treatments. I was required to take a handful of different pills as well, which I always took with breakfast. I channeled my passion of being the best swimmer into creating the best college experience for myself. I played in intramural soccer leagues, I got a job at the school gym, and I created lifelong friendships. I stayed relatively healthy all through college. Every summer when the campus would close down, I would return to my hometown where I would do IV tune-ups for the summer. These allowed me to remain healthy during the school year."

At the age of twenty-one, as a senior at SDSU, her health worsened yet again. "I began to notice signs and symptoms of a CF illness making an appearance in my body. For all of my college years, I had only been seen at Stanford for my CF. I was still being followed by the team that I had started working with during that first hospitalization. I could tell that I was declining. Not enough for a hospitalization, but enough to get set up with a CF team in San Diego. I reached out to the CF team at UCSD (University of California San Diego) and began seeing them. I explained to them that I could feel myself getting more fatigued and producing more sputum. They placed me on oral antibiotics several times throughout the year and I began to feel better. I had a full social calendar and was enjoying my remaining days as a college student.

"One night, I came home from a late-night class with a 105-degree fever. I self-admitted myself to the hospital." Erinn was diagnosed with pneumonia. After about three nights in the hospital, Erinn got up one night to use the restroom and fell from passing out. She was rushed to the ICU where she was placed on a ventilator.

"The fear truly set in when I had nurses running my bed down the hall," says Erinn. "I still can see the face of the nurse placing a giant oxygen mask over my face saying, 'Don't worry, you are going to make it.' At that point, I realized he was saying that because there was, at some point, a chance I was not going to make it."

Erinn spent the next seven days in the ICU, "terrified. Although, my memory of everything that went on is vague—my feeling of fear for my life is still vivid in my memory." Eventually Erinn was transferred from the ICU to the step-down unit, where, now in stable condition, she carried on with her school assignments. "I still had to finish all of my final exams in order to graduate college on time," says Erinn.

Erinn was always able to motivate herself when there was a problem in front of her and she knew she would need to again in order to graduate. "I remember being in sixth grade and working out a math problem on a test. I was silently, and under my breath, discussing with myself how this problem would be solved. The teacher snapped at me and told me to be quiet. I was confused on why this angered her so much. It was something I always did. Before every race, as I was approaching the swim block or sometimes on the block, I would talk to myself. I would give myself mini pep talks or reassurances. It was just a way to remind myself that I could do it. I could conquer whatever race or task was in front of me.

"As I stared down at the final exam in front of me, I slowly began to talk to myself in the same manner. 'It's only five pages of an essay and then you can graduate . . . you have written pages much longer.' And then I remember telling myself, 'There she is . . .' What I meant by that was that I was still me. I was alive. I had made it out of the hardest part—the ICU. I was a fighter. The same one who had fought in the pool, fought to get into college, fought to stay healthy, and I was going to fight now."

Erinn did fight. "I was still in the ICU five days before I was set to graduate," she says. "Early that week, I had been intubated—unable to speak or breathe on my own. I was using a bed pan to go to the restroom. I felt like a shell of a human. I had recovered enough to be able to be transported to the step-down unit. In the five days after the ICU in which I spent in the step-down unit is where the fight to graduate took place. They were going to have to physically restrain me from not walking at graduation. I had worked hard for four years at San Diego State. I had worked on my health and my education. I had gone four years without a hospitalization. I didn't think one hospitalization out of four years should hold me back—regardless of how serious it was.

"I was transported back to high school me who also landed in the hospital in the fourth quarter of the game. I retreated to the denial and believing that if I fooled others into thinking I was okay than eventually I would be. The school, just like my swim coach, allowed me no leniency. I was required to take all of my finals. They were, of course, modified, as I would be taking them in a hospital instead of a classroom. In between breathing treatments, hospital rounds, IV courses, and all-around hospital life, I managed to finish them all in the required time frame to graduate. I was released in the late afternoon the day before graduation. The next day, I walked across the stage with an IV in my arm and received my diploma for earning a degree in criminology while minoring in sociology. I fought and won that battle.

"Post-graduation, I began sleeping with oxygen every night," says Erinn, "but other than that I was able to return to a semi-normal life. I moved home to my parents' house the summer after graduation to rest and recover. By fall, I had moved back to San Diego and into an apartment with my two best friends. I got a job working behind the counter at Torrey Pines Golf Course. It was a challenge to get them to understand my disease and that I needed certain allowances.

Erinn continues, "The first day on the job, I was scheduled to open the pro shop at six a.m. This meant I had to wake up at four a.m. in order to do my vest treatments and get ready for work. This felt unreasonable and left me feeling paralyzed by oxygen. The next day I had the same task of opening the pro shop at six a.m., I would be off of work by one p.m. and decided to wait to do my vest until the shift was over in an attempt to score some more sleep in the morning. However, this didn't work either. My chest was tight, and I was overproducing sputum because I hadn't had a chance to clear it in the morning. I decided to ask my boss to only be scheduled to close the pro shop. It would give me time to vest before work and overall be better for my health.

"Unfortunately, the individuals I worked for were not understanding. They instead accused me of wanting to stay out late with my friends and that's why I did not want an early shift. I went as far as to have my CF doctor write a letter to them educating them on cystic fibrosis and why I needed certain allowances. Once I was able to establish a decent work schedule, with the help of my doctor, my life resumed as normal. I recovered shockingly well and went back to living a 'normal' life. Full of friends, work, and a full social calendar.

"However," says Erinn, "after about two years of working in the pro shop, my health began to decline again. I believe it was a combination of things—being overworked and forced to stand on my feet for eight hours a day, working in an environment where I dealt with the public (increased exposure to germs), and the unavoidable fact of aging and cystic fibrosis being a progressive disease. About five months before being listed for a transplant, I went on temporary disability through the state. I found myself unable to keep up with the demands that a job required."

Still, she couldn't quite catch a wave of consistently good health. "I was told I would need a port-a-cath when I was twenty-four years old. I stayed up the whole night looking at pictures of myself in a bikini and focusing on the one area I didn't have a scar—my chest. I ultimately backed out of the surgery placement the next day. I told the doctor I just couldn't bear to mark up my body more than it already was. [Eventually], I had no choice but to get a port placed. I cried the whole day knowing that I would be adding another scar to my body."

Erinn's lung function had decreased to only 15 percent, and just two months prior to receiving a double-lung transplant, she was living on full-time oxygen. "I knew that my old lungs were done," says Erinn. She was listed for transplant at the age of twenty-five and three short months later she was flown in on a medical plane from San Diego to Stanford hospital, preparing for a double-lung transplant.

"The most shocking part about my thoughts on the medical plane to Stanford is that I wasn't having any medical thoughts," says Erinn. "My thoughts were consumed with my life outside of my CF. I had just moved into a new apartment with roommates I loved. I had just adopted a cat. I was in a semi-new relationship, and I had a close circle of friends who I loved. I was in the process of truly building a life that I loved and was proud of. I was devastated to leave that all behind. I was scared that the transplant would take all of that away from me and that by leaving San Diego, my friends I left behind would forget about me. They would move forward and continue to build healthy lives while I was stuck living with my parents, awaiting a transplant."

Erinn received her new lungs at Stanford Hospital on February 1, 2016. The surgery was deemed a success and, after seven months in the hospital, where she began a program of recovery that included twice-a-week respiratory and physical therapy, she moved back to San Diego.

"I always find it difficult to answer the question of how long it took me to recover after my transplant," says Erinn, "because . . . are we ever truly fully recovered? I still feel myself healing daily."

Erinn admits that one of the most difficult parts was her body insecurity. "After my transplant, I didn't look at my chest in the mirror for seven days. I would turn around when I walked past a mirror. I didn't want to see what my scar looked like." Slowly though, Erinn's perspective changed. "I slowly grew to love my scars. Especially, my transplant scar. The one that runs right down the middle of my chest. I began to wear clothes that showcased it."

In the following years after her transplant, Erinn became a big advocate. "I always enjoyed making video compilations. I had always made them for friends for their birthdays and anniversaries. I had been asked by family and friends to make a few for different memorial services. I loved putting images and videos to music. While I was in the hospital awaiting my transplant, my cousin was recording everything. At the time, she just wanted it for her personal memory. I realized that I was so lucky to have that footage and decided to put together a video somewhat documenting my transplant experience. I used footage from the day of the transplant and included some of my favorite memories with friends and family that I had collected over the years on tape. I ended the video by urging people to become donors. My goal was to show viewers what a full life I had led and how having a transplant was my hope to improve my quality of life. I also wanted to honor all of my beloved friends and family and showcase so many amazing memories that I had kept.

"I posted the video on my Facebook page and the response was overwhelming. I had multiple people messaging me to let me know that my video had led them to sign up to become a donor. I had others messaging me that it encouraged them to quit smoking, live life to the fullest, or be more appreciative of their health. What started as a fun project for my cousin and I became something bigger than I could have dreamed. The response to that video showed me that my voice has influence. People responded positively and passionately to my video that I decided I wanted to do more in the way of advocacy. That is when I began posting more on social media and presenting speeches for patient advocacy for UCSD, as well as a speech in Hawaii for the Mauli Ola (which means "the breath of life" in Hawaiian) Foundation, on the importance of getting kids in the water for exercise."

Something else happened following her transplant. "I discovered the Transplant Games as I was in the waiting room of one of my weekly transplant appointments at Stanford," says Erinn. "There was a pamphlet casually tossed on the table in front of me. I picked it up and started to read. I noticed that they offered swimming. At the time, I was attending physical therapy twice a week. It was required by Stanford. I enjoyed physical therapy. It gave me something to do twice a week. They set goals for you each week and I enjoyed working toward those goals.

"Physical therapy was coming to an end, and I realized I would need something else to become a motivator for me. What people do not talk about post-transplant is the depression and emptiness. You have just undergone this major lifesaving surgery. And now what? You are not allowed to drive yourself anywhere or be more than two hours away from your hospital. You no longer can hold a job because your focus is taking care of your new lungs. I was often home alone all day while my sister and parents were at work. It can be lonely and isolating. I needed a goal and something to work for. Even while on the waitlist for a transplant, my goal was to be strong enough to undergo the procedure. When I saw the pamphlet, I didn't see a sport I loved, because I had given that up at age seventeen. I saw what my parents saw when I was only five years old and they originally introduced me to swimming—a goal, and that goal was to make my new lungs stronger."

Erinn first started in the pool in her parents' backyard. "It is approximately fifteen yards and by no means straight. But it was a start. I was slow and weak at first but as I built strength, I eventually got back into a competition pool. It was not until about six months into training that I began to feel a passion for the competitiveness of the sport again. I had reached the point in my training that I felt I had a chance to compete and win. That is when the passion returned."

Erinn went on to compete in the World Transplant Games in July 2017 in Malaga, Spain, and later in July 2019 in Salt Lake City. Combined, she medaled in every event in which she competed and amassed a total of thirteen medals. She also became the current American record holder in the fifty-yard breaststroke for women in the Transplant Games of America with a time of 39.45 seconds. Erinn's success resulted in earning her the distinction of Athlete of the Year for the Boomer Esiason Foundation in 2019.

"I was just excited to watch her compete again . . . after everything she had endured," says Anne. "It was just an added bonus that she was so successful."

Kristen knew her sister would be successful again. "Honestly, I never thought anything of it. It seemed like a natural progression for Erinn. She likes to compete, and she likes to win. It all added up for me."

As a result of her great comeback and her newfound confidence, Erinn posted a photograph for a competition that the *Sports Illustrated Swimsuit Issue* (also referred to as *SI Swim*) was holding, and her photo was chosen and featured on their social media page as she became the first CF/transplant patient to be featured.

"I realized that growing up I had no positive role models of women with scars," says Erinn. "They were never featured or glorified in beauty magazines. I began to wonder that if I had seen them in the media, if I would have felt a different way. So, when I saw the open casting call for *SI* swimsuit models, I knew that I had to not only do this for me but for girls everywhere. I did not want another little girl to feel the same insecurity I had felt. I wanted her to know that both she and her scars are beautiful.

"The photo that *SI Swim* chose to feature on their social media platforms was one where I chose to wear a pink blazer to match my pink scars. Unfortunately, I did not make it to the final round of being in the actual magazine. However, the photo was posted on their platform that is followed by over two million people. If I could influence one of those people, then I have done my job. I also received dozens of positive personal messages thanking me for my courage and saying that it gave them the confidence to no longer hide their scars."

Erinn goes on to say, "I have been through so much in my life to make it to where I am today: healthy and alive! [My scars] are a sign of that. They represent strength, beauty, and a second chance at life. I want to continue to spread my message of scar positivity and beauty. I plan to do this through the power of social media and auditioning again to make it to the final rounds of the *Sports Illustrated Swimsuit Issue*. There is a major void in the media of celebrating women with scars. I want to help fill that void. I want to be an advocate for women and girls with scars. To help them gain confidence through their stories. I fear that the biggest issue in our society and the CF community with the developments of social media is the art of comparison."

"Erinn is naturally beautiful," says Anne, "but I know she has had some insecurities about her scars throughout her life. She has overcome those insecurities and she wants the same for others."

"My parents never allowed me to blame my cystic fibrosis for flaws in my life or if something did not go my way," says Erinn. "They would remind me that I am more than my CF and not everything that happens is a result of that. I learned to take responsibility for every aspect of my life, including my health. I believe that this shaped my outlook on life and what contributed to me having such a life outside of cystic fibrosis."

Today, Erinn remains stable, having moved back to San Diego once her doctors deemed it safe following her transplant. She dreams of getting married someday and eventually having children through surrogacy. In order to keep those dreams alive, Erinn continues to take amazing care of herself. "My current treatment includes twice daily transplant medications," says Erinn. "These include a variation of anti-rejection drugs and steroids. Because I was placed on steroids after the transplant, this caused my blood sugars to rise. I now must manage what is called 'transplant-related diabetes.' I wear an insulin pump and a Dexcom monitor. The combination of the two helps me monitor my blood sugars while administering the correct amount of insulin."

Like many, Erinn was impacted by the pandemic, but it hasn't slowed her down. "All of the pools in my area closed for a year," says Erinn. "During that time, I purchased a treadmill for my home. This allowed me to be able to work out safely and stay healthy and strong inside my home. I just recently began swimming once a week in a public pool while I rebuild my endurance. I also play soccer once a week through an adult team in San Diego. It is a co-ed team that I have been playing on for about three years now."

Erinn sees sports as a metaphor for life. "In swimming, we often say that many will start the race fast but very few finish strong," says Erinn. "I think it's safe to say that in life, I was quick off the blocks. I slowed down significantly in the middle of my race, but I have every intention of finishing the race stronger than I started it."

DYLAN MORTIMER

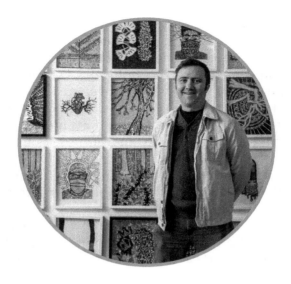

Age: 42
Resides: Los Angeles, California
Age at Diagnosis: 3 months

THE ART OF BEATING CF:
FAMED ARTIST SURVIVES TWO TRANSPLANTS

Dylan Mortimer not only brings art to life. He also tells about his life through his art. Dylan was diagnosed at three months old with cystic fibrosis in 1979. He was doing pretty well in elementary school and began taking a liking to art in the third and fourth grade when he started watching other kids draw cartoon characters.

Dylan's passion appeared to be basketball though—his prize possessions were his Air Jordan sneakers—but his choice form of self-expression would emerge as adversity reared its head.

About the time he entered middle and high school, Dylan's lung function began to decline, and he had more exacerbations. In fact, he was in a hospital room in 1989 when the CF gene was discovered, and Dylan thought this was a cause for celebration. "The news was so big,

I thought a cure for cystic fibrosis would occur in the next five to ten years," he says. "Of course, that did not happen."

Viewing his CF as a source of pity, Dylan often hid his CF from everyone around him. "I felt insecure and unseen in middle and high school, initially," he says, "largely because of CF. I wasn't able to do things most other kids were doing by that time. And honestly, I wasn't very interested in what others were doing. So, I channeled all that energy into creating things. I was very introverted and at times felt very alone. I did not tell many people I had CF. But creating things was, firstly, a way for me to engage, cope, and eventually stand out and gain an increasing sense of identity and purpose both within myself and outside to others."

As he became more introverted, Dylan began taking his art to the next level and, as a senior in high school, began producing bigger pieces.

He went to the Kansas City Art Institute, where his passion continued to grow, and received his bachelor of fine arts. He then pursued his master of fine arts at the School of Visual Arts in New York. Meanwhile, he was working as a pastor at his church, the same profession his father had for many years.

In 2004, four days prior to leaving for graduate school in New York, Dylan met a young woman at his church named Shannon. Dylan, twenty-four at the time, admits he was not looking for a relationship. "I saw CF as a burden, and I didn't want to put that on anyone else," he says. Still, Dylan says that the two of them seemed to click immediately. "Shannon actually seemed excited about being on my cystic fibrosis journey."

"When I found out Dylan had CF, it was an obstacle I felt we could overcome together in faith," says Shannon. "Rather than a hindrance, I saw it as a battle he had been fighting that I wanted to join."

Dylan was suddenly reluctant to move so far way but his calling remained strong, and he made the big move. "We kept in touch via email and phone," says Dylan. "This was long before the days of the social media craze." He and Shannon were married the following year.

Shannon joined Dylan in New York until he finished graduate school. A year later, they moved back to Kansas City where Dylan returned to work as the church pastor. They soon began trying to have children through IVF and "were blessed with Noah," he says. Two and a half years later, after another round of IVF, their second son, Liam, joined the family.

While Dylan primarily worked as a pastor, art was relegated to a moonlighting endeavor. As he was selling more pieces, he began to see that art could be his full-time profession. But while Dylan was enjoying his family and his art, his health was beginning to decline, and once his lung function was at 25 percent, the talk of a lung transplant became a reality.

Dylan's response was to, for the first time, begin consciously making art that referenced his CF journey. "As my health worsened, it began to feel right exploring so many aspects and symbols of CF and transplant scars, cells, DNA, bronchial trees, masks . . ." he says. "And people really seemed to respond emotionally. My earlier artwork was about faith and prayer in a more academic way. I didn't consider that I was trying to avoid CF, just thought I was moving beyond it. I don't regret that work but I'm glad I transitioned to incorporating more of the health journey."

Dylan knew that he had found his niche, but more than that he realized his work could be therapeutic to others battling CF and the possibility of lung transplantation. "I was always showing art in galleries and museums," he says, "but the work around health brought a more personal and emotional response: people crying, extreme joy, sending messages, etc. It became my way to transform a seemingly hopeless diagnosis into one of hope."

Dylan's lung function was in the forties when Noah was born but had slipped into the twenties by the time Liam arrived. At thirty-five, he was evaluated and his lung function hovered around the mid to low 30-percent range. Two years later, he was listed, as his lung function had plummeted into the low 20-percent range. Two months later, after four embolizations, he received his first transplant on January 18, 2017, in St. Louis.

"I felt the best I'd ever felt," says Dylan just months after his transplant. The family prepared to move back to Brooklyn so that Dylan could focus on his art.

Just prior to moving back to Brooklyn, Dylan's lung function began to plummet from PFTs in the 90-percent range in June to the 20-percent range in November. He was in chronic rejection. "Climbing up the stairs on the subway was so difficult," says Dylan. "I knew I could do it, but it was definitely challenging." Dylan would need another transplant.

Shannon remembers his toughest days prior to each transplant. "Through all the health challenges," she says, "Dylan stayed as present as possible with the boys, finding ways to run and play football with them when it was nearly killing him. It's been hard for our boys to watch him go through all this. And incredible for them to see him work through both transplants and thrive. He was committed to providing for us, emotionally, financially, and spiritually, even down to ten-percent lung function."

Dylan was listed for a transplant donor through Columbia University. He was told that because of the antibodies developed from the first transplant, it was very unlikely they could find a match, and they suggested he try Duke University which had a larger reach with regard to donors. Then, just prior to getting listed at Duke, Dylan received a strange phone call from a nurse in Kansas City who had seen Dylan's work.

"Her cousin just passed," says Dylan, "and her family wanted to donate his lungs to me because not only had the nurse seen my work, she had read about me on Instagram and wanted to help me." Dylan didn't think a transplant could work that way but, while very rare, it turns out it can. "It is called a 'deceased will donation,'" says Dylan. Still, the likelihood of the lungs being a match were slim. It was far less than a one-percent chance to get matched a second time for me. Because of the antibody issues I had, I was screening out seventy-one percent of potential donors." It seemed so unlikely to him that he didn't even tell Shannon.

"The doctor at Columbia called me the next day to say they were a match," says Dylan. The hospital flew a doctor to Kansas City from New York to inspect the lungs. They approved them and hours later, on April 13, 2019, Dylan was in the operating room.

After a seven-hour surgery, Dylan was breathing again with new lungs. "It was surreal to go through a transplant once and now to do so twice," says Dylan. "A month after surgery, I was jogging and even completed a 10K."

Still, he says that the person who doesn't get enough credit is the woman he married. "Shannon has been inspirational from the moment I told her [about CF]. Rather than seeing it as any reason not to further a relationship with me, she was inspired by the fight and eager to join it. She was my caretaker through both transplants and simultaneously parenting two boys with me. She is proud of me, but I get more attention. She is a true hero, one who chose to enter this life. I am eternally grateful for her!"

"Both transplants were very difficult on our whole family to say the least," says Shannon. "We were so supported in prayer and love and had faith and hope in spite of the circumstances. Love and faith carried us through to be able to take the next step at each point in the journey."

In June 2022, Dylan and his family moved to Los Angeles for new opportunities, for both his art career and Shannon's fitness career. Now living on the West Coast, he has taken advantage of his new lungs by creating more art pieces and previewing them all over the world. His pieces can be found in medical centers, hospitals, and pharmaceutical companies, and, specifically, are big attractions in CF clinics at New York-Presbyterian Hospital, Children's Mercy Kansas City, and at Barnes-Jewish in St. Louis; Vertex Pharmaceuticals, the leader in CFTR modulators around the world, in Boston; and, of course, museums, including the KC Jewish Museum, Longwood Arts in New York, and the Nerman Museum of Contemporary Art in Kansas. His incredible story has been featured in the *New York Times*, the *New York Post*, the *Chicago Tribune*, the *Kansas City Star*, the *Baltimore Sun*, and the *Washington Post*.

Dylan now has an art studio in Los Angeles. "I work primarily in collage and sculpture," he says, "inspired by all this to transform situations and symbols of trauma into those of hope."

He creates glittery interpretations of scars, lungs, and operating rooms, and says his work often starts as a feeling he is experiencing, a memory, or even a situation and soon becomes a sketch. Eventually, he buys glitter by the pound to illustrate this experience with his battle with CF. Many of his sketches include bronchial trees that he contrasts with actual trees and even Air Jordans, with which he is still fascinated, reflective of both his love of basketball and mostly because of the fact that there is air on the bottom of every shoe. "Air is something that people with CF hope for," says Dylan who hopes to one day write a book that features his work. "Art has allowed me to tell about my journey," says Dylan.

"I love how his artwork reflects the struggle and joy both in the journey," says Shannon, to whom Dylan has now been married for two decades. "I love the use of glitter and shiny materials as a way to reveal hope amid the pain and struggle."

Dylan, who makes time to volunteer at the Boomer Esiason Foundation, Rock CF, and the Bonnell Foundation, says his dreams are to see his children as adults, to do some serious traveling, "and to create more art!"

ALEX PANGMAN

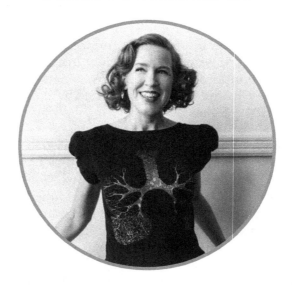

Age: 44
Resides: Toronto, Ontario, Canada
Age at diagnosis: 18 months

CANADA'S SWEETHEART OF SWING: SINGER FACES THE MUSIC

"**C**anada's Sweetheart of Swing" Alex Pangman was diagnosed with CF when she was eighteen months old, prior to which, "the doctors thought I was being overly concerned," says her mom, Connie. "But Alex was never happy, was salty to kiss, and got bad pneumonia." Finally, by virtue of a sweat test at eighteen months, a doctor confirmed the worst of Connie's fears: Alex had CF.

"The doctor said to [me], 'Aren't you happy you know what it is?' and [I] said, 'No. I'm not happy!' The bottom fell out of my stomach." Still, the doctor tried to comfort Connie by telling her the outlook for patients was so much better and more hopeful than when Connie was a nurse in the 1960s.

As postural drainage became less possible for Alex due to pernicious and tenacious hemoptysis (coughing up blood) around the age of twelve, a gentler way of agitating her chest secretions was desired.

"How about pony physio?" Alex, who had been taking riding lessons since the age of nine, suggested to her mom. Despite a lack of evidence that riding horses was beneficial for lung clearance—"Pony physio was *my* term," Alex says—doctors agreed to let Alex try, and Alex's parents let her get a pony, but only on the condition that she wore a body vest to protect her enlarged CF liver and spleen in case she fell.

Alex, already under her spell of equines with her exposure to her mother's and grandmother's horses, kept active with her new pony Gypsy, which the family purchased for Alex the week she turned thirteen. The beautiful chestnut mare helped with her fitness and, indeed, with mucus clearance. Most importantly, perhaps, Gypsy helped keep Alex happy.

"Gypsy has always played an incredible role in my life," says Alex. "She was more than just my daily physiotherapy. She gave me something other than chest physiotherapy to wake up to in the mornings. Gypsy was also my best friend and constant companion."

Alex describes herself as "scrawny" when she was growing up. "Thanks to CF," she says. "I was always trying to take on calories. I also dealt with many bouts of hemoptysis, which was often brought on by postural drainage performed by my family. Eventually, I had to give up on this form of airway clearance and depend on pony physio, which I admit is probably not the most effective route when trying to clear the lungs."

Alex missed a lot of school due to hospital admissions and says her CF scared away friends and boyfriends, but she always felt fortunate to have the support of her family and, of course, Gypsy. "Gypsy was not scared off by CF," says Alex. "She was steadfast. She knew when I was feeling well enough to enjoy a gallop in the field, and she likewise could sense when I was feeling poorly and needed her to be solid and slow beneath me. Her gifts at assessing my health were something akin to magic. Sometimes she could almost pre-cognitively sense things, slowing down moments before I began to spit up blood. Gypsy came into my life as my angel, and nanny." Twenty years into their partnership, not only were Alex and Gypsy competing in and winning jumping competitions, but Gypsy was even carrying Alex's oxygen tanks.

Connie credits Alex with her uncanny resilience. "It's just the way [she was]: brave; gutsy. We tried not to make our house a house of sick people. John [Alex's dad, now deceased] and I tried to make it fun for [Alex], but [her] positive, gutsy outlook just came from [Alex]."

The successful therapy opened Alex's lungs, and the door to another one of Alex's passions: singing. "I gravitated to my parents' record player as a child and would practice singing into a hairbrush," says

Alex. "I loved to sing. Much like with the pony, my parents had a hard time telling me no. I clearly remember my mother voicing concerns to the doctors at SickKids in Toronto about singing in smoky nightclubs (at the time), and the fact that I had lung disease in general might be thought of as stressful and her being told that singing could be good for me, delivering air into the base of my lungs."

Alex notes that her career started when she landed the title role in *Annie* her junior year of high school. "Having red hair didn't hurt my chances," jokes Alex. "Singing gave me a purpose and an anchor. It fed my soul. I was so happy when I was singing, and that is really all the encouragement [my family and I] needed. In a life studded with hospital visits and postural drainage, music seemed like a panacea, and a way to thumb our nose at the CF gene. As it turned out, all that breathing into a microphone taught me very good breath control, which served me well as the scarring began to take over my lungs. CF patients are hyper aware of their lungs. A CF vocalist? Even more so!"

As the years went on, singing became her identity. So much so that she decided to become a professional singer when one too many hospital admissions caused her to lose a year at university. "When I got out of the hospital, it had become clear to me," says Alex, "I was going to do singing because that is what I loved."

Alex's first big fan was Gypsy. "I stumbled onto my nascent career while playing guitar and singing to my pony," says Alex. "A fellow equestrian took my guitar and played some jazz to me, right there sitting on a hay bale. I'd never heard this music form before. In the months that followed, he encouraged me with old records which I'd learn tunes from and perform with him at the local schnitzel house, of all places.

"I was soon falling in love with songs and artists from the 1920s and '30s. I fell in love with the beautiful melodies and found the lyrics to be so poetical. I began singing in my small town and incubated there, learning more songs and confidence. Eventually, I went to the big town, Toronto, where I would meet more and more musicians my age to work with who also loved this music from a bygone era. Through many, many performances in dance halls, nightclubs, and concert halls, I learned my trade. I never went to music school, I just listened to a lot of records and learned on stage. I feel like I grew up on a stage surrounded by musicians. Eventually, larger and larger bookings came, records happened, videos, recording contracts. I was working with world-renown musicians and was dubbed 'Canada's Sweetheart of Swing' by Dan Barrett, a trombonist who played at the Toronto jazz festival."

One fall afternoon at Toronto's Cameron House, during the intermission at one of his Country Bluegrass concerts, Alex made the acquaintance of mandolin player Tom Parker. "I was out on the town to hear some mandolin," she says, "and knew that Tom Parker played one. I'd always loved country music, and had a mandolin that I was struggling with, so I thought I should go hear some country music played by this popular band with a good reputation for old-school country.

"In a small room, it isn't hard to 'fraternize' with the musicians on set break. Tom and I had met once many months before, so he knew who I was and about my reputation as a jazz singer, and we struck up a chat as he was passing the tip jar. Conversation was easy and he offered to help set up my mandolin, which had some questionable intonation. Looking back now, it probably seemed like a preconceived pickup line, but it wasn't. I really was out on the town to hear some music. I'm not complaining that I got more than I bargained for!" Alex says she was dating someone at the time but that it was falling apart. "When it did," she says, "Tom was there with heart in hand."

The two began dating, and not only did he not balk at the discovery of Alex's CF, he also embraced it. "A realist, but an eternal optimist," says Alex describing Tom, "he came to the hospital to see me [during an admission]. There he was, magazine and CDs/radio in hand for me at the hospital, and me in my blue gown looking like hell. He knew what he was getting into from the start, but he so clearly saw me and not merely the trappings of my illness. He is a very special man. Others before him had left me for fear of the CF."

Alex and Tom were engaged by the next spring. "We walked up the aisle with a PICC line in my arm in 2006," says Alex. "I feel very blessed to have found a partner as truly strong and special as he."

"Thinking about seeing Alex struggle through the bad times makes me realize how strong her life force is and always has been," says Tom. "Her perseverance is a testament to her take on life. She doesn't let hard times destroy her spirit, and she is happy to put the most difficult times behind her and to live as much in the present as she can."

In 2008, Alex was struggling more than ever. She was told by her physician, Dr. Stevenson, that she had a 50/50 chance of surviving more than a year if she did not "hurry and get listed for a lung transplant," says Alex. "At this point, I was already resistant to most IV antibiotics and was getting smaller, and weaker, and less able to do the things that defined me: singing loudly, galloping on ponies, and having a social life outside of pills, tubing, and oxygen tanks."

Antibiotic resistance happens because bacteria change in ways that eventually reduce and often eliminate the potency of drugs used to treat infections, thus the bacteria can now survive the drugs that could destroy them. When a patient takes an abundance of antibiotics, resistance is, unfortunately, a common result. Alex and Tom hung in there for six long months of waiting for new lungs as Alex's health continued to deteriorate. She was warding off one infection after another, enduring endless courses of IVs, oxygen hoses, coughing fits, and panic attacks. She was flirting with numbers like 25 percent FEV1. That number ceased to rebound after a course of antibiotics, which became scary because she didn't know when or if lungs might arrive. And yet, in her darkest hour, Alex found herself part of a special group of people.

"It was interesting to be part of the community at the transplant hospital," says Alex. "Three times a week, everyone on the list had to show up at the 'treadmill room' and walk on the treadmill, do our stretches and squats (to be strong for after transplant), and pedal that dreaded stationary bike. I hated the exertion, but I met so many friends there who were in the same boat as me. They were all seeing their numbers diminish, all hoping for 'the call.' Once in a while, someone would get a transplant and come back to the treadmill room reborn, and we'd all get inspired and happy and feel our morale reinvigorated. I tried not to concentrate on the what-ifs and negatives. I just had to get it done and stay positive. But honestly, I was exhausted. I was helpless and very dependent on other people for help. My coughing muscles ached. I was scared of bleeding out from hemoptysis, and I was out of breath . . . and almost out of time."

Alex's first call about a possible new set of lungs turned out to be a false alarm. "A calm voice tells you, 'We may have a set of lungs available for you and you need to come to the hospital right away,'" says Alex. "The lungs and the heart that day went to another patient who was ahead of me on the urgent list. Had the heart not passed muster, it would have been my chance at the lungs. It was a very emotional thing, to be waiting and hoping and fretting in one room, only to hear the celebrations in the next room when the other needy person won the coin toss. Driving home that day in the sunshine was something else. Deflated, in shock, I sat in the backyard and the waiting recommenced. I know the false alarm meant I was reaching the top of the list, so we tried to stay hopeful with that tidbit of inspiration. You grab onto any hope in that instance."

In November of 2008, a donor came to the rescue. "The day I got my lungs I was awoken in the morning," says Alex, "not by my pager, as I'd expected, but by my telephone. It interrupted a dream where I was washing my hair without an oxygen tank (a task that had become arduous in the months leading to transplant). It all happened rather quickly this time— heart thumping, I got in touch with Tom who was teaching at the Toronto District School at the time and said, 'Round two!'"

"I don't remember what I was thinking at the time," says Tom. "I just knew I had to get to the hospital ASAP."

"And off we went," says Alex. "This time things moved much more quickly, and before we knew it, I was in a blue gown saying tearful so-longs to my close family.

"Before the surgery began," says Alex, "I remember telling the team in the OR who was busy all around me in the bright room, 'Please watch out for my vocal cords when you intubate me. I'm a singer.' The team said not to worry—in fact, the anesthetist told me, 'I'll look after you like you were my own sister.' I remember her smile. I didn't know her name, but she calmed me in those final moments."

After her eight-hour transplant, Alex remembers being in a darkened room that was quiet except for beeping and blinking machines. "I was still intubated and that panicked me a little," says Alex. "The nurse sang a hymn to me, and it calmed me down. I never knew her name, or if I did, it was quickly absorbed in the blur of postoperative meds. Her presence was warm and caring. She was near the bed. Panic and pain are not uncommon after transplant surgeries, so I suspect she knew that some patients need calming. I wish I could remember the hymn, but it, too, was obliterated by my mental state. Sometimes good people come into and out of your life and you never know their names. I never knew the name of my first donor either, but they gave me an incredible gift. This nurse also gifted me some calm in that dark room of beeping machines.

"I suspected I was alive because I was feeling things! I remember family near the bed, and scrawling down on a piece of paper, 'Is it over? Did it happen?' It was happy news to know I was on the post side of the lung transplant. Even happier news when they told me to exhale, and out came that tube. What a relief."

Alex knew that a return to her singing career was not a given. "The greater risk to my singing career," she says, "was if I didn't get the transplant. So, I knew that any hope of survival (and singing) depended on a transplant. Of course, I worried about my career, but I worried more for my life in the lead up to the pager going off. Singing had taken a backseat but singing and horses were the prize I kept my eye on."

The nurses in the ICU played some of Alex's music from YouTube to remind her of her passion. "I don't think I personally sang for at least a week," says Alex, "just a few notes in the hospital, and then not really a full song until I got home when I discovered that I was able to make phrases so much more easily than pre-transplant! Only thing was, the stitches were still in and my chest was tight, and that kept slowing down my phrasing. Still, I could do it!"

It took Alex a while to get back to professional singing. "I had a lot of healing and med changes to adjust to," she says. At first, the anti-rejection medication gave her a slight tremor, which included her vocal cords. "I had a very fancy vibrato for a few months," she says, jokingly. "As the dose was lowered, I got control of my voice back and sounded more like myself, and it felt excellent. It was as if someone had replaced my broken-down tricycle with a shiny new Ferrari! In fact, my career really took off after my transplant when I was well enough to tour more and make more recordings. I think the doctors were delighted too.

"It really was so much easier to sing without constantly coughing. My lungs filled with so much more air supporting my voice. I could sing louder, longer, stronger. I could finally sing how I'd always wanted to; it was amazing! I think it was most touching for my CF doctors to hear since they'd known me so long and watched me get so sick. For them to see me reach my potential without lungs ravaged by CF meant a lot. That being said, some of my biggest fans are transplant doctors, and I have to say, the feeling is mutual!"

One of Alex's first orders of business was to, quite literally, get back in the saddle. "I remember that first time swinging my leg up over and into the saddle post-transplant," says Alex. "It had been several weeks, but my legs found their place in the leather like no time had passed. I think I did some walking around, grinning from ear to ear, and then gradually tried some trotting. It was so much easier now than before the transplant. What a joy! Now I just had to get fit again, and in time, Gypsy and I even competed in some jumping again. Me, the double-lung recipient, and my (by then) very old pony, Gypsy. It was a double triumph to win a first-place ribbon that summer together."

Returning to sing after her first transplant was a slow thing for Alex. "I had too much vibrato for a time from the medications," she said, "and I was shy to go out without full control, but also scared of being in public as I'd struggled for a time with low white cell count and was sheltering from germs. I can't quite recall how it happened, but I'd gone out with Tom to hear a friend play some New Orleans music at a small club in town. As is not uncommon, I was asked up by my friends to sit in. I did. I sang. It was great fun, and it was also when I learned that adrenaline mixed with high med levels gave me an even more tremulous voice, but also [my] legs and hands shook too. Nonetheless, this small jam session with me in a small club was a giant leap for post-transplant! I was back!"

But in 2012, it became clear when her lung function dropped off for no obvious reason that she was experiencing chronic rejection. "I was re-listed for transplant," says Alex. "I was fighting off infections so often that it contributed to the rejection, we think. I learned about the balance between rejection and infection firsthand. I have to admit, chronic rejection felt way more suffocating than end-stage CF had. It just felt different. In CF when I felt short of breath, my oxygen SATS were always low. Not so with rejection. I'd feel so short of breath, but the SATS would be normal. It was a mind game as much as a body game."

In June 2013, while battling chronic infection, Alex also had a wonderful opportunity to open for legendary country music artist Willie Nelson at Massey Hall, a famous performing arts theatre in Toronto. "I was twelve minutes away from the transplant hospital. My pager was on. My game face was on. When I woke up that morning, all the humidity left Toronto, which is saying something for midsummer. What you need to know is that without the humidity, I could breathe and sing so much more easily. Seated on stage on a lovely tall stool loaned to me by Willie's crew, I pulled the biggest fast one of my life: a jazz singer, who was waiting for a lung transplant, opening for a country legend, and wasn't about to let on. Yes, I needed the stool to keep from being breathless, but I did it. Jazz singers have purred on bar stools for a century now! What they didn't know didn't hurt them. Massey Hall is a jewel of a venue, and I thought, *Well, if my pager never goes off, at least I'll go out on a high note!* at one of Canada's best venues. My voice in that room? Those boys in the band? It was magical. And for one hour, I was 'Alex the star,' and not 'Alex the patient.'"

Two months later, in August 2013, a second donor's lungs presented themselves. "This time, things went a little smoother," says Alex. "I'm grateful to my second donor as well. Honestly, transplant life is not a cure, but it sure is a life raft, and I'm so grateful that it has come into my life.

"Post-transplant the second time around, I came home after a couple of weeks recovery, but I'd been struggling to find a substitute vocalist to fill in for me at a jazz festival we were supposed to play at in Port Hope, Ontario, later that month. Well, with no understudy in sight, I decided to just play the gig. I mean, it was only a one-hour-long concert, and I was on lots of prednisone which made me feel like a super woman, so I just sang the gig. Ha! I hadn't even opened my mouth to sing with a band until sound check. I couldn't even wear a bra yet because of the stitches . . . but there I was, on stage in front of hundreds of people. It was not just that I was still on opiate pain killers, that gig was one of the thrills of my life! So many good feels! The audience, none the wiser to my condition, responded to the amazing energy on stage between my friends, the musicians, and I. [They] stood up and gave us a standing ovation. I was in tears of joy! Amazing. The music just poured out of me!"

Alex was soon singing ten to fifteen songs per show before her voice and body would become exhausted. Six months after the operation, she was able to sing thirty songs in a night and, by March of 2014, Alex was in the recording studio again for her album *New*, which she recorded about six months after her second transplant. She was nominated for a JUNO, Canada's version of the Grammy. Tom is just happy to hear Alex sing. "Either on stage or singing in our kitchen!" he says.

Along with her singing career, Alex returned to something with which she has been involved since 2006: organ donation. "Since 2006, well before my first transplant in 2008, I've been an advocate for the cause," says Alex. "I did a Christmas CD and each copy had a donor card in it, which was a perfect launch point to sell the idea of donation. There was even a Christmas song I rewrote about waiting for transplant."

Today, Alex routinely gives PSAs from stages across the country. "I've spoken at the mass memorial service/award ceremony for donors and their families twice, played shows for the Lung Association and Oxygen companies, written a song at the Toronto Jazz Festival that benefited the Lung Association called 'Breathe In' and spoken on national radio, television, and print multiple times over." Sixteen hundred individuals in her home province of Ontario are waiting for a lifesaving organ transplant, and one of them dies every three days because they failed to receive their transplant on time. "Now, after having two transplants because of the kindness of strangers," says Alex, "of course I feel even more compelled to support the cause."

Post-recovery from Alex's second transplant, thirty-plus-year-old Gypsy was showing her most obvious signs of aging. "She tore a tendon, not from any real accident but just from old age," says Alex. Now, the tables turned, it was Alex's turn to look after her ailing pony. "I gladly erected the recovery pen, gladly walked beside her in the long months of recovery when she could not be ridden, gladly bent down and dressed her legs in poultices and bandages for months and months, gladly grated her carrots into mush when her teeth became problematic. She was the most deserving creature; I would do it all again."

Gypsy did make a recovery of sorts, and Alex was able to accompany her for measured daily rides through the woods that they both loved so dearly. "She knew the sound of my voice in the stable and would call out to me when she heard me arrive." In December 2015, after a short illness, Gypsy passed at the age of thirty-seven. "Sure, we won awards in our youth," says Alex, "but her being my caretaker is better than all of our showing wins put together."

As of this story's publication, due to the pandemic, Alex only performs in virtual concerts. "Singing during the pandemic has been limited to mostly online gigs," she says. "This is amplified in my case because my anti-rejection medications make me immunosuppressed which increases the risk of contracting COVID-19. Singing livestreams has kept me musically engaged and alive! I joke that it's 1930s music using 2020s technology! I also joke that this music has seen folks through the Great Depression, wars, and previous pandemics—it's perfectly designed to lift the spirits and console us again. Mostly, making music is what I do—I am a singer. Bringing music to people, connecting to them, even when I can't see their faces, has been very fulfilling. Sometimes people are listening from across the globe. I've never met them, but they are hearing us play music online. So, just like strangers saved my life, or the nameless nurse sang at my bedside, I feel like I can pay it forward by bringing music to other strangers that I may not know. And there's something that feels great about that. To bring beauty to people and joy and happiness. Seems like the right thing to do, especially now, because transplant has brought joy and happiness back into my life."

7

RUNNING FOR OUR LIVES: THE CF RUNNERS

MICHAEL CARUSO DAVIS

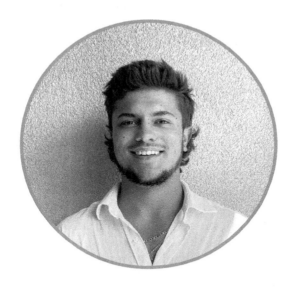

Age: 19
Resides: Townsend, Delaware
Age at Diagnosis: 3 weeks

THE RHINO: AGE IS NO EXCUSE

Michael Caruso Davis lives life by what he calls the *rhino mentality*. "Whatever is thrown my way," says Michael, "I put my head down and go straight through it."

In June of 2021, Michael completed the Ironman 70.3 Eagle Man in Cambridge, Maryland, becoming the youngest male in the United States with cystic fibrosis to do so. Quite an accomplishment for a man who's spent his whole life in and out of hospitals, being admitted about three times a year for about four to six weeks at a time.

"When Michael was first diagnosed at three weeks old, as a new mom I was devastated and scared," says his mom, Jen. "Scared wondering what the future would hold, scared I was going to lose my sweet baby boy. But our family quickly rallied behind us, and together we tackled everything that had come our way with strength and grace."

Michael does over two hours of breathing treatments and swallows forty pills daily. "I have always been very compliant with doing my treatments and taking my medicine," says Michael. "I've been told I was going to die young, not be able to be physically active like others, need a lung transplant, and many more things that no child nor person should have to hear. But my family has always tried their best to make my life as normal as possible despite having this harsh disease."

When he was in the fourth grade, he discovered a love for running through the Boomer Esiason Foundation and was inspired by older CF athletes, such as sixty-five-year-old Jerry Cahill, and signed up for his first 5K. He finished in first place! "Back then, a 5K was a lot for me and I was extremely proud of myself," says Michael. "Ever since then I have been chasing that feeling which I get at every finish line." Jerry has been inspired by young Michael as well. "Michael Davis is an amazing man who is living, breathing, and succeeding with CF," says Jerry, "and in the game of life. Michael is committed to his health, nutrition, mental well-being, and above all, his loving family and friends."

At the age of twelve, Michael had an unusual request with each tune-up. "Each admission I would request a treadmill to be brought into my room and I would run daily," says Michael. "I found running as a way to strengthen my lungs and keep me healthy and hospital-free along with the new medications on the market." Michael has taken full advantage of CFTR modulators as he has gotten older. He started Orkambi in August of 2015, Symdeko in April of 2018, and Trikafta in November of 2019.

His scariest moment came in 2015 when, at the age of twelve, Michael's lung function plummeted from the mid- to high-nineties baseline into the mid-sixties as he was diagnosed with acid-fast bacillus, or AFB—a type of bacteria that causes certain infections like tuberculosis. He says his doctor told him he was going to die young and that, to rid him of the AFB, he'd need a nine-month treatment with side effects that included a loss of hearing.

"As crazy as it sounds," says Michael, "I am so thankful for that doctor, because that was the moment I decided to give everything I've got into fighting this disease even harder." Michael and his family made three big adjustments: they moved down by the beach so he could regularly breathe the salt air, he officially made running a lifestyle, and he added surfing to his list of hobbies. The result was that his lung function rose into the mid-eightieth percentile, which got his AFB under control and relieved him of the need for the nine-month treatment.

"I could use having cystic fibrosis as an excuse to sit on my butt and feel sorry for myself," says Michael. "Instead, I use it as fuel to live each and every day to its fullest. I view life very differently because of having CF. I enjoy the little things and live more in the moment than many others, because tomorrow truly isn't promised."

In 2016, at age fourteen, during another hospital admission where his lung function had dropped into the low-seventy percent range, Michael was determined to fight and trained for the next eight weeks for his next athletic achievement. Michael signed up for and completed his first half-marathon, which took place in New York City. "When I crossed that finish line, I knew anything I set my mind to, could be done," says Michael. He ran another New York City half-marathon as well as the Rocky Run half-marathon in Philadelphia before diversifying his résumé to include two sprint triathlons, a forty-mile bike ride, and an Olympic triathlon. Then, in October of 2019, he completed the Chicago Marathon, making history as the youngest person (age sixteen) with CF to complete a full marathon. To mark the achievement, his picture was placed on a billboard in the middle of Times Square in New York City.

Michael wakes up two hours before his peers to do his treatments so he can be ready for an early lacrosse practice and either doubles his treatments from two to four when he is sick or just finds more time to exercise. "Exercise has helped my lungs so much," he says.

For the Ironman, he trained six days a week for twenty weeks. "The seventh day was a recovery day, meaning yoga, foam rolling, ice baths, etc., so I really didn't have any days completely off," says Michael, who supports the Boomer Esiason Foundation as a member of Team Boomer through his endurance events by raising both funds and awareness. "I did three runs, three bikes, and three swims a week. The weekends were my longer training days, being over an hour or a brick workout, which meant biking followed directly by a run."

"When I first met Michael, I knew close to nothing about cystic fibrosis," says Michael's girlfriend, Kayleigh. "I remember early in our relationship we watched the movie *Five Feet Apart* together. It wasn't until then that it hit me how much work went into fighting this disease. I always do my best to make him feel comfortable about being open with me, especially concerning his CF. We've gone from him being nervous to do treatments in front of me to it being our every night routine to watch TV together while he does them. Seeing firsthand all the hard work he puts in every day to stay healthy has only made me love him more. He is the most determined, dedicated, and inspiring person I have ever met. Watching him set goals and accomplish them motivates me to be the best version of myself every day. Michael's light shines over anyone he is around, and I'm so grateful to know him and his amazing family."

"Being Michael's mom has brought with it worry and heartache," says Jen, "but most of all, it has brought me the greatest joy in life, which is being his mom! I am so incredibly proud of how he has handled this journey and thankful for all the support from his friends and family along the way."

"My "why" is what keeps me going on a daily basis," says Michael, who recently was named the 2022 Wishes & Dreams for CF Shining Star. He is now a student at the University of Delaware and aspires to complete an *ultra*marathon. "I strive to inspire others with and without CF. I get my strength from those who have lost their battle to CF. I also think about the people close to me who have passed away. I know they are all watching over me, cheering me on. I am not wired differently than anyone else. I am not special. I have no natural talents. What I am is determined. Nothing beats hard work and there is simply no substitute for it. I am where I am today due to teamwork with my family and doctors, new medications on the market, and my passion for endurance sports like running and triathlon. I know that all the late nights and early mornings will all pay off at the finish line. I think of it like building my own empire: every training session, I lay down bricks to build this empire, and when my time comes to go to heaven, I will leave behind an empire. And it starts with my breathing."

BRADLEY J. DRYBURGH

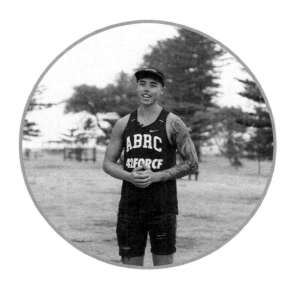

Age: 25
Resides: Wollongong, New South Wales, Australia
Age at Diagnosis: 3 weeks

#42FORCF: THE STORYTELLER SHARES HIS OWN STORY

"**A** person's only real obligation in life is to find their purpose and relentlessly pursue it for the rest of their days," says Bradley Dryburgh who left his lucrative real estate career to be a full-time "storyteller" through his fundraising initiative #42forCF and *A Lot To Talk About*, an audio and YouTube podcast on which he interviews inspiring people around the world with the intent of helping listeners in their twenties and thirties as they navigate the trials and tribulations of life. He refers to it as his "pride and joy."

"Real estate isn't my purpose, and money isn't my motivation. At a young age, I told my family that I would change the world. My goal is to be a world-class storyteller. I am on a journey to realize that."

Bradley's résumé is chock full of tangible successes, from athletic to entrepreneurial, and yet it's an intangible quality—his relentless positivity, the kind that inspires action—that seems to make him so unique.

"I was incredibly [fortunate] that I had the best dad, mum, and sister any kid could ask for," says Bradley. "Encouraged to be whoever I wanted to be, my childhood was full of athletic endeavors and good health. CF, liver disease, [and] diabetes weren't going to hold me back or dictate what was possible for me."

When Bradley was diagnosed with cystic fibrosis through a standard procedure called the Guthrie Test at just three weeks of age, a doctor told his parents that CF would ruin his life. "You will never see our son again," his parents said in unison. After a deep search, they found Dr. John Morton at Sydney Children's Hospital who joined them in embracing a positive outlook for Bradley's future.

"I was extremely outgoing and confident as a child," says Bradley. "I still am. I was even vocal about my CF. For me, it was a badge of honor to be beating my circumstances on a daily basis." Bradley's routine in his early years, up until the age of five or six, included postural drainage twice a day; however, the introduction of the pep mask replaced that routine. He used Pulmozyme and hypertonic saline through a nebulizer while occasionally using tobramycin. His digestive enzymes were taken with each meal in the amount necessary and every day included some form of exercise.

"I competed in sports seven days a week," says Bradley, who took a particular liking to rugby and track, which not only kept him in tiptop shape, but, at the age of nine, resulted in state one-hundred- and two-hundred-meter track titles in the state private school system in New South Wales. At the age of twelve, he expanded his interest in physical activity to include a disciplined gym regimen which he says was inspired by his father. "My dad has always been really fit and looked muscular my whole life, so I always wanted to be like him, and that's what inspired me to step foot in the gym."

From sixteen to eighteen, Bradley was in the gym Monday to Friday. He ran a few kilometers during each weight session until he left for university at the age of seventeen. Over the next two years, he focused on weights but regrets stopping the cardio activity because of the benefits it had on his lungs. He also spent a lot of time bodyboarding in the ocean which he says was great for his lung health due to the saltwater. "I never missed out on anything due to my CF. That was a credit to my attitude and healthy endeavors."

Bradley says that, at a young age, he became very educated about his cystic fibrosis. "Whilst I've always been motivated to stay healthy, I believe this comes with a great understanding of health and how cystic fibrosis works. My early understanding was through asking questions at my clinic appointments and doing my own research to further develop that understanding. I studied some level of human physiology in my fitness career and that helped me to understand the exercise that would have real impact on good CF health."

At eighteen, Bradley was watching a movie with his father when he suffered from his first bout of hemoptysis and he was rushed to the emergency room. "I called my mum and sister who were working together at the time," he says. "I was quite worried. To experience your first bleed and not understand what is happening inside your body is terrifying. I'm never pessimistic but for the first time in my life I wondered whether I would see my mum and sister again and whether Dad would have to experience the loss of his son firsthand." He spent the entire trip to the hospital managing his mind, trying to keep it from spiraling to the worst-case scenario, which is to say a fatal diagnosis. "Within a few hours, I knew I was going to be okay." Fortunately, it turned out to "just be" pneumonia and was treatable with a three-week-long stay in the hospital.

Though he had subsequent hospital visits to address similarly dire circumstances, Bradley had developed a tried-and-true way of processing the fear and anxiety that can accompany such critical states. Since the pneumonia episode, he's had three more lung bleeds that led to hospitalization.

"Every good story presents the main character with a new challenge to disrupt the triumph," says Bradley, "and at eighteen years of age, pneumonia was mine and it wouldn't be the last. For the past seven years, I have had my ups and downs. Lung infections and lung bleeds being the major culprits of my trip to the ward and ED [emergency department]. While they present a hurdle to overcome, I believe my greatest asset in my fight against CF is the strength of my mind and character." Bradley says that he did not have a single watershed moment. "It took three to four watershed moments—mostly through lung infections that led to ten- to fourteen-day hospital stays before the final moment that changed my perspective for good. That would be the bleed in 2020 that inspired #42forCF and a lifestyle I wanted to share with the world that now feels like second nature."

The hashtag refers to Bradley's quest to run a marathon (42.2 kilometers), which he started training for to raise money for Cystic Fibrosis Australia. Bradley says that quest likely started when he was a young child. "I wrote and illustrated little books often about the hero's journey and the discovery of life. As the years went on, that process became more about sharing my own story in hopes to inspire others. As they say, a picture speaks a thousand words, and I know the image of a CF patient overcoming lung bleeds to cross the finish line of marathons is a form of poetry in motion that will strike a chord in the CF world more powerful than that of the spoken word."

Bradley says he always hated running long distances. Then in June and July 2020, "I started doing slow 5K runs with mates just once a week for three weeks before I had my three lung bleeds." Rather than ditching the effort, he doubled down, recognizing the inspirational message he'd be sending if he were able to run a marathon in the wake of three lung bleeds. On December 12, 2020, Bradley conquered his marathon and raised $56,000 for CF Australia.

"#42forCF is proof that no challenge is too big to overcome if you believe in yourself," says Bradley, "and I hope it inspires CF patients the world over." His podcast began on February 12, 2020, and just two and a half months in, he had walked away from his career in real estate. "I believe that my purpose is to be a world-class storyteller. My CF message in all honesty isn't a part of my purpose. While CF is part of my life, it is not who I am nor how I define myself. I see it more so as a blessing and great teacher—the reminder that life is not meant to be easy and that's what makes it so beautiful. However, I am glad that on the journey of fulfilling my purpose, being a positive role model for CF patients and their families will come with the territory."

On October 16, 2021, Bradley ran another marathon for CF Australia and expected from himself a stronger showing than his run in December 2020. His training consisted of several days filled with cardio. "I run three to four mornings a week," he says. "One of those is always a long run, often a half-marathon. The others are more moderate five to fifteen kilometers or interval work, depending on what stage of my training I am in." He also lifts weights two to three days a week, in the evenings, at a gym. "Purpose fuels progress," says Bradley, "and I believe that's where the love for running began—as a purpose outside of myself."

The run on the sixteenth did not go as Bradley had planned. "I began cramping at the thirty-kilometer mark," says Bradley. "My lungs struggled a little and I found myself shivering on the ground. I asked my team to go ahead and finish strong, but they refused to leave me, and I cannot thank them enough for that." Bradley intends to use the setback to motivate his comeback for his next marathon on May 14, 2022.

Bradley's quick to cite his father, mother, and "little sis, Shania [two and a half years younger and a CF carrier]" as his first orbit of support. "They are my everything," he says. "They ingrained the belief in me that I would go on to do incredible things in this world. It's the reason I do what I do today, and without them, I know my life would be very different."

Bradley also mentions the boost he gets from his running companions, the "Active Boys Run Club," founded by two other guys who wanted to create a guys' group for the creation of healthy habits. "Since I started running with those guys," says Bradley, "it has grown to be a large group of men *and* women who love challenging each other and being alongside each other on that journey. A lot of the crew ran #42forCF alongside me."

Bradley continues, "I hope to inspire not just people with CF but the world to live life to the fullest. To find purpose and relentlessly pursue it for the rest of your days. That is the meaning of life."

Bradley says his routine today is pretty consistent. "Mid-afternoon, after I return from my podcast studio, I do my nebulizers and physiotherapy. I take most of my tablets when I wake up or get out of bed and my digestive enzymes as needed with meals." Bradley qualifies for Trikafta and says Australia expects to have the drug approved by the end of 2022.

But his *perfect* day includes diving into the ocean, grabbing a coffee with mates, hanging with his family—"whom I adore more than anything"—watching a game of "footy" (Australian rules football), and sharing an inspiring story with his listeners.

Bradley qualified for Trikafta and recently received the exciting news that the drug was listed on the Pharmaceutical Benefits Scheme (PBS) for the first time in Australia, beginning on April 1, 2022. "On the twenty-seventh of March, 2022, I woke up to news of Trikafta's PBS listing," says Bradley. "With a new sense of hope, my life flashed before my eyes. I could see the kid who was told he never had a chance but fought for his life anyways. I watched the young man with bleeding lungs who gave everything he had to cross the finish line of two marathons. I could see a man whose armor had been banged up, whose skin showed the battle scars of the life he has lived, yet here he is, standing tall despite it all, and my life is about to change forever."

Bradley's story has certainly had its share of ups and downs but he believes it's the difficult times that make it a story worth telling.

"Remember the great movie where the main character faced no challenges and cruised through life?" he asks. "No? That's because it doesn't exist. [CF] has challenged my character like a weight would a muscle, and I know I'm bound to be stronger every time."

KATIE O'GRADY

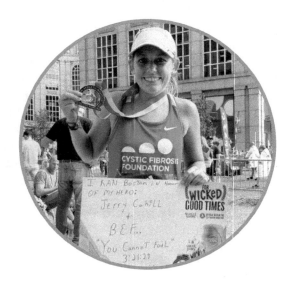

Age: 26
Resides: Boston, Massachusetts
Age at Diagnosis: 6

KATIE'S RUN: A MISSION TO BREATHE AGAIN

Unlike many of her fellow CF warriors, Katie O'Grady's perceived adversity didn't start until her freshman year in high school, after she had already established herself on the local, regional, and *national* levels of the high school running circuit.

"I found out how scary CF was when I had done a biology project and how some people with CF are much sicker than me," says Katie. "It changed me mentally. I started putting limits on myself instead of pushing through workouts or runs when my breathing was hard. I felt like my naïve young self had vanished because now I had this life-threatening illness that was worse than I had imagined. My narrative changed from thinking 'CF can't stop me' to 'I am sick and will always be sick.'"

Not long after, her mom, Jackie—one of the two people to whom she always turned to in a time of personal difficulty (the other being her dad)—was diagnosed with stage-four colon cancer. "My mom and I always had this weird connection, slightly spiritual maybe," says Katie. "We would both get intense feelings where we knew what would happen in the future. She especially had some deeper connection with life. She always said I would do something great with my life."

Katie made it to the age of six before digestive issues began to surface and cause discomfort. "I saw so many doctors and none could figure out what was wrong with me," she says. "I got checked for lactose intolerance, Crohn's disease, and a number of other issues. Eventually, a sweat test would determine that I, in fact, had CF."

"When Katie was diagnosed, my wife and I were devastated" says Katie's dad, Kevin. "But my wife and I pushed her to follow her interests and made sure she was vigilant with her treatments."

"At an early age, my parents had gotten me into sports," says Katie, the oldest of three children and the only one with CF. "They never held me back or told me that I couldn't do something because of having a disease. So, I always believed I was normal and could keep up with the other healthier kids."

"I didn't have to keep Katie active at all," says Kevin, who insists that Katie was self-motivated. "As a young child she was very active by running, swimming, biking, et cetera. She loved being physically active, which is great for CF children."

In terms of organized competition, Katie started with soccer at around five years old because her cousin, who she admired, was a very successful player. "I was horrible at it," says Katie, "but I loved running up and down the field. Looking back now, I know I wasn't meant to be a soccer player because I wasn't aggressive enough, but back then I thought I was the star of the team despite never making a goal."

Around the time Katie started playing soccer, Katie simultaneously found her passion. "I would go on runs with my dad here and there and even ran my first 5K with him, a charity run called the Emerald Society 5K, which I did each year until seventh grade when I joined the middle school track team."

Katie played soccer up until the eighth grade, when she decided to switch it up and join the middle school cross-country team.

"In my first race, I came in first by about two hundred meters or more. I fell in love immediately," says Katie. "I loved the rush of the win. I loved a shiny trophy or medal that I could hang on the wall and show them off to family and friends." During her eighth-grade season, Katie won the county championships for her age group, broke the long-standing county record, and continued her undefeated season. "After the race, when we were all celebrating," says

Katie, "Coach Diglio, the high school head coach, came up to me and pulled me aside to talk about potentially running for his team come winter track. I was very surprised and wondered if he could do that considering I went to a whole different school and would be the only eighth grader on the team."

After talking it over with her parents, Katie joined the varsity high school team at North Rockland. "I went on to become All-American my eighth-grade year with my 4 x mile relay [four runners who each run a mile and pass the baton to the next individual until all four team-mates have completed the race] team in 2009 when my team finished sixth out of approximately twenty-four teams at the Nike Nationals." Besides achieving All-American status and a scorching-fast 18:49 in the 5K that year, Katie earned a medal at the competition which she still considers one of her most precious awards.

Still, Katie says that while she competed early on in high school, she had a sense of loneliness because of cystic fibrosis. "When I first started to experience how reactive my lungs were to pollen in the eighth grade, I started reaching out to people on Facebook like pro runners," says Katie. "They didn't have the lung issues to the extent that I did. I continued looking for runners who had CF, but I was always coming up empty. I felt very lost, but I eventually learned my body through trial and error."

Her parents helped the best they could. "My mom was a physical therapist, and she would do physical therapy on me if I had any tightness or pains and would give me exercises so that I would stay strong and fit during my intense training," says Katie. "My dad was my running partner over winter and summer training. We did a lot of miles together and he would actually end up running marathons, which he says was a product of *me* pushing *him* to come running. When I was sick, oftentimes with either GI issues or a sinus infection which would drip down to my lungs and cause excessive coughing, or after returning from a rare hospitalization, [my parents] were always there to comfort me but also always ready to push me when I was mentally down. My parents wanted me to know I wasn't limited by my disease but instead I just had a few extra steps in my life, like doing my treatments and seeing doctors every three months or sometimes more if I was sick."

It was around this time that Kevin introduced Katie to Jerry Cahill of the Boomer Esiason Foundation (BEF), a CF warrior now in his sixties who stresses the importance of exercise through his *Cystic Fibrosis Podcast* and who inspires many in his audience with his powerful slogan, "You cannot fail."

"Jerry has and continues to inspire me because of his unwavering determination to live and exercise regardless of where he is in his CF journey," says Katie. "I vividly remember watching him running on a beach with an oxygen cylinder strapped to his back and I was inspired by his relentlessness. He made me believe that if you want something bad enough, you will do what it takes to get it done, no matter what life throws at you."

Katie says that her mom was her primary caretaker especially around four to six years old. "She was the person who mostly brought me to my appointments. She was the one who taught me how to do my treatments. In the mornings before school, she would wake me up, carry me downstairs, and would set me up to my nebulizer and vest as I continued to sleep. There would be nights I would wake her up because my stomach would be hurting so bad. She would take me to the bathroom so I could use the toilet and sometimes I would be there for an hour, and she would just sleep on the floor next to me so I wasn't alone. She would also be there when I was coughing at night and would lay in my bed and rub my back to help me relax."

Katie's cross-country success continued into her freshman year but then came the biology project that alerted her to the disease that threatened to consume her body. And soon after, she'd find out about the one that threatened her mother. "When I found out my mom was diagnosed with stage-four colon cancer, I felt broken," says Katie. "I cried but also felt like everything was going to be okay. Weirdly enough, my mom felt the same. We used to talk about our symptoms together and I know we didn't fully understand what we were both going through, but I always hoped I helped her feel okay when I would say 'I feel that too, at times.'"

Soon, a role reversal began to take place between Katie and her mom. "I started to become her caretaker more than she was mine," says Katie. "After her first cancer treatments, her cancer had all but vanished. My mom's doctor, who was cold at times, had actually given my mom the look of surprise and happiness. A look this doctor didn't seem to possess before. Her health would continue for a while and even when her cancer seemed to slowly come back, my mom would always be strong and say, 'I got this.'"

In early January 2013, Katie worked on her first podcast with Jerry Cahill at her house, which would eventually be posted on YouTube in May 2013. "[My mom] was starting to decline around then," says Katie, "but just like Jerry, she was still determined to fight and live life as normal as she could. During my podcast with Jerry, I was dealing with a lot of illness. I was underweight and getting sick almost every other week. In hindsight, this was probably due to the stress of watching my mom get sicker."

Jackie's condition worsened right as Katie contracted a severe case of pneumonia and would receive IV antibiotics for the first time, which resulted in her missing four weeks of school. "My grades did not suffer. All my teachers were aware of what was happening, and they would let me make up exams and, in some cases, just let me skip them. Katie's health had been relatively well compared to a lot of young adults with cystic fibrosis who had experienced bouts with IV antibiotics at some point during their childhood. "I had gone from running fast and far to barely being able to run a few feet without feeling like I was going to pass out due to not being able to breathe," she says. "I now had to be stronger for my family and my mom than my body wanted to allow."

Katie still had her PICC line in when Jackie went into hospice. Then, in April, two months before Katie graduated, Jackie passed away at the age of forty-nine. "She was my best friend, we did everything together," says Katie. "I was stuck to her hip, probably more than she would have liked at times. I believe the bond between a mom and a daughter or son with a chronic illness grows so strong because they are who care for us day in and day out (at least in my life).

"When I was sick, she cared for me. We would spend countless hours together at doctor appointments and tests, and as bad as they were sometimes, my mom and I would always make the best of it. When I was younger, I had to go through many rounds of allergy shots. I have very severe asthma/allergies caused by my cystic fibrosis and we had hoped this would help my lungs, especially in the spring when running would be so hard because of how tight my lungs got from the pollen which often led to a CF or sinus infection. During the many months of getting allergy shots, my mom would pick me up early from school and we would drive thirty minutes to get my shots. I may be crazy, but I would get so excited for her to get me on these days, not because I wanted needles in my arms but because I would get to spend time with her. She would also always get me back to school in time before practice. She was a miracle worker."

"When my wife died, and Katie had pneumonia, it was difficult and scary," says Kevin. "I just tried to focus on Katie's health and kept my other two kids positive about Katie's health. I kept focus on Katie's health by reminding her of the positive things that would happen if she maintained good health through vigilant treatments, nutrition, and exercise." The result of this perseverance was a scholarship to compete in Division II athletics at St. Thomas Aquinas College in New York.

"Some days I just wanted to sleep," says Katie, "but my dad pushed me to go for my runs and do my meds to get better. I know my dad was just scared for my health during that time because he couldn't lose me too. He was a huge part in getting me back after pneumonia."

Katie says another person played a big role: "Coach Diglio was a big part of my life during this time and helped structure a running plan that I could follow despite the fact that he was no longer coaching spring track as he had other responsibilities."

Katie found the strength after her mom passed to take care of her siblings. "It wasn't a role I was told to do," says Katie, "but more something I just did. I was my dad's go-to person to take care of things at home because my siblings were still younger and needed my help, especially when my dad was at work."

"Katie was the rock of the family that kept everything in check after my wife died," says Kevin. "I never had to push Katie to run and take her meds," says Kevin. "Katie lives to run and runs to live. It's simple. Her love for running and trying to get better at her skills made her realize the importance of her maintaining her health."

"I had to learn how to live a life without my mom," says Katie, "but in the last year of her life, I knew she wasn't meant to be here for long. In the final months of her life, when I began helping her at home because I stopped going to practice as much, because I was getting increasingly sick, she said, 'Don't let anyone tell you how to live your life,' and I had the presence of mind to internalize those words and the way she said them. Though my body felt rigid from the pneumonia and running felt almost impossible, those words helped me keep the faith as I fought to keep and make good on my scholarship."

In college, Katie was competing in races most weekends, much the same as when she competed in high school. Katie's first year in college would be a growing point for her as she found herself finishing last on the team quite frequently. "I was nowhere near my capabilities, but each race slowly brought me closer to who I used to be," she says. "I was used to being a top finisher in races, sometimes even breaking records while doing so. Now I was finishing last in races; in some cases, during track, I would be lapped by the whole field of runners in the race, and when they would finish, I would still have a lap or two to run all by myself, and I would get what they called the 'pity' clap from all the spectators when I would run by.

"My self-confidence during this time would slowly decrease. Each race became mentally harder as it did physically as well. I would be gasping for air, my legs would burn, but my stubbornness was what would keep me pushing through. It's a very slow process and I had to be happy with every little mental win or personal-time win. I knew I wouldn't regain my strength overnight, so I had to be patient."

Katie continues, "I ran my first collegiate 5K in 21:47.7 and finished third to last out of fifty girls in September 2013. My patience paid off though, because by the end of my freshman year, I ran a 5K in 19:12 at the conference championship in May 2014. I worked so hard the summer going into my sophomore year. I honestly didn't even know how fit I was until practice started back that August. That was the beginning of an amazing year for me. I ran my best 5K in 18:39 in October 2014 and broke our school's cross-country 5K record and became All-Conference. In outdoor track, I got the school record and meet record in the 10K by coming in first and running 41:40. I earned the Smiley Award for succeeding despite hardship and was named MVP for the first time." Katie not only earned MVP of her team her sophomore year but helped St. Thomas Aquinas qualify for NCAA Division II Cross Country Championships in Joplin, Missouri, for the first time in their school's history.

Katie majored in biology in hopes to become a physical therapist like her mom but that would change after graduation when she developed a passion for coaching. "After I graduated, I got the opportunity to work as a distance coach back at my college," says Katie, "and after a year there I decided to make the biggest move of my life. I got the opportunity to coach at Boston University (BU) where I got to learn about how to be a coach at a big Division I school."

After a year at BU, Katie got the opportunity to coach at another prestigious school, Tufts University, where she's been for two years to date and coaches thirty young women for both cross country and track, with focuses on the girls running from the half mile (eight hundred meters) to the 10K (6.2 miles). "I am there to motivate them when they are having a bad workout or race," says Katie, "as well as coaching them strategically to help them run well and gain points at meets. But more than anything, I love helping others, so I put my love for running into coaching." She also does both teams' social media.

Katie continues to run daily. "On my easy days, I will run between two to five miles and on my harder, long-run or workout days, I will run between six to eighteen miles," she says, "depending on where my training is at." Katie runs approximately fifteen to forty miles per week and sixty to 120 miles per month and, as a member of Team Boomer, competes in two to five races per year. "I love how they promote exercise to the CF community as a way for us to fight CF," says Katie who, in 2011, at the age of seventeen, came in second in her age group at the New York City Half-Marathon with a time of 1:38.33 and raised over $5,000 for the Boomer Esiason Foundation.

This was Katie's first half-marathon, but she remembers the run for other reasons. "My mom was battling cancer during this time," says Katie. "I am grateful I was able to run and have her watch because this was the only time she got to see me race in a big road race. This was also the first time I ever raced for something bigger than just myself. I was running for other people with CF and the money I had fundraised would be going to all of us."

In June 2019, Katie reunited for another podcast with her inspiration, Jerry, who is also a big fan of Katie. "Katie is an amazing young woman who is relentless, committed, and a true hero who respects all people," says Jerry. "Besides being an amazing runner, Katie is always smiling and lighting up people and the world around her."

In October 2019, Katie started taking Trikafta and what a big difference the CFTR modulator has made for her. "I was hospitalized in September 2019 and received IV antibiotics for two weeks," says Katie. "Pre-Trikafta, my health was starting to decline. I was getting sick a lot more and I was starting to see that it was getting harder to fight off infections even with the help of antibiotics. Even after two weeks of IVs, two weeks later I got another infection and was put back on oral antibiotics. [A month later], my life completely changed.

"Pre-Trikafta, I was getting sick once a month. I have been on Trikafta over two years now and I have been sick maybe four times where I needed antibiotics. I once thought my running career was over but, apparently, it's just starting. I am able to stay healthy long enough to see all the hard work I have put into my running. Before, it was hard to gain anything when I was getting sick every few weeks. My PFTs are the highest they have been since middle school. I never thought I would see numbers like that again. Lastly, I can take deep, deep breaths, and I was able to gain weight and put on muscle. Something I really struggled with pre-Trikafta was being underweight." Katie, who at four feet, eleven inches, weighed around ninety-five pounds, but since starting Trikafta she is a much healthier 110 pounds.

Katie has also noticed one more incredible change. "I don't cough anymore!" says Katie. "Especially in a time of COVID, I'm so thankful I'm not coughing like I used to. I would definitely be getting a lot of stares if I still had my CF cough."

In October 2021 just five months after completing the Providence Marathon, Katie joined a fundraising team created by her doctor at Boston Children's Hospital. "It was an amazing experience from start to finish," says Katie. "The crowds were electric, and it really helped push me along. I felt unstoppable. I went into Boston with a goal that I knew was achievable, which was to qualify for the Boston Marathon while running it [because Katie was fundraising for the Cystic Fibrosis Foundation, she did not have to qualify to run the race].

"I never believed that I could run a marathon and feel amazing from almost start to finish. I didn't truly start to struggle until mile twenty-three when my legs started to cramp up. The last 0.2 miles, I actually had a mild asthma attack. It wouldn't be me without my lungs giving me some sort of issue."

Katie raised nearly $7,000 for the Cystic Fibrosis Foundation while competing and ran the race in 3:21.26, which was about nine minutes ahead of the qualifying time for her age group. After the race, Katie held up a sign created by her father which read, "I ran Boston in honor of my hero Jerry Cahill & BEF . . . 'You cannot fail' 3:21:29, 10/11/21."

Katie says that while the accomplishment ranks among her greatest achievements, she is still not satisfied. "I am already ready to try and improve on that time," says Katie. "I will be returning to Boston in April 2022."

Katie says her biggest inspiration is still Jackie who loved watching Katie race. "Sometimes I still think I hear her yelling 'Kate' from within the roar of the crowd," says Katie. "She is one of the reasons I'm going at marathons the way I am. Trikafta has given me a second chance at running. I thought the days of me running to my potential were over but now they aren't, and I know my mom would want me to do something great with this newfound potential."

In addition to coaching, she's also started her own virtual coaching business, called Mission Breathe Again, to help others with chronic illness through running. "When I was younger, no one understood what I was going through," says Katie. "I scoured the internet looking for someone who would understand what it was like trying to run while also having a disease that would hold me back more times than not. Unfortunately, I never found that person who could keep me motivated when I was not. I wanted to be able to share my experiences with running and living with CF to help others succeed without having to be confused and frustrated when no one understands them."

"Katie is my hero, and she pushes me every day to be better," says Kevin, who has worked in law enforcement for over thirty years and says of all the heroes he's met, and he's met many, Katie tops the list. "Katie has shown her team members that everyone has hardships in life, but you can overcome them if you work and believe in yourself. I have always said, 'Katie was born with fifty percent lungs and 120 percent heart.' I believe she is an inspiration to many who look at her and if she can break records, win honors, and work hard, ask, 'why not me?'"

"Have faith when life gets tough," says Katie, echoing the sentiments of her mom. "When I get sick or find life is just not going my way, I try to remember that things will get better if you believe. Everyone is on their own journey through life, and the good and bad days you experience are just part of your story. I believe everything we go through in life opens doors to where we are meant to go and makes us into who we are supposed to be."

BRADLEY POOLE

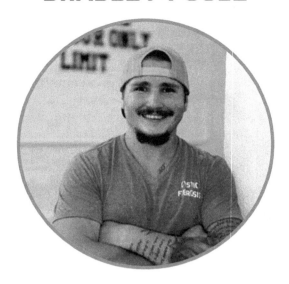

Age: 34
Resides: Salamanca, New York
Age at diagnosis: 6 days old

IN THE LONG RUN: RUNNER MAKES THE IMPOSSIBLE POSSIBLE FOR A GOOD CAUSE

B radley Poole, who has raised over $100,000 for the Western New York Chapter of the CF Foundation, is known for the publicized trek he took around Western New York. Bradley hit his goal by raising a grand total of $65,000 by running and walking his way to 266 miles in just seven days. Some would argue that his journey to get there was more difficult than those scorching seven days in July.

Bradley was born in Olean, New York. Over the first few days after his birth, he was constipated and his stomach was bloated. His mother, Ruthann, also noticed he had very salty tasting skin and felt like something just was not right with her son. "You could call it mother's intuition," says Ruthann. "The day Bradley and I were to be discharged from the hospital, a nurse came into my room and told me I'd be discharged but not Bradley. I freaked! Doctors came into the room to tell me and Jim (Bradley's dad) that Bradley did not pass his first stool and they suspected he may have cystic fibrosis."

Bradley was mercy-flighted to Children's Hospital in Buffalo where they performed surgery on his abdomen and ran a bunch of tests. Six days after he was born, Bradley was diagnosed with cystic fibrosis. "I said my prayers and then got to work," says Ruthann. "I decided to immerse myself into learning all I could about CF to keep my son healthy."

"Growing up with CF was difficult at times," says Bradley. "Childhood wasn't too bad as I didn't really know what CF was or why I had to do all these treatments. As I approached my teenage years, things started to change. I started caring about what people thought of me. I hid my illness from everybody because I was worried I would get picked on and lose friends. I was embarrassed I had CF. When friends would come over to my house, I would hide my pills and breathing treatments because I didn't want them questioning anything. I also began diving deeper into what CF really is. I remember looking up the life expectancy and seeing that it was in the early thirties. I became fearful, scared, and questioned, *Why me?*"

Bradley's family made sure he was involved in sports from a young age and played all through high school. "I played soccer, football, and basketball from childhood through high school," he says. "My family encouraged me to stay positive and always told me I would beat this disease. I was hospitalized for the first time at thirteen. I remember that being a wake-up call for me as to how serious this disease is. But it also scared me because, in my mind, I was going to die young, and I rebelled."

In his late teens, Bradley started abusing alcohol as a way to cope with his CF and mental health. "I was sad, depressed, lonely, anxious, scared, and the list goes on. I was having racing, suicidal, unwanted, and irrational thoughts. I slacked off on treatments despite my family pleading with me to not sway from the right path. I just wanted to be a normal kid. None of my friends had to do anything like I did, and I guess I wanted the life they had—as in, a life free of breathing treatments and pills. I also was very embarrassed that I had CF. So I didn't really tell anyone I had it. Only a few close friends knew I had it. But as I continued to slack off, the harder it got for me to breathe, especially during sports."

Ruthann remembers this time and the helplessness she experienced vividly. "Young adults, at times, feel they know everything," she says, "and won't listen to a dang thing their parents try to tell them."

"I remember coughing all the time in school and people thinking I was sick all the time," says Bradley. "That led to frequent two-week hospital stays. I was partying like a rock star instead of taking care of me." All told, Bradley says his alcohol abuse lasted into his early twenties. "I was doing that to cope with my CF and my undiagnosed mental health issues at the time. That led me down a dark and scary path as I was hospitalized frequently due to lung decline."

Bradley says he's struggled with mental health issues most of his life. "I was fourteen years old when I had my first suicidal thoughts," he says. "They played on repeat in my mind. No matter what I did, I couldn't get them to go away. The thoughts scared me, and I told my dad what I was experiencing. He suggested I talk to the school counselor, and so I did. I met with her for a few months, and she said it was just a part of adolescence. She wanted another opinion though, as I was struggling with suicidal, intrusive, irrational, and unwanted thoughts. She sent me to a psychiatrist who told me the exact same thing. I got put on medication and it seemed to start working after a while. However, the thoughts came back full force around the age of seventeen, and I started playing around with alcohol.

"I used alcohol as a coping method for my CF and mental health struggles. I got to the point where I was drinking five to six days a week to the point of blacking out most times. When still in high school, I would only drink on the weekends. But after my senior year is when I started drinking more often. But the partying led to slacking off on treatments, which led to more hospitalizations because I wasn't taking care of myself. My number one priority was partying to help cope with my struggle."

Despite struggling with alcohol at the time, Bradley did manage to meet Stephanie at a party when he was twenty and she was nineteen. "I remember seeing her for the first time and thinking, *Holy cow I [have to] talk to this girl*. But I need liquid courage first before I could. After a few hours, I managed to talk her into playing beer pong with me and we chatted for a bit at the party. The next day I remember looking her up on Myspace and sending her a message. For some reason, I just let her know everything about me as far as the CF goes. I had multiple girlfriends in the past who never knew I had CF and that's because I was embarrassed to tell them. I didn't want to hide it anymore, so I made sure to tell Steph right off the bat. She knew what it was because she babysat a girl who had it. So, we chatted and got to know each other better through Myspace and we ended up getting together and hanging out.

"Whenever I got hospitalized, Steph was right by my side. She stayed at the hospital with me even when she was going to college. She would wake up early, drive two hours to school, and drive back after she was done. She was just always there to help and really put up with a lot of [my issues]. The only thing I failed to tell her was about my mental health. I never told her I was struggling, although I was the entire time we were together. I guess I never told her because I was afraid she'd leave had she known the type of thoughts I was having."

Bradley was not the only member of his family to struggle with alcohol. Bradley's father, Jim, was in a terrible train collision which caused him to witness the death of two of his good friends and, subsequently, caused him to develop PTSD. "This led to excessive alcohol abuse for years and years," says Bradley. "I was only three months at the time of his accident. He would get help from a psychiatrist for fifteen years but continued drinking his nightmares away. He was thirty-nine at the time of the accident and got diagnosed with cirrhosis at fifty-eight."

Bradley points out that despite his father's battle with drinking, it did not define the man. "He was an amazing father who loved all his kids dearly. He just had his own battles he was fighting inside. After being diagnosed [with cirrhosis], my father quit drinking cold turkey and started getting healthier." Bradley also points out that his father, who was divorced from Bradley's mom, Ruthann, took custody of Bradley's older sister's son, Eli, when Eli was just three years old.

Bradley says a few things helped him to break the vicious cycle. When he was twenty-three, he was on his fifth hospitalization in two years. "I remember a nurse coming into my room and saying this may be my new normal," he says. "She meant me being hospitalized frequently. Again, I was hospitalized often because I slacked on my treatments and made partying and drinking my number one priority over my health."

The nurse's comment motivated Bradley. "I wanted to prove her wrong," he says. "That wasn't going to be my new normal."

It was also when Bradley's father passed away from cirrhosis at the age of sixty-two, just three and a half years after the diagnosis, that Bradley was compelled to take charge of his own life. "I decided to change my life around," says Bradley. "I knew if I kept on that path, I wouldn't make it another five years, or, at best, I would be waiting on the transplant list. I was sick of being sick and wanted to prove that nurse wrong. I had new responsibilities on my hands. My father had custody of my nephew at the time and I took him after my dad passed after my sister agreed. He was my blood, he was my nephew, and I wanted to take care of him. Getting custody of Eli helped me get on the right path. And I also had a loving girlfriend who helped me through some of my darkest days.

"So, at twenty-three, I really started to change my life around and get on the right path. I wanted to be around for my friends and family for as long as possible. I wanted to be able to live a normal life. It was [during] that hospital visit where I promised myself I'd start taking better care of myself and make my health my number one priority."

Bradley continues, "My mental health issues would be good for a while and then come back full force at the age of twenty-eight. I would have to perform rituals daily to help alleviate the anxiety of my thoughts. An example of one of my rituals is turning a door knob a certain amount of times until it feels right. I have many different rituals. But the thoughts that really got to me were the suicidal and violent thoughts of harming myself or someone else. I battled through the worst thoughts ever—too dark to even mention. But, deep inside, I knew I never wanted to really act on those thoughts. I struggled with these thoughts from an early age."

This time it was different though, for one big reason. "Now I had a good support system to help me through," says Bradley. It was Stephanie who helped Bradley to keep searching for answers. "When I had my breakdown at twenty-eight," says Bradley, "she was the first one I went to. I told her I needed to talk to her about something and just let it out. I was afraid to speak up but knew I had to say something. I used to talk to my father about all my issues, but he wasn't around anymore to talk to. So I went eight years without saying a word to Steph [about my mental health issues] and I hit another breaking point to where I had to tell someone. She was encouraging and supportive and suggested I see a counselor. She went to school for social work and was a counselor herself at one time. So I listened to her advice and that's when I was diagnosed.

"In 2015, at the age of twenty-eight, after having experience with a variety of counselors, two misdiagnoses, and another breakdown, I was finally diagnosed with obsessive compulsive disorder (OCD), which I had lived with all my life but was unfortunately misdiagnosed a couple times."

Since being diagnosed, Bradley began working with a counselor to prevent relapse and his life has done a 180. He has only been hospitalized one time in the past ten years. A bad cold caused his lung function to drop significantly. But Bradley's new mental fortitude allowed him to even bounce back from that without chronic repercussion. "You never know how strong you are, until strong is the only choice you have," says Bradley, who tattooed those very words onto his wrist.

In his new quest to get his life on the right track, Bradley went back to school. "I knew I wanted to do something sports or fitness related as I enjoyed sports and fitness helped me stay healthy. So I figured why not have a career in that field? Bradley received his bachelor of science in sports management, in 2014, from the University of

Pittsburgh at Bradford, his master of sports administration, in 2015, from Canisius College in Buffalo, and his bachelor of science in exercise science, in 2016, from the University of Pittsburgh at Bradford.

"During my master's program, I did an internship with the strength coach at St. Bonaventure University and had the opportunity to train and work with all the Division I athletes. That really piqued my interested and helped me find out the direction I wanted my career path to go. After my third degree, I started working out of a gym as a personal trainer and fitness instructor and fell in love with it. I saw how fitness impacted my health physically and mentally and wanted to help others become better versions of themselves."

On August 15, 2015, Bradley married Stephanie. "We have our ups and downs like all married couples," says Bradley, "but we still love and support each other through the good and bad. Steph and I had talked about trying to have children after our wedding. We knew we probably had to do IVF. So we started that process a couple of years after our wedding. The whole process was nerve-racking. We made a six-hour trip to and from clinic for meetings and procedures. We ended up with four embryos. Two of them were miscarriages. The third time was a charm as we introduced Sadie into our lives on September 18, 2020. We have one more embryo left to use and will do it when we feel the time is right."

Bradley continues raising his seventeen-year-old nephew, Eli, of whom he got custody in April 2011 after Bradley's father passed away. "Signing those custody papers," says Bradley, "was one of the best days of my life. Stephanie and I lived at my dad's house, so we really have been in Eli's life since he was a baby," he says. "But Eli was six when my dad passed. He passed away two weeks before Eli's birthday. I told my father that Eli would be fine and in good hands. Eli is now a senior in high school. He is very smart, athletic, and in the top of his class. I'm glad Steph and I could give him that support system he needed."

Bradley wanted to do something big for the Cystic Fibrosis Foundation when he came up with the 266-mile run in seven days. "I had been doing CF fundraisers for seven years prior to my big run. I did basketball tournaments, cornhole tournaments, and exercise for CF events," says Bradley, "but in 2020, I wanted to do something different. I wanted to do something that would challenge me physically and mentally. I also wanted to show those fighting CF what's possible. I had been running for four years prior to this event. I did half-marathons, 25Ks, 10Ks, 5Ks, 50Ks, and trail races. So I wanted to do something with running.

"My younger sister, Lauren, came up with idea of running through every town in Cattaraugus County (which is where I live). I thought that sounded like a fun and challenging idea. From there it blossomed into putting together the 266-mile run, finding a coach, getting the course together, and finding a team to help."

Bradley soon met Mark Wilson when he was preparing to do the long run in seven days through every town in Cattaraugus County, New York, in September 2019. "I put a post on Facebook that I was looking for a running coach," says Bradley, "and someone tagged him in [the] post. I contacted him and met him in person. I told him what I wanted to do, and he offered to train me for free since it was for a good cause."

They would talk on the phone every Monday and give Bradley the plan for the week. But Mark didn't always think this run was a good idea. "Well, at first, I thought it was insane," says Mark, "but then, I started doing the math and realized it was possible as long as we had a good plan. So, I agreed to coach him." He started off with what Mark and Bradley considered low mileage of twenty to thirty miles per week, but as the months progressed, Bradley's runs increased to the point where he was running about five days per week with an average pace between eight to ten minutes per mile. Once a month, he would run forty-two miles, the distance he would have to run each of the first six days of his seven-day trek to reach his goal.

By July 5, he was ready to go. "I did forty-two miles per day for six days beginning July 5, and fourteen miles on the last day, July 11, 2020," says Bradley, who, it turned out, happened to choose the hottest week of the year when it was sunny and over one hundred degrees on the pavement every day.

"Cattaraugus County is very hilly, so I had lots of big hills to climb up and down which made the task even tougher. I would run forty-two miles and then stop. I would go home to rest for a very short period of time. I was only getting four to five hours of sleep. Then my wife would drive me back out to where I left off and I'd go another forty-two miles. It took between ten to twelve hours each day to complete the forty-two miles.

"I had a car ahead of me and one car behind me the whole time. I just needed someone to be there in case something happened. But I also needed food and drinks, so we kept those in the cars as well," Bradley continues. "I went into the event with a strategy, but that strategy changed a few times as I needed to listen to my body. I had originally planned to just do all forty-two without any rest, which I did on the first day. But after the first day, I was totally drained and couldn't stop puking on the way home. I was also suffering from severe body cramps. The heat and humidity took a lot out of me. So, after that first day I didn't want to continue on, but I forced myself out of bed the next day, got to the location, and put one foot in front of the other.

"On the second day, I had decided to stop at twenty-one miles to rest, go home, and come back out in the evening. That seemed to work decently, but then I was getting done too late at night and was getting even less sleep and less recovery time. On the third day, I started dealing with severe shin splints. Every time my feet hit the pavement, I would get shooting pain from my ankles to my knees. It hurt even worse when going down hills. I had to continue to just block out the pain and keep moving forward and decided to run twenty-one miles, but then only rest for one hour where I stopped. I would eat, rehydrate, and then continue on for the next twenty-one miles. That strategy is the one I stuck with, as I was getting done earlier and had more rest time before the next day.

"By the fourth day," Bradley says, "my right leg from my shin down to my ankle swelled right up. It eventually got to the point to where it kind of went numb. Which, looking back, wasn't a good thing. So from days four to seven, I was in severe pain, shin splints, body cramps, completely fatigued mentally and physically, and I just wanted to be done. But what helped me through were the people who were there with me every day. I had runners with me every day and also the people in the towns holding up signs and cheering me on as I ran through. It was the adrenaline rush from the support I was receiving that powered me through. I was drinking lots of water, Gatorade, and Pedialyte. I was eating fruits, lots of carbs, and proteins to help with muscle recovery. I wouldn't eat a lot as I didn't want to run on a full belly, but I ate enough to give me the energy I needed."

One of those people along for the ride was Shannon Collins, a mother of a three-year-old boy named Lucas who also has cystic fibrosis. "I did a loop while pushing my jogging stroller with Lucas," says Shannon. "We ran with Bradley because I have been following him on Facebook, and he is so passionate about raising money to find a cure for cystic fibrosis, which is near and dear to my heart because my son has it. I told Brad I thought he would be an amazing advocate for Lucas, especially as he gets older and has more questions and concerns about his condition. Bradley has a very caring personality, but also shows how strong and how much of a true fighter he is. That's what my son will need as he grows up."

"This event did get a lot of local attention," says Bradley. "It didn't get national attention, but it was awesome to see the local news stations reporting on it as it brought in more awareness of what I was doing. I knew if I did something off-the-wall crazy that this event could attract some attention, which it did. It also helped to raise sixty-five thousand dollars for the Cystic Fibrosis Foundation, during a pandemic none-theless. After the event was over, I took some time to relax, recover, and enjoy myself. I had put myself through the toughest thing I've ever done, and I just needed to rest and be happy for what I had just accomplished."

Bradley worked out of a gym for a couple of years before becoming an independent-contractor personal trainer out of another gym. He did that for a couple of years before opening up his own fitness center, Warrior Fitness & Wellness, LLC, on January 4, 2021. "I named it this because I am a warrior and I've been through so much in my life. I could have given up many years ago, but I never gave up on myself, found my purpose, and pursued my passion. I want everyone to know that we all have that warrior within us. At my facility, we can help you out, push you out of your comfort zone, and to not stop until you achieve what you want to achieve. CF means the world to me, and I wanted to display that in some way in my facility . . . so I decided to go with the colors of it—yellow, purple, and blue."

"He goes above and beyond to raise awareness for CF," says Ruthann. "My son is awesome! He is motivated by his caring heart and dedication to his and others' health and well-being. I am beyond proud of him. And I know his dad is too."

Bradley also developed a run called "300 Miles for CF: Running for a Cure," which he attempted in June 2021. The entire course is a four-mile loop in a town nearby to Bradley's home. His mission was to run a remarkable seventy-two hours (with restroom breaks) and his goal was to make it three hundred miles within that time limit to raise more money to benefit the Cystic Fibrosis Foundation.

"As of May 2021, I was putting in between forty to fifty miles per week of training," says Bradley. "That number increased as the event got closer. I also lifted a couple days a week and threw in some HIIT [high-intensity interval training] workouts."

"Brad has no fear," says Mark, who continued coaching Bradley and trained him for the 2021 New York City Marathon in November 2021. "He truly steps into practically impossible situations and finishes. It's a personality trait that most people will never understand, not to men-tion experience."

Bradley gave the three-hundred-mile trek a shot at five a.m. on June 9, 2021. "I started off doing well," says Bradley, "but it was extremely hot and humid. I hit the sixty-mile mark at nine p.m. Throughout the day, I started developing minor body cramps, but they wouldn't last long. When I hit mile sixty, I was pretty exhausted. The body cramps became more severe. I felt very weak and fatigued. I took a shower and ended up sitting down in the shower due to severe cramps that brought me to my knees. After my shower, I tried eating some food and drinking but I puked it all back up. I decided at that point I was going to take a little nap before getting back out there. I dozed off for four hours and started running again at two a.m.

"By four a.m., I put in another twelve miles which put me at seventy-two. I felt even worse at this point and decided to take another quick nap to sleep it off. I got back out there at seven a.m. and ran another eight miles which put me at eighty miles. By the end of that, I knew I needed help. My body felt like it was giving up on me. I had a crew with me, and we decided to call the ambulance. I was hoping they could just give me some fluids and I'd be off running again."

Bradley continues, "After running tests on me, they found that I was very dehydrated, as my resting heart rate was in the one hundreds when it's usually low forties. After agreeing to go to the hospital, I knew I wouldn't hit three hundred miles, and I was bummed. I was hoping the hospital would just give me IVs and I could get back out there. The doctor did some blood work and found out that I was suffering from rhabdomyolysis. It's when the proteins break down in the muscle and get into the bloodstream, which can lead to kidney failure. I was bummed to hear that I had to stay in the hospital for at least twenty-four hours so they could monitor me and pump me with fluids."

Bradley was disappointed and assumed his trek was over, but his amazing community came to the rescue. "While I'm sitting in my room," says Bradley, "I start getting tons of pictures and videos sent my way of people doing my miles for me. Over one hundred people from all over came and put in miles of their own to help me hit three hundred. It was very cool to see the support."

One of those people was, once again, Shannon Collins. "I didn't want him to feel like he was in this fight alone. I ran an extra four miles on my own route while he was in the hospital," says Shannon. "I love the fact he runs for a cure as well because I love to run. It's very amazing what he does."

"I ended up getting out of the hospital the next morning," says Bradley, "and put in twenty more miles, as I still had one more day left. I wanted to at least hit one hundred on my own. So I hit my one hundred, and with everyone else combined, we finished with over one thousand miles."

Bradley sees the importance of leading by example. "The best thing I can do is keep pushing through," says Bradley, who, when he's not in intense training, spends his time with Stephanie, Eli, and Sadie. And his family will be growing as Stephanie and Bradley used their last embryo to make one more IVF attempt and were blessed with the news that a baby boy will be joining them in July 2022. "It's truly a blessing," says Bradley, "to be able to have biological kids when you have CF. Growing up I was always told I couldn't have kids of my own. To now have a second one on the way is a miracle."

He also completed the New York City Marathon in just three hours and forty-seven minutes in November 2021, finishing among the top 20 percent of finishers. "To complete the New York City Marathon while living with CF is incredible," says Bradley. "It's such a great feeling. I never thought I'd be able to do what I do today. I always thought by this time in my life I'd be waiting on a transplant or be gone. So to go out there and crush it was awesome."

Bradley didn't stop there. He completed his 24 Hour Fitness Challenge for Cystic Fibrosis on June 4, 2022, at his gym, Warrior Fitness & Wellness. The competition consisted of a fifty-mile run, three thousand pushups, three thousand squats, three thousand sit-ups, two hundred tire flips using a two-hundred-and-fifty-pound tire, and a fifteen-mile bike ride. As of the publication of this book, the event has raised nearly $20,000 for the Cystic Fibrosis Foundation. "That was extremely grueling and taxing on the body and mind," says Bradley of the twenty-four-hour challenge, "but I'm a warrior so I had to push through."

Bradley says the secret to his success is learning from the past and making the most of the present. "I won't quit. I won't give up. I fight like hell," says Bradley. "I stay as positive as I can, and I surround myself with positive people. I've had many tough times, but those things have helped me to work through them. Tough times don't last forever."

EVAN SCULLY

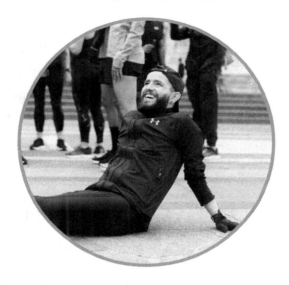

Age: 35
Resides: Navan, Meath, Ireland
Age at Diagnosis: 5 months

THE RECORD-BREAKER:
A PASSION TO BEAT CF . . . AND EVERYONE ELSE

Ireland native and CF warrior Evan Scully was a runner before he can even remember. "I was always running around," he says. "If it was in football [soccer] or playing [chase], I knew I could run all day. One of the first memories of running I had was when I was about four. The organizers of the summer camp had a 'Run 'Til You Drop' challenge. They had to tell me to stop so they could go home."

Evan was diagnosed with cystic fibrosis at five months of age after having symptoms of failing to thrive, chest infections, and being unable to keep any of his food down. "I was given ten years to live," says Evan, now thirty-five. "Thankfully, my parents worked endlessly to try to give me the best ten years of my life. Their discipline with regard to my CF and focus on giving me a great life presently, as opposed to focusing on simply a long life, laid great foundations for the life I now have. Both my parents showed me that hard, smart, and present work always wins. I've carried this on with whatever happens in my life."

As a child, Evan would administer his nebulizers and physiotherapy five to six times a day for airway clearance and take enzymes to digest fats. He also used inhalers to help with his exercise-induced asthma.

Evan was not exactly shy as a kid. "I would like to say 'mischievous,'" he says, "but I'm sure I was just cheeky and tried to get away with everything."

Evan says he first ran a race at the age of eleven while in the fifth grade. "My whole class was [told to run it]," says Evan. "I ran the cross-country race in my school uniform, and I won it. So that qualified me to run the race against all schools in the area. I figured out I was quite good at it. The more I ran, the more I loved it. The running community has some great people in it. It's like a big family. Running being good for my CF was just a byproduct of running. It wasn't until later on that I realized I have to run for my health even if I don't want to. That is the driving force when I really don't want to run."

When he was seventeen, Evan went on his own to Ethiopia to live and learn from two-time Olympic gold medalist and Ethiopian long-distance track and road-running athlete Haile Gebrselassie. "Haile was a huge inspiration to me as a runner, so to live with him in his house was something I will never forget."

Evan says his competitive fire is something he's had all his life. "I always felt I could not just be good at something; I have to be the best I can be," he says. "This could be making a cup of tea or trying to break a world record." Evan's running exploits are legendary in the CF community. "I have run too many races to count," he says. "My notable achievements would be running for Ireland while also being the world record [holder] as the fastest person with CF in the 5K, the 10K, and the half-marathon (1:07:31)."

The most important impact of his passion has been its effect on his health. Evan says that while he still takes thirty to forty pills a day, mostly digestive enzymes, and still uses inhalers to help with his asthma, his competitive running exploits inspired a fitness nutrition regimen that he believes has precluded him from ever being hospitalized.

Evan, who is formerly an Under Armour ambassador and currently an ASICS ambassador through the ASICS FrontRunner program, says his entire world is about competition and sports. "I have visited thirty-four different countries, working as a therapist and strength-and-conditioning coach to thirty-six Olympic medalists and three hundred Olympians."

Evan says his passion for helping others to accomplish their goals just happened. "I've always tried to help people be better," he says, "even if it meant they become better than me. I worked very hard and endlessly to sharpen my skills until I got my break. Once you get your break and get your name out there, then it becomes much easier to work with world-class athletes. You become a part of that world."

Evan says there was a moment in his life when the disease made him ponder his future, especially meeting his future wife, Yasmina, who he met at a Jay-Z concert. "We nearly fell in love immediately," he says. "When you know, you know. Explaining about CF was made easier as she is a very understanding person. She didn't really care [with regard to the concerns about cystic fibrosis]. But leading up to telling her, I had all these scenarios in my head. Turns out love is greater than certain flaws that you might have. Yasmina knows that I need to run. She encourages me, but also, she tells me to go running because I can be a pain when I don't. Those are her words. I do remember a time when I was thinking about life expectancy. Was it fair or wise to get married when there is a huge possibility that I won't be around for the normal life expectancy of someone who doesn't have CF? I let other people's stories infiltrate my mind and I didn't look at my own story."

"Better to have loved and lost than to not have loved at all," says Yasmina, "but the worst thing you can do is Google CF."

"The internet outlook is fairly bleak," says Evan.

Evan uses #BeatCF on all of his social media posts, which he started a few years ago to show that everything you do to nourish your body in fitness, nutrition, and mindset is "beating CF." He has also recently started the magic drug "Kaftrio." "It has changed everything I've known about my CF. I can't describe how it has worked so well! I never really feared CF, but with Kaftrio, I know that I don't need to fear CF for much longer." He says that he loves getting old and proving the statistics wrong. When he turned thirty-two, the median life expectancy in Ireland was the same number so Evan celebrated the feat of hitting that number and each year after pushing that number higher. "When I reach forty and when I reach fifty, that statistic is always going up," says Evan. "I love that I'm getting wrinkles. I love that I have gray hair."

Evan says his hobbies are cooking, making coffee, and making videos on his YouTube channel for his nearly 3,500 subscribers, but "I'm obsessed with running," he says. "I run six times and approximately fifty to seventy miles per week, mostly on country roads." He says he has run as much as 128 miles in a week, "though I prefer to listen to my body rather than my head to decide how far or how often I should run." Evan sometimes uses a treadmill, which has especially helped him keep his distance during the pandemic. Evan says he also practices meditation at least once a day to keep his mental strength.

Once the pandemic is over, Evan has one goal in mind. He is targeting a sub-three-hour marathon in a bid to reclaim the European best by someone with cystic fibrosis. The record is two hours, forty-seven minutes, and forty-seven seconds. He recently did an unofficial 2:55:27 in a time trial during lockdown—three weeks after partially tearing his Achilles tendon. "It was quite enjoyable to be honest," he says. "This was my third marathon, my fastest but my easiest."

Evan knows he is not supposed to be able to do what he is doing but he doesn't follow the stereotypical CF narrative and he doesn't think anyone else should either as long as they do one thing. "You need to work harder than everyone else," says Evan, who is an ambassador for Cystic Fibrosis Ireland. "Don't ever take a step back and think CF is under control. Prove everyone wrong and work your ass off! I try to simplify everything in my life. For instance, if I run and eat well, then my CF is under control. If I don't run, then CF will 'run' me. It's not that complicated. Running stabilizes and grounds me. It gives me energy and keeps CF at bay. In my youth, I ran to be the best. I took pride in beating people in sports who did not have CF. Now I run more to keep healthy, in body and mind, but also to keep a routine in my life."

MATT BARRETT

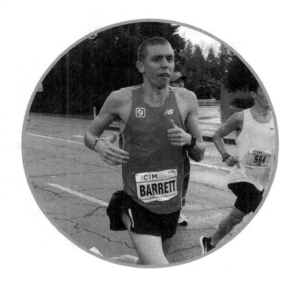

Age: 35
Resides: Verona, Wisconsin
Age at Diagnosis: 9 months

ALWAYS ON TRACK: MARATHON MAN HAS OLYMPIC DREAMS

C F warrior Matt Barrett—who has completed six marathons to date, has broken several course records, and has many top-five finishes in races of various distances—discovered running when he was fifteen. Prior to that, from the time he was in elementary school, he struggled with feeling undersized. "Everyone grows and develops at different rates," says Matt, "but there were definitely times I didn't understand why I was always one of the shorter, skinnier kids."

Then, in high school, he met cross-country and track coach Dave Hirsbrunner. "Coach Hirsbrunner was the ultimate motivator and knew how to drive me and get the best out of me each day," says Matt. "I then went on to run cross country and track for Coach Steve Plasencia at the University of Minnesota. Coach Plasencia was a two-time Olympian, and he also found ways to push me to achieve more and get faster and stronger each day."

While at the University of Minnesota and running seventy to one hundred miles per week, Matt was working with Dr. Robert Kempainen, a pulmonologist who also happened to be a two-time Olympian and top-ten finisher at both the Boston Marathon and New York City Marathon, and he really helped Matt understand how much running was benefiting him and his lung function. "And my ability to fight CF," says Matt, "and how it was the best form of therapy I could do."

Matt says his parents, Jamie and Julie; his brother, Michael; and his sister, Taylor, have been a major source of motivation. "They'd always come watch me run races over the years no matter how far the drive," he remembers. "I don't know where I'd be without my family. They mean everything to me." Matt says that growing up he learned the importance of keeping a healthy regimen. "I do feel that I've been fortunate over the years," says Matt, "that following the plan prescribed by my doctor (daily nebulizer treatments and medication), along with running for airway clearance, has kept me on the healthier side. Knock on wood, I have never had a major lung event in my life. I thank my parents for instilling that routine in me of nebulizers and medications, as well as just being active my whole life."

As far as CF's effect on his performance, Matt says, "CF has impacted my running at times, mostly when I get a sinus infection. Having to go on an antibiotic would drain me a bit, aside from the side effects of the sinus infection. Doing harder workouts with a sinus infection, I always have to temper my expectations of that workout and be okay with adjusting the paces of the workout if necessary." But though Matt says he has to "temper" his expectations, especially during the fall and winter months when he is more prone to sinus infections, he still strives to join the elite of his sport. "My dream is to compete in the Olympic trials."

Upon graduating from college, he moved from the 5K/10K distance on the track to running half and full marathons and completed his first 26.2-miler, the Chicago Marathon, in 2014. "I think the unique thing about the marathon is that for the Olympic trials, there isn't a limit on how many people can be in the race," says Matt. "If you hit the qualifying time standard (at virtually any official marathon), you [qualify for the Olympic trials], and have a shot at the Olympics, whereas for the US Olympic trials for track races, it's only the fastest twenty-four people in the country who get in. Now, for me, I realize that getting to the Olympic Games would be a real long shot (only the top-three runners in the US at the Olympic trials make it), but for me, to say I was one step away from the Olympics is something I've always strived for. And I think with the marathon not capping the field at a certain number of entrants, it has always kept me motivated and driven to try and reach that qualifying standard."

Matt's wife, Jess, an endurance athlete herself who has competed in the Ironman 70.3 World Championships and has completed six full Ironman competitions and has qualified for the Ironman World Championships, "is so supportive of all I do to stay healthy," says Matt. "She's always by my side doing what she can to keep me healthy as well. She inspires me daily. I'm forever grateful for Jess for everything she takes on as a spouse of someone with CF." Ironically, Matt met Jess when going to buy running shoes as his wife was working at the store. "We are a good pair," he says. "It's nice we each have our own thing—me running and her doing triathlons—but also good we can support each other."

"We are driven people, and we work together each day to help Matt defy the odds of his disease," says Jess. "Even though I am not the one living with the condition, I know that my life choices and level of support contribute to his overall health. Matt's high level of activity motivates me every day to be active. We eat nutritious food together, get plenty of sleep for recovery, and make healthy living a lifestyle."

Jess says, when she initially learned about CF, "It was scary. The worries decreased pretty quickly when I saw Matt's strong will to overcome the adversity in his life. My anxiety does go up when Matt gets sick. Going through the COVID-19 pandemic with a spouse who has a pulmonary disease has been exceptionally hard, but we were able to adapt to it."

Matt seems more concerned with his racing results and Olympic aspirations than the disease he's spent a lifetime fighting. "The pandemic put a damper on competing in races and improving on my time," he says, "but I will rise to the occasion when it is safe to do so. As race opportunities come around again, I'm excited to keep chasing that standard."

During the pandemic Matt continued to run eighty to one hundred miles per week. Sometimes he'd run in the brutal cold due to him living in the frigid winter climate of Wisconsin, but he was helped in the coldest months by his access to an indoor track, membership to which he obtained with a Cystic Fibrosis Lifestyle Foundation (CFLF) Recreation Grant he received in 2015. He has also been a Great Strides participant to benefit the Cystic Fibrosis Foundation.

Matt says his current running schedule is easy runs on Monday and Friday, two runs each day on Tuesday and Thursday, a harder workout on Wednesday, and then on the weekend, an easy run one day and the other day would be a long run with some harder miles included in that run. Despite all the time put into his running, he still finds time to administer his nebulizers, take his enzymes, and take his Trikafta. He also admits he is careful about one thing in particular. "I have always been aware of the health of those around me," says Matt, "whether it be coworkers who sit in close proximity (pre-pandemic, of course), friends, and also family members around the holidays or gatherings. Obviously, the last year has highlighted the importance of that for all of us as humans with the pandemic."

Though the pandemic canceled all in-person events, Matt celebrated his thirty-fourth birthday by running his own marathon. "My wife, Jess, biked alongside, and some family members and close friends came to support me along the way," he says. "I also had a friend of mine jump in and run about half of the marathon with me. My coach, Jason Digman, and I work every day to get me closer to that Olympic trials qualifying standard. As of now, the qualifying standard for the Olympic marathon is 2:19:00 (5:18 per mile). My personal best in a marathon to date is 2:23:09 at the Chicago Marathon. On my birthday, I ran 2:19:49 (5:20 per mile)."

Matt says that while he feels extremely blessed to have had three great coaches over his years of running competitively, it's the words of his late friend Gabriele "Gabe" Grunewald that still serve as a reminder to keep defying the odds: "It's okay to struggle, but not okay to give up."

Gabe ran at the University of Minnesota, on the women's team, at the same time as Matt . She was a four-time cancer survivor before, unfortunately, passing away in 2020 at the age of thirty-two. "Gabe was, and still is, an inspiration to me," says Matt. "For four years, I ran countless miles with her husband, Justin, and the men's and women's cross-country and track teams at the University of Minnesota were very close, so there were a lot of times we all got to interact. After college, watching her continue a very successful professional running career while battling cancer was beyond inspiring. Seeing her do that gave me and so many others hope that anything could be overcome, and anything is possible."

Matt says that running has brought him so much more than race results. "I'm a naturally competitive person and I will always chase personal bests," he says. "But more importantly, it's brought many amazing people into my life, including my wife and many close friends. Running changed my life in countless ways, but I would not be where I am at today without the support of my family, doctors, coaches, and friends who have been by my side throughout this journey.

"Medals are nice, but what I want most is for someone who is going through a tough time, CF or otherwise, to find hope in my story."

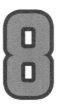

8

CF STANDS FOR
"CELEBRITY FOUND":
FAMOUS CF ADVOCATES

COLTON UNDERWOOD

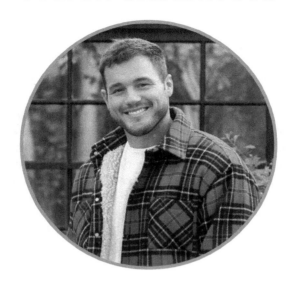

Age: 29
Resides: Denver, Colorado
Connection to CF: Cousin to a CF warrior and founder
of the Colton Underwood Legacy Foundation

COLTON'S LEGACY: THE "VEST" WAY TO HELP

Many people know Colton Underwood from his days on season 14 of ABC's *The Bachelorette* and later as the leading man on season 23 of ABC's *The Bachelor*. In the cystic fibrosis community, though, Colton is known for starting the Colton Underwood Legacy Foundation.

"I started the Legacy Foundation to serve individuals living with cystic fibrosis by providing help and hope," says Colton. "I wanted to focus on wellness and overcoming daily obstacles to pursuing goals and dreams. So many organizations are working on raising funds for research—which is critical and effective in extending the lives of people living with CF—but I wanted to be able to impact the quality of individual lives as they pursue their dreams, knowing that they have longer to live than ever before."

Colton, a former American football player who played defensive end for Illinois State University as well as professionally, started the foundation largely in support of his cousin Harper, who has cystic fibrosis.

"Harper was in the NICU for about a month following surgery for meconium ileus after she was born," says Colton. "We knew that she was going to be born with CF [his aunt Shannon was tested just prior to Harper's birth]. This was the first family member that was born with a preexisting condition. No one else in our family has had CF, that we are aware of, so her diagnosis was a surprise and there was a very quick learning curve for all of us. We come from a very close-knit family. We were going to help and support. We started educating ourselves as a family about the disease. I'm so proud of her parents, Shannon and Jason, not only for taking amazing care of her but making sure she learns to advocate for herself too."

Harper was born during Colton's junior year at Illinois State. "I just had an All-American year," says Colton, who was one of only three players in school history to be a two-time finalist for the Buck Buchanan Award which went to the most outstanding defensive player in the Division I Football Championship Subdivision of college football. "My family came to every single game, especially my aunt Shannon, and I would spend time with Harper during the offseason. During my senior year, after my last game, my hometown of Washington, Illinois, was hit with a tornado and Harper's house was destroyed. The only thing left standing was her crib and her CF equipment. She lost a lot of meds but the Cystic Fibrosis Foundation in Peoria, Illinois, helped out." Colton said this was a scary time for the family, but it wasn't until he left for the NFL that he wanted to get more involved.

"In the weirdest way, I accidently fell into it," says Colton. "One year during the offseason with the Chargers, I wanted to start a football camp. I wanted to blend my passion for fitness with my love for Harper and others with CF, so we held some football camps in my hometown of Washington, Illinois, and raised funds to support patients at the local CF clinic at the Children's Hospital of Illinois. We accidentally raised fifty thousand dollars for the Cystic Fibrosis Foundation.

"We had four kids with cystic fibrosis sign up for the camp. They wore stickers so we knew they had CF and we had to keep them on opposite sides of the field to keep it safe (due to cross-bacterial contamination between patients). The parents were really appreciative that their kids could have fun in a safe environment. I knew the Cystic Fibrosis Foundation does a great job with research and medical and providing big dollars—taking care of everybody. I want to impact families and specifically change the lives of kids and young adults with CF. I wanted to encourage them and stay on with them for discipline as they get older with regard to doing their treatments. I wanted to impact individuals and impact families with cystic fibrosis. I just wanted to simplify it. I may not be able to change the lives of everybody with cystic fibrosis but I can help bit by bit and person to person."

Around this time, Colton visited a kid with CF in Peoria, Illinois. "He was a soccer player, and he was showing me his vest," says Colton, "and it had duct tape on it, on the hoses. He had to hold the hoses to the side of the vest to make the air and the machine work properly. Insurance wouldn't approve him for a new one. This equipment for him would cost ten thousand to twelve thousand dollars. My heart was broken. I reached out to the CF clinic in Peoria. They just had an AffloVest rep come in. They gave me their contact info."

Colton connected with International Biophysics Corporation, the parent company of AffloVest, shortly after establishing his foundation to see if they could help him get an AffloVest to the young man in Illinois. "I shared this remarkable family's story, and they not only agreed to meet that request, they also invited me to come visit the facility in Austin, Texas, and get to know them and their product," says Colton.

"We immediately hit it off—I was impressed by their technology and the generosity of the team. Our discussions grew from the single AffloVest donation to David Shockley, their CEO, surprising me and suggesting the fifty AffloVests in fifty states concept. That's how the legacy project was born. I've never known more generous, genuinely good people. I am so grateful for that partnership."

Colton is well aware that Trikafta is helping some to minimize their vest usage and he is thrilled. "Now, fortunately, we are racing against the clock, as Trikafta is working so efficiently they don't have to use their vests as much. We are trying to get out as many vests as we can to people especially the ten percent that Trikafta doesn't cover."

"I have a special relationship with Colton because he's my cousin and he does so much to help people with CF," says Harper, who, at the time of this book's publication, is nine years old. "I think it's really thoughtful that he would do that for me and other people who need it."

"Harper is a sparkplug of sass," says Colton. "She is strong and sweet and funny. She is someone who can hold her own at such a young age. She loves gymnastics, and she and her parents make sure she stays very active. She may not always like it but she takes all the pills, does all her daily treatments, and has a great relationship with her CF clinic. She's doing really well. Harper is the definition of CF.

She was forced to grow up quick. Kids with CF are forced to understand things that others don't have to. They take this perspective that their lives are everything. They don't wake up knowing that they don't have to fight every day. For me, that's what's so inspiring watching Harper go through. For Harper, it's like 'Yeah, I have CF but watch this.' We don't treat her any differently. She's such an inspiration to our family."

Soon, the Legacy Foundation was growing in support. "After we launched the Legacy Project in partnership with AffloVest, we quickly grew to reach people across the country," says Colton, who earned his way onto the practice squads of the San Diego (now Los Angeles) Chargers, Philadelphia Eagles, and Oakland (now Las Vegas) Raiders before an injury cut his career short.

"While I was grateful for the platform the NFL gave me," says Colton, "our visibility grew exponentially when I was cast in *The Bachelor* franchise. There were a lot of deciding factors to go on *The Bachelor*. I was just coming out of football and didn't know what I was going to do. I was going on [*The Bachelor*] to have a good time. If love happened, good for that. At the core of it, though, raising awareness for an underdog illness for me was a motivation. CF is important to me, so it was natural that I would talk about it with a prospective partner. I am hopeful that those conversations helped to raise questions among people who didn't know anything about CF. And, with an increase in social media followers for the foundation, we were able to share facts and stories and broaden the community to include people who are inspired by CF warriors."

Colton, who is currently working on an unscripted Netflix series, says that life after *The Bachelor* has proved to him that he has made a difference in the CF community. "I can't tell you how many people reached out saying we don't see cystic fibrosis on a national stage like this. CF doesn't get enough publicity," says Colton. "It's one of those invisible diseases. I think it is important for me to bring a little more visibility to [CF] because it needs attention."

Since its inception in 2015, a year prior to the foundation becoming a 501(c)(3) organization, the Legacy Foundation raised $10,000 for the Cystic Fibrosis Clinic at the Children's Hospital of Illinois to purchase aerodynamic bikes and medical equipment for patients. They also welcomed four hundred children of the Legacy Football Camps and raised a total of $60,000 for other CF organizations during three football camps to support clinical studies and research.

The Colton Underwood Legacy Foundation has given nearly $500,000 in equipment, which includes donating fifty AffloVests to CF patients across the United States and other donations to CF patients as well as clinics focused on treating people living with cystic fibrosis.

This year, with the help of American Biophysics Corporation, they will have donated twenty-nine vests in total to people in twenty-five states and hit the halfway point with the goal of reaching all fifty states. A majority of the vests were handed out by Colton himself.

The Legacy Foundation has a partnership with the Joyce Family Foundation and American Airlines, and their support allowed Colton and his team to make the trip and add an "experience" with the vest donation. Colton had to limit his appearances due to the pandemic but hopes to return to handing out vests when the pandemic comes to an end.

The foundation has now received more than one thousand nominations and applications for the Legacy Project. They have visited children's hospitals with NFL players to brighten the day of patients. They have purchased more than $6,000 in toys, crafts, and other items for hospitals to provide to their CF inpatients.

"I am inspired by every single individual I meet. I read all of the applications and nominations for our Legacy Project and each one inspires me," says Colton. "I know and have seen the routine of a warrior with meds, treatments, check-ups, tune-ups—and it's a lot. I know that many fight feelings of isolation, anxiety, and depression. Nevertheless, they fight on, they support each other, they advocate for themselves, and they go after their dreams."

JUSTIN BALDONI

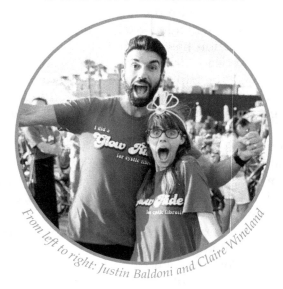

From left to right: Justin Baldoni and Claire Wineland

Age: 37
Resides: Los Angeles, California
Connection to CF: Friend to a CF warrior and
director of *Five Feet Apart*

FIVE FEET APART: HOW AN UNLIKELY FRIENDSHIP TURNED INTO A HUGE, GROSSING FILM

While Justin Baldoni is perhaps best known for his starring role as Rafael in TV's *Jane the Virgin*, the cystic fibrosis community know him as the person who brought cystic fibrosis to the big screen in 2019 with the movie *Five Feet Apart*. *Five Feet Apart* tells the complicated love story of CF patients Stella and Will who are not supposed to be within six feet of each other due to bacterial cross-contamination.

Justin does not have a DNA connection to CF, but he became inspired by the friendship he developed with CF legend Claire Wineland during filming of his 2016 documentary series *My Last Days*. The series depicts the inspiring stories of individuals living with terminal illness, and Claire's episode, "Meet Claire," opened the second season. On the set, Justin asked Claire if she had a lot of CF friends that came by to see her. "She told me that two people with CF have to stay six feet apart," says Justin. "I thought how interesting that the very person that should be able to understand you more than anybody is the one person you have to stay away from. That gave me the idea for *Five Feet Apart* and Claire was the inspiration."

Justin says he could talk about Claire for hours. "Most people recognized something unique about Claire within the first few minutes of getting to know her," he says. "She wasn't normal in all the best ways. She was so young but had so much wisdom. She was like an eighty-year-old monk in a frail eighteen-year-old body. She was so life-affirming, passionate, and introspective. She was infectious. You could feel that you were in the presence of an enlightened being. She just made you feel good. I tried to capture that feeling in *My Last Days*. We became close through that show. She taught me how lonely and isolating of a disease cystic fibrosis was, and I set out to create a commercial film that could do justice to her CF experience and raise awareness at the same time."

Claire and Justin developed *Five Feet Apart*, and CBS Films gave Justin $7 million to make it. The movie grossed more than $90 million and raised tremendous awareness for cystic fibrosis. Sadly, Claire never saw it.

"I was almost done with my director's cut of the film when I found out she was getting her new lungs," says Justin. "Following the transplant, she suffered a stroke when a blood clot cut off blood flow to the right side of her brain, and she was put into a medically induced coma but never emerged from life support."

Justin got a call from Melissa Yeager, Claire's mom, that Claire was not going to make it and invited him and his wife, Emily, to the hospital to say good-bye. "I was absolutely devastated, and heartbroken . . . it just didn't seem real. Yet I was honored to be one of the few friends Claire directed her mom to invite to the hospital to say good-bye." Justin raced to the hospital with his wife and promised an unconscious Claire that he would do everything in his power to make sure as many people knew her name as possible, and that he would always continue to support her legacy and her foundation.

While Claire never saw *Five Feet Apart*, "She got to hear the movie at the table read—I surprised the cast and the studio by bringing her to the table read," says Justin. "After the table read, she gave an incredible speech where she teared up and said that she never thought she would see the day that a movie would be made for the big screen inspired by her life, and that celebrated the unique experience she has had living with CF."

Justin, who attended the 2016 Glow Ride bike ride fundraiser for the Claire's Place Foundation, never forgot his promise and attended the first annual Clairity Ball for Claire's Place Foundation in Santa Monica, California. The foundation's mission is based on Claire's hope to "provide heartfelt assistance to the families of children and to individuals diagnosed with cystic fibrosis." Claire's mom is grateful for Justin.

"Justin has been an incredible supporter of Claire's Place Foundation," says Melissa. "He is always available to use his fan following to get the word out about our fundraisers and other charitable initiatives for the CF community. Justin has been a key asset to build awareness for CF."

Justin says he often quotes Claire, whose beautiful words can still be found all over social media, to his young children so that they can learn about the girl who he considers a "beautiful piece of art in my own life."

LARRY WAYNE "CHIPPER" JONES JR.

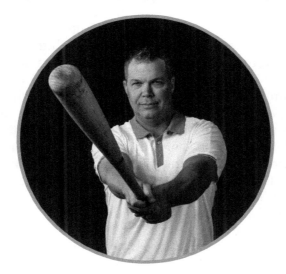

Age: 49

Resides: Atlanta, Georgia

Connection to CF: Loyal supporter of the Cystic Fibrosis Foundation

THE INSPIRATION OF MATTHEW: HOW A HALL-OF-FAME BASEBALL PLAYER HIT HIS BIGGEST HOME RUN OFF THE FIELD

Larry Wayne Jones Jr., who was born in DeLand, Florida, in April 1972, was just like his father Larry Sr., a teacher and high school baseball coach—so much so that many of his family members often referred to him as a "chip off the old block." Eventually, his family and friends began calling him "Chipper" and the name stuck.

Most people know Chipper Jones as the Hall-of-Fame third baseman who played all nineteen seasons of his career with the Atlanta Braves. Chipper is one of the few players to be drafted first in the MLB (Major League Baseball) draft and elected to the Hall of Fame. He won a World Series in 1995 with the Atlanta Braves (the first in the team's history since moving from Milwaukee to Atlanta) and, among his personal achievements from his illustrious playing career, is an eight-time All-Star; was the 1999 National League Most Valuable Player; was a 2000 NL Silver Slugger Award winner for third basemen; was the MLB batting champion in 2008 with a .364 batting average; ranks second-in-career RBI for switch hitters after Eddie Murray (another Hall of Famer); is also the only switch hitter in MLB history with a career batting average of .300 or more from both sides of the plate and four hundred or more home runs; is also the only switch hitter to accumulate five thousand at bats and finish with at least a .300 batting average, .400 on-base percentage, and .500 slugging percentage; is also one of two MLB switch-hitters in history to have at least five thousand at-bats and hit over .300 from each side of the plate; is top-three all-time in the following categories in Braves history: home runs, RBI, bases on balls, on-base percentage, at-bats, WAR, total bases, singles, doubles, slugging percentage, extra base hits, runs scored, hits, and games played; and finished his career in 2012 with a .303 career batting average, 468 home runs, and 1,623 RBI. In 2021, he became the Major League hitting consultant for the Atlanta Braves who would go on to win their second World Series since the team moved to Atlanta in 1966.

Chipper loves deer hunting. He was once a co-owner of Outdoor Channel's hunting show *Buck Commander* and is currently co-owner and cohost of the television show *Major League Bowhunter*, which airs on the Sportsman Channel.

Chipper had just won his first World Series and was preparing for the 1996 season when he was asked to appear at the Buckmasters National Deer Classic in Selma, Alabama, to surprise a young fan, who perhaps was as enamored with Chipper's hunting exploits as he was his baseball career!

"[My son] Matthew [Bowles] loved life," says Matthew's mother, Linda Caldwell. "He never took anything for granted. He loved to do things that everyone else was doing and just feel like a normal kid. He was passionate about hunting and happy to be hanging out at the hunting club as just one of the guys. Matthew was also an avid Braves fan. He thought Chipper was so cool and just knew that he was going to be more than just a great player."

Laura smiles when she thinks back to when Matthew saw Chipper arrive at the event. "He was a little shy at first but very quickly realized how easygoing and approachable Chipper was," she says. "The bond was almost instantaneous! They were talking nonstop about hunting and baseball both. Lots of jokes were passed around. Like a big brother-little brother vibe." Laura says that Matthew knew all of Chipper's stats which were much more difficult to locate prior to the social media age. Matthew also collected baseball cards and, of course, had several of Chipper's, a few of which he brought to the event and which Chipper graciously signed.

"I met Matthew when he was eleven years old and I think I was twenty-three," says Chipper. "He was part of the Make-A-Wish Foundation initiative and had CF. He touched me so deeply and I was looking for something to give back charity-wise. His passion and spirit were something that immediately impacted me. To know that this was a disease that primarily affected children, because at the time, not many people that had CF lived past childhood."

"Matthew loved baseball as much as hunting," says Laura. "He took it very seriously and would get frustrated at times when he didn't feel like his teammates were trying their best. He always played shortstop [the same position Chipper played predominantly in the Minor Leagues]. Because he was so much smaller than his teammates, sometimes the [umpires] would question if he was supposed to be on the team. He would let them know real quick, 'Yes, let's play ball!' We made a special pocket over his port-a-cath to add extra padding for protection. He would sometimes need to put his oxygen on after sprinting around the bases but that was just extra equipment to him. No big deal!"

Matthew was doing four breathing treatments a day while taking about fifty pills yet still he was able to hunt with his idol and even instructed Chipper where to find what is referred to as a "ten-pointer," which means a buck whose antlers have ten total points. The ten-pointer is considered a prized kill. Chipper and Matthew had made a special agreement. "I'll tell you about an ideal deer stand," Matthew said, "if you sign the rest of my baseball cards!" The two young men went together. Chipper made the kill and, more importantly, they developed a special friendship. "Unfortunately," says Chipper, "our relationship was brief. Matthew passed away a few weeks after we met."

Chipper, who, with his wife, Taylor, now has six sons of his own, says he kept up with Matthew's family for a while after that and thinks of them to this day. "When I tell the story of Matthew," says Chipper, "it still touches me that this young man knew he was likely going to pass away soon and had such a bright personality and passion for life."

The role Matthew played in Chipper's life was instrumental in him doing more for those with cystic fibrosis. "Chipper said that as his career first started," says Laura, "he was approached by many organizations and charities seeking an endorsement from the upcoming and talented baseball player. He told me that he asked his mom about which one to choose. She told him that when the time was right, he would know which charity would be the right fit for him. Fast forward to 1996, and the special bond he formed with Matthew at the Buckmasters National Deer Classic, and Chipper knew that supporting the Cystic Fibrosis Foundation was where he was supposed to be. His mom was right. He knew then that this was a charity he could endorse wholeheartedly. His bond with Matthew that week made it personal. Chipper saw in Matthew not only a face but a beautiful, enduring spirit and personality that instantly brought light to the foundation and the many people who live with this disease. I admire Chipper for his continued support, time, and tireless effort to support the foundation for more treatments and ultimately a cure for cystic fibrosis."

Chipper has served as the chairman of the 65 Roses Foundation and has held an annual golf tournament for over a decade that benefited those with cystic fibrosis. When he won the Marvin Miller Man of the Year Award (created by the Major League Baseball Player Association and given annually to the player who inspires others through his on-field performances and contributions to his community), Chipper's monetary award also went to benefit those with CF. He has hosted numerous kids at the ballpark and on hunts and he has visited dozens in the hospital. "It captured my heart and still has today," says the first ballot Hall of Famer. In all, Chipper has contributed upward of $1 million to benefit those with CF. "I am thankful of every young child and family I have met along the way."

"Chipper visits young CF patients in the Children's Healthcare of Atlanta hospitals as part of one of the Georgia Chapter's events," says Linda Murphy, Senior Development Director of the Georgia Chapter of the Cystic Fibrosis Foundation. "He does so without fanfare and specifically asks that it not be publicized outside the CF community. I've had the pleasure of accompanying him on these visits. Chipper's face breaks into a genuine smile as he meets the kids and their parents. He talks privately and passionately with each young patient about their hospital stay, their health, and their hobbies. He hands each an autographed baseball and poses for photos with them and their families. The smiles of the kids, their parents, the healthcare providers, and Chipper's own smile show his love for and commitment to the CF community."

In the late fall of 2012, after Chipper had retired, he was honored by the Cystic Fibrosis Foundation, who thanked him for his many years of support and presented him with a book of photos of children and adults with cystic fibrosis thanking him for all he had done for the CF community. "We had reached out to Laura and the inspiration behind Chipper's commitment to the CF community," says Linda, "to ask her to attend the presentation. She agreed and came to Atlanta as our guest to surprise Chipper. I picked up Laura at her hotel and we drove to the presentation event together. I will never forget Chipper's face lighting up when he saw Laura for the first time in many years . . . he immediately remembered her and began talking about Matthew and his memories of [his] time with him."

Laura is not only grateful for what Chipper meant to Matthew but for what he has meant for the CF community. "Chipper's dedication to the Cystic Fibrosis Foundation means the world to me and my family," she says, "and to so many others who are fighting this battle. He helps bring light to the disease, which consequently helps to raise the funds that will help to not only find a cure but help manage the disease until the cure is found. He has the biggest heart of anyone I've ever known, especially to make the Cystic Fibrosis Foundation his charity."

Chipper, who, along with his best friend and agent B. B. Abbott, started the Chipper Jones Family Foundation—which has donated hundreds of thousands of dollars to repair and refurbish ball fields both in Florida and Georgia—remarks on the impact his association with the cystic fibrosis community has on his own approach to life. "My fondest memories involve spending time with the kids like Matthew," says Chipper. "They are fighting such a terrible and unimaginable disease, and through it all, they remain vibrant, loving life to the fullest. We can all learn something dear from them: never, ever take life for granted."

LEWIS BLACK

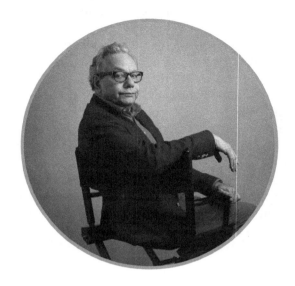

Age: 73

Resides: New York City, New York

Connection to CF: Loyal supporter of the
Cystic Fibrosis Foundation

TURNING FUN INTO FUNDS:
COMEDIAN TAKES ON SERIOUS MISSION

"He was a sweet and loveable kid," says world famous comedian Lewis Black about Gio Villani, son of Pat Villani. "He shined with light. And he was a wicked good golfer. I played with him—he beat me, not that it's hard. He was competitive and not afraid to show it. He was tough as he gave his all to survive that horrid disease. He passed away way too young [age fourteen]. The trophy we give to the winner is named for him.

"His passing had a huge effect on me, one I don't think I realized at the time, but I am sure it is what strengthened my commitment to finding a cure [for cystic fibrosis]. I also have had the great joy of getting to know Mary-Elizabeth Huggins and Wells Clark who both have CF. Along the way, after performances, I have been able to meet with a number of folks who have CF. They are all as extraordinary as they are inspirational."

Originally from Silver Spring, Maryland, Lewis Black is known as the "King of Rant." Whether he's discussing politics, religion, or anything else that gets under his skin, he doesn't hold back during his stand-up comedic performances. Lewis, whose comedic idols include George Carlin, Bob Newhart, and Richard Pryor, tours all over while maintaining a residence in both Manhattan, New York, and Chapel Hill, North Carolina.

A graduate of the University of North Carolina, undergrad, and the Yale School of Drama, Lewis is one of the most successful comedians of all time and has done more than a dozen stand-up specials, including performances on HBO (one of which received an Emmy nomination) and Comedy Central. His weekly, three-minute segment for Comedy Central's *The Daily Show* in 1996 evolved into *Back in Black*, one of the most popular and longest-running segments on the show throughout its history. Lewis's appearances on Comedy Central led to him winning "Best Male Stand-Up Comic" at the American Comedy Awards in 2001.

Lewis, who won a Sports Emmy for his work on HBO's *Inside the NFL*, has had three runs on Broadway: in 2012 with *Black on Broadway*, 2016 with *Black to the Future*, and 2018 with *Celebrity Autobiography*. In addition to performing for audiences all over the United States, he has toured throughout Europe, New Zealand, and Canada and done three tours with the USO to support the United States military overseas. He was the voice of "Anger" in the movie *Inside Out* and has played Santa Claus numerous times on *SpongeBob SquarePants*. He's also starred in films such as *Accepted* and *Man of the Year*; appeared on television shows such as *Law & Order*, *Law & Order: SVU*, and *The Big Bang Theory*; and received five Grammy nominations and two wins in his illustrious career. Lewis also hosted a two-hour documentary, *History of the Joke with Lewis Black* on the History Channel, is the author of three best-selling books, which spent numerous weeks on the *New York Times* best sellers list. He is also a playwright who has penned more than forty plays and has appeared on talk shows *Late Night with Jimmy Fallon*, the *Late Show with David Letterman*, *Late Night with Conan O'Brien*, *The Late Late Show with Craig Ferguson*, *Larry King Live*, and *Piers Morgan Tonight*.

Lewis's first encounter with CF happened by chance in 1994. "I was asked to perform stand-up at the first annual Ultimate Golf Experience (UGE), [located in Pinehurst, North Carolina]," says Lewis. "In exchange, I could play golf at Pinehurst [a world-famous golf course]. I knew nothing about cystic fibrosis or the [Cystic Fibrosis] Foundation but I did know about Pinehurst and that I really wanted to play golf there, and actually do a little good.

"So I was standing around, waiting to go out and play the first round of golf, and was smoking a cigarette. Someone approached me and told me I couldn't smoke. I said why not—North Carolina, where we were was a tobacco state. They said I couldn't smoke because cystic fibrosis was a lung disease. You think I might have read up on it before I went, but I didn't. I put the cigarette out immediately."

Lewis continues, "After the three days of the tournament, the presentations at the dinners about the disease, the history of the foundation and what it was doing, and meeting an extraordinary group of wonderful people who were deeply dedicated to finding a cure, I was hooked. When they asked me at the end if I would join them again next year, I leaped at the opportunity, and I have been dedicated to the CFF and the UGE ever since. No one at that point knew who I was, I was one of a lot of comics working clubs around the country. The interest the foundation had in me was not my celebrity but who I was. The friendships I have made with those who gather together each year have been an important part of my life."

Lewis remains a staunch supporter of finding a cure for CF and has hosted the UGE twenty-five times since first attending the event and learning about the disease. He has also done a couple of events in Baltimore to raise funds, most recently at the Lyric Theatre, and a golf tournament, put together by Dave and Sherry Mount, and one for Pat Hitchcock O'Connell. Lewis and his huge team also produced *Lewis Black Presents: Big Stars, Big Cure*, which featured celebrities including Whoopi Goldberg, Joy Behar, Kathleen Madigan, Chris Bliss, and Jon Stewart and featured special video performances by Meryl Streep, Joel Grifasi, Larry David, Robin Williams, Stephen Colbert, and Will Ferrell. The event raised around $1 million to benefit the CF Foundation.

Lewis says that while the CF Foundation developed a relationship with him, he has stayed supportive because of the strides the foundation has made. "I believe that what they have done in terms of their search for a cure has a profound effect on medicine in general," he says, "and also the way in which they have gotten drug companies on board through the type of funding created by Joe O'Donnell [O'Donnell's Joey Fund in memory of his son has raised $250 million for the Cystic Fibrosis Foundation]. I also believe that it is important to find a cure for a disease in my lifetime, the way in which I saw polio cured. It would mean a great deal to all of us. And no one should have to suffer at the hands of this disease. I also support the CF Foundation because it shows what we can do as a people when we set our minds to it and leave politics behind and realize all that matters is a better world for all of us."

9

THE "REALITY" OF HAVING CF: REALITY TV STARS

BRIANNA COLLICHIO

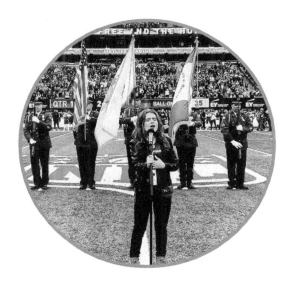

Age: 16
Resides: Spencerport, New York
Age at Diagnosis: 2 months

VOICE GONE VIRAL: BRIANNA'S BIG BREAK

Season 19 *American Idol* contestant Brianna Collichio has been performing publicly since age six.

"She used to try and sing with me even as a newborn, she would coo when I would sing!" says her mom, Colleen. "But the first time I heard her really sing is when I was putting up the Christmas tree. She was six years old. I was playing Céline Dion's song, 'O Holy Night.' Brianna began belting out the same notes that Céline was hitting! I said, 'Sing that again!' I cried. It was amazing. I called a vocal coach I knew about getting her some lessons for voice. He said, 'She's too young.' I said, 'But listen to this!' Brianna sang through the phone. His reply was, 'When can we meet?'"

Brianna began working with vocal coach Richard Fink IV who specializes in a vocal technique called "throga"—a science-based approach to developing a strong, healthy, and balanced instrument for any style of singing—and after a short while, the two teamed up with singer-songwriter Johnny Cummings to produce Brianna's first original song, "On My Hands."

"The song exposes the struggle of cystic fibrosis," says Colleen, "but declares that Brianna will be 'unstoppable' by faith, even if she has to walk 'on her hands.'"

Brianna was diagnosed with CF at two months of age but says that growing up she did not realize that CF was supposed to prevent her from singing. One of her biggest fans, her older sister, Sentina, who is CF-free and was learning about CF alongside Brianna's development, was the one holding her breath.

"My whole life before Brianna, I wished every year on my birthday before I blew out the candles that I would have a little sister," says Sentina. "I was twelve years old when she was born. It was hard for me being such a young age, seeing the little sister I wished for my whole life be sick with this thing called 'cystic fibrosis.' I knew that I didn't wish for *that*, and it was extremely difficult for me to comprehend what was even happening. It was sad to see her as a baby being so small and having to shove enzymes down her throat with apple sauce before she ate her food. It didn't seem real at the time. I didn't want it to be real."

Sentina says she spent so many years being sad and upset that Brianna had this horrible disease. "I didn't want to accept it," says Sentina, who struggled with being a "normal" teenager while forging a bond with her young sister, who needed more urgent attention than most other babies. And yet Sentina says this not only made their bond stronger, but it ultimately gave her a perspective on how to deal with supposed adversity. "I saw how many people she started inspiring with her story and her voice," she says. "She would sing out somewhere and people would know her story and would come up to her and be like, 'Wow, that really touched me in ways I've never felt before.' It started to inspire *me*. I realized that this disease doesn't define her, it's just *part* of her. Because of her disease, I feel like I personally can get through my own struggles and obstacles, and I truly hope to, likewise, inspire others."

But Brianna's inspiring message doesn't make her forget the physical challenges of dealing with CF, and in fact, the message is a bold confrontation with those challenges. At fifteen, about nine months before her *American Idol* audition, Brianna began the drug treatment Trikafta, and she immediately noticed better health. "My lung function level is about 150 percent [anything above 100 percent means higher than the expected value for someone with the same age, height, and sex]—that was all the machine was able to record," says Brianna.

"Smaller things have changed as well, like not waking up with stomachaches every morning or nearly throwing up from laughing due to coughing spasms. I still take enzymes, but ever since starting Trikafta, I've been able to give up a lot of my normal routine; things like my [vest] and inhaled antibiotics included."

Brianna's aspiration to use her voice to send a message of hope surfaced long before American Idol. At nine years old, just before the release of "On My Hands," she was named junior ambassador for the Starbright Foundation, a foundation that helps rescue trafficked and abused children and a cause that remains close to her heart. And when Brianna was eleven, she sang the national anthem in front of seventy thousand people at a New York Jets game—with a cold!

But what she sees as her big moment started with a TikTok video, posted by Sentina, featuring one of Brianna's singing appearances. Sentina made an agreement with Brianna that if the video went viral, Brianna would try out for *American Idol*. The video reached viral status with over 2.1 million views. "I was floored and overjoyed," says Brianna. "Nobody expected the TikTok to go viral. But it was when I read through the comments that I realized the impact I had on people."

Brianna would make good on her promise, but not without some emotional trials quite literally days leading up to her audition. First, there was the loss of her friend, supporter, and fellow CF warrior Jenna Simonetti, whose family started the Just Breathe Foundation in 2013 and who, at thirty-two, died exactly one month before the audition. "Jenna was very special to me," says Brianna. "She always looked out for me and was an incredible source of support for my mom."

Then, the evening prior to the audition, Brianna collapsed and had to be hospitalized for a bacterial infection and operated on for kidney stones. Sentina stepped in and once again tapped the TikTok community for support by tagging *American Idol* while revealing a video of Brianna sitting up in her hospital bed, with the words, "Let's get her voice and story heard" as Alessia Cara's song, "Scars to Your Beautiful," played in the background. This video garnered over 3.3 million views, giving Brianna a second chance.

"They had rescheduled twice for her due to kidney stones on both sides," says Colleen. "Peter Cohen from *American Idol* said, 'Brianna's health is what is most important. We have more auditions scheduled for the end of the month. She can audition then.' I was humbled."

"I was sitting in pre-op getting ready for a procedure for a kidney stone when Sentina called me and told me the news," says Brianna. "I was ecstatic! It was so amazing to hear literally moments before they put me under."

Then came the moment of truth. "I was very nervous before I stepped into the audition room," says Brianna. "I had to keep remembering who I was and what I was there for; it wasn't all for me that I was there, it was for everyone who needed to hear my message. I can only describe the experience as the best moment of my life."

Brianna's audition aired on Sunday, March 14, 2021, and shows her nailing "Scars to Your Beautiful," garnering *wows* from the judges and earning her a ticket to Hollywood. Brianna's run on *Idol* ended during Hollywood week but the experience and the public response further confirmed for her, quite literally, the power of her voice and how she could positively affect people and move the CF needle. Among the CF ambassadorial endeavors closest to her heart is singing at the Christmas Ball for the Just Breathe Foundation for her friend Jenna.

"My family has taught me to trust God and to take excellent care of my body," says Brianna, whose gratitude is evident. "They taught me there is always a plan in the pain!"

Brianna enjoys dancing, writing, inline skating, hiking, and playing the piano, but it's her voice that she understands can help inspire others. She plans to return to *American Idol* in 2022 in the hope of going even further in the competition and giving her an even larger platform to help CF warriors in waiting and all those who need a voice to help find their own.

"Keep pushing through by faith," says Brianna. "And keep breathing!"

ETHAN PAYNE

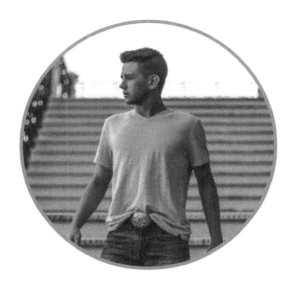

Age: 18
Resides: Nashville, Tennessee
Age at Diagnosis: 18 months

ETHAN'S GUITAR: FROM MAKE-A-WISH TO *AMERICAN IDOL*

Singer-songwriter Ethan Payne's journey to music began at the age of eight when he started playing the guitar as a hobby. His journey with cystic fibrosis began six and a half years earlier when, at eighteen months old, he was diagnosed along with his older brother Chris.

"My parents found out they were both carriers when my mom was pregnant with me," says Ethan, "so when my older brother Chris had gastrointestinal issues and [his weight plummeted] to forty-seven pounds at the age of seven, they insisted on genetic testing for all of us. That's when we found out we had CF." Ethan's oldest brother Joshua is a carrier of the Delta F508 gene but does not have the disease.

Ethan says his early days were difficult. "I was hospitalized several times for respiratory infections as a toddler and would get IV antibiotics. One time I was admitted for a bowel blockage." After that, Ethan was not hospitalized again until the age of fifteen. Ethan was fascinated with trucks and the weather and was never shy about discussing CF with his friends growing up. "I am a social butterfly," says Ethan "so it's never been an issue for me disclosing CF. Having CF is all I have ever remembered."

At the age of ten, two years after picking up the guitar, Ethan started singing. "I took vocal lessons for about a year when I was twelve after my voice started changing," he says. "I knew right from the start that I wanted to make a career out of music." Ethan says that singing has been more than just a passion or even a career ambition; it has benefited his health. "My PFT's before singing were in the seventy-percent range," he says. "Now my PFTs are in the high nineties. My physicians do believe that my singing has definitely improved my lung function."

He has already shared the stage with some big names, including Luke Bryan, with whom he got to perform in Dallas, Texas, in 2016 as his Make-A-Wish. At the end of the performance, Luke gave Ethan his guitar, which he brought with him to his audition for *American Idol* season 17 in 2019. When Ethan appeared before the judges, which included Lionel Richie, Katy Perry, and Luke himself, Ethan boldly invited Luke up to participate in the audition. Luke admitted on air that he was nervous but grabbed a guitar from offstage and joined Ethan in a duet that brought Lionel and Katy to their feet. "I was physically nervous when I started," said Luke as he returned the guitar to a production assistant during the televised audition. "I don't know how these kids do it, y'all."

Lionel, Katy, and, of course, Luke enthusiastically sent him through to Hollywood. "The fact that you're attacking life full speed ahead," said Luke, "you're not waiting around for [CF] to affect you in any way, is very inspiring." Ethan went on to have success during Hollywood Week, and of the eight songs he's released since on various platforms, one is called "Luke's Guitar." He is currently an ambassador for the Make-A-Wish Foundation and helps raise money so other kids have the opportunity for their own life-changing experience.

But it was right after his *Idol* journey that he started having some respiratory issues. "I ended up in the hospital for a tune-up," says Ethan. "That's when I realized I was not invincible and how my disease was real. I really felt like I was not going to make it." Ethan says the silver lining was that he realized he had to take better care of himself. "To that point, I honestly tried to pretend that I didn't have CF and would sometimes not do what I was supposed to do. So going through the difficulties at that time helped me change." Ethan also started Trikafta in May 2021. He says the biggest difference he's noticed so far is a "decrease in the amount of sinus infections."

Ethan, who was named Georgia Country Teen Artist of the Year in 2020, says his family has played a big role in his success. Not only are his parents both medical professionals who keep him on top of his medicine regimen and treatments but his mom and grandmother actively support his music interests by helping him balance his life around lessons, performances, and recording obligations. He also notes the strong support of his brothers, Joshua and Chris. Chris is now twenty-four and, unfortunately, along with frequent sinus infections, still struggles with gastrointestinal issues and weight gain.

"Live life to the fullest," says Ethan, who relocated to Nashville in May 2021 shortly after graduating from high school to pursue his dreams of securing a record deal. "Don't let anything or anyone get in the way of your dreams."

LAUREN LUTERAN

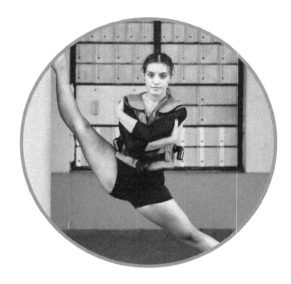

Age: 22
Resides: Orlando, Florida
Age at Diagnosis: 5 months

LET'S DANCE: DANCER MAKES HER DREAM COME TRUE

In 2015, at the age of fifteen, Lauren Luteran's Make-A-Wish was granted when *So You Think You Can Dance* (SYTYCD) legend and Emmy-winning choreographer Travis Wall worked with her on a contemporary solo routine. She loved the routine so much that four years later, in 2019, she used a modified version of it as a contestant on season 16 of the hit show.

A bad cough when Lauren was five months of age pushed her pediatrician to order a sweat test. "When we first heard Lauren *could* have cystic fibrosis, we had no idea what that was," says her mom, Maribel. "We had only one week from her screening/testing to research CF. We took to the internet and became overwhelmed and kept seeing one thing: 'death is inevitable.' We then tried to find articles that gave us hope but, unfortunately, all of them said the same thing — *no cure . . . fatal . . . life expectancy*. We tried to remain positive as neither of us [Lauren's parents] wanted to make the other worry. That in itself made things harder since we basically didn't lean on each other for support—we were each on our own."

Armed with a wealth of alarming information, Lauren's parents returned for the results. "The appointment with Lauren's pediatrician was one neither of us will ever forget," says Maribel. "She wanted to speak with us and discuss the results of the sweat test. The look on the pediatrician's face said it all, and the moment she verbalized it was positive for CF, the room became eerily silent. I dropped to my knees as I felt the weight of her words drain me. Yes, we questioned the results, as we knew of no one in our family that had ever been diagnosed. However, after the blood work confirmed the initial test results, we resigned to what our calling was. We put our advocate hats on a few weeks later and enrolled at our first Great Strides walk and began the work by raising money. We haven't really stopped since."

Lauren began dancing at the age of five. From that moment on, she fell in love with it and found it to be a great way to cope with cystic fibrosis. "It is my escape from all that I had to endure," says Lauren in retrospect. "It is my safety net. Something to lean on when everything seemed to be falling apart with my health. They say home is where the heart is, and mine is definitely on the dance floor."

In fact, with a combination of finding her passion so early and her parents' positive attitude, she admits to not feeling overly burdened by her challenging circumstances. "Growing up with CF my whole life, I never understood what it was like *not* to take thirty-plus pills a day, do chest therapies at least three times a day, and spend days and sometimes weeks in a hospital bed," she says.

While Lauren was falling in love with dancing, she felt challenged with trying to handle cystic fibrosis. "I was very introverted when it came to discussing anything about my disease as a child. I wanted to fit in with others so badly that I would almost pretend like my CF didn't exist. It worked for a while; however, years later it started to become more noticeable because of my declining health. As a kid, I never let CF get in the way. It was quite the opposite actually. I was determined that this would not hinder my success and life. As I grew older, CF definitely started to [have] an effect on my dancing abilities, which really would bum me out since it was something I was supposed to use as an escape. Even with limitations in dance, it fueled me to work harder, stronger, and smarter. I became so in tune with my body and its needs at a young age, which has been a huge help now."

Lauren was apprehensive about sharing her story initially. "I think having that platform on the show [SYTYCD] really inspired me to be vulnerable and open up. The producers told me how inspiring my story was and wanted me to give them all the information I could to make my story something remarkable. In that moment of being frightened, I decided to let go and share my story in depth from multiple perspectives. I wanted the world to know, even though I might not get to live a long life, I still get to live. My story was a reminder for all to not take moments for granted and to keep going even in the face of adversity. The platform provided me with that little push that I needed.

"From when I was eight years old, I dreamed of dancing on that stage in front of those judges," says Lauren. "After going through the producer round, there was a lot of waiting around before I heard if I was moving forward to the next phase of the audition. Once I got the green light that I was moving onto the next round, I packed my bags and flew out to LA.

"After going through the whole televised process, I came to find that I truly enjoyed getting to experience not only the dance portion of it but also the interviews and press," says Lauren, who around that time was also featured in *People* magazine to discuss her experience on the show and her journey with cystic fibrosis. "After getting to dance on stage, the adrenaline rush came to me. It was such a surreal experience to say the least, to dance on a stage I always dreamed of dancing on. After doing my performances, getting a standing ovation, and all yeses from the judges, I felt so overwhelmed with joy and excitement. Once I received the feedback from the judges and was moving onto the next round, I couldn't even believe it." And lest she harp on her public success, she was acutely aware of the benefit of appearing before judges who suggested improvements that could be made to her performance. "The constructive criticism *as well as* compliments really helped shape me as an artist and person."

The bigger issue, though, was that *while* Lauren was auditioning for SYTYCD, she says, health wise, she was never in worse shape. "My lungs were rapidly declining. I was having to go in for tune-ups at the hospital every three months. My days were numbered. I was scared that none of the antibiotics were working and my lungs were just rapidly declining. I have never been scared of death, but in those moments, I just remember thinking if I will ever get to live out any more monumental milestones."

Still, Lauren says that despite her health she was able to compete. "Walking on the stage, I was extremely nervous," she admits. "I was a bit shaky honestly. I finally mustered up the strength while performing to stop and keep moving. It was almost like a light bulb clicked inside and I felt so incredibly free. I just enjoyed my time getting to perform on such an iconic stage in front of thousands of people and judges. At that moment, it all felt so surreal. Afterward, my body did feel like crashing and like every last drop of energy was drained."

Lauren was eventually eliminated from the show. "I felt defeated in that moment because it was a harsh reality. I couldn't make it through because my health didn't allow me the chance. It was deteriorating so rapidly, and I felt very weak." It was at that moment that Lauren's life path changed. "I realized, after this experience ended, that dance wasn't something I wanted to pursue professionally," she says. "Instead, it inspired me to be an advocate for CF and take on a bigger role in the CF community. I wanted to be someone people looked up to and can relate with. I wanted to be someone who wasn't afraid of what CF was going to do but instead used my scars to persevere through hardship."

In October of 2019, Trikafta, the "miracle drug" as Lauren calls it, was approved by the FDA. "Trikafta has been a complete game changer for me," she says. "After getting it in November of 2019, my lungs have never been in better shape than they are now. I am breathing better and able to move air more efficiently. I feel like I can finally live a quality life. I have never seen a future so bright. I feel more hopeful than ever that there is a cure on the horizon."

The result of envisioning a life beyond her personal CF struggle, and even dancing, has paved a way for even greater purposes. "I am a big advocate for the CF Foundation," says Lauren, who has helped raise thousands of dollars over the last twenty years for her team, Team Lauren Luteran. Lauren currently has a store where she sells clothing and accessory merchandise, each embroidered with the phrase "Breathe easy," which matches the tattoo inscribed on her ribcage, accompanied by a red rose representing 65 Roses. "It's good advice," says Lauren of her tattoo inscription. "It's really simple but it goes a long way." The proceeds she makes from her sales go toward CF research.

Lauren's parents are both extremely supportive of her goals and dreams. "They know that I am a fighter, and my personality is very ambitious. Therefore, they are very good at helping me pace myself and stay organized while living with CF."

"Lauren was always at the center of our fundraising efforts," says Maribel. "We are proud to say that, eventually, she began taking on a more independent role with her entrepreneurship skills and campaigning efforts. She now is the lead on most of our campaigning and has been fulfilling our mission to the tee."

Lauren—who has her own book, *Breathing Easy Through 65 Roses*, which was released November 2021—continues taking and teaching dance classes in her spare time at different dance studios around Central Florida. "I am not a professional dancer, as I am choosing to take a different route career wise," she says. "I am pursuing a profession in communications and journalism in hopes that one day I can continue writing articles and advocating for cystic fibrosis any way I can."

AMBER DAWKINS

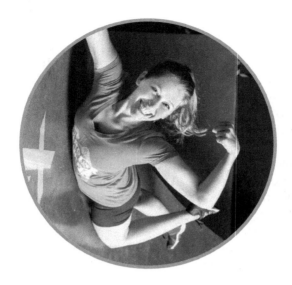

Age: 37
Resides: Olathe, Kansas
Age at Diagnosis: Birth

PICTURE PERFECT: PHOTOGRAPHER BECOMES CF WARRIOR NINJA

C F warrior Amber Dawkins had always loved the show *American Ninja Warrior.* She got to attend the setup in 2017 when the show was in Kansas City, and she watched them test the course and met some of the athletes she so admired. Then she found herself wondering, *Could an everyday person like me train to test the course next time? Is this something I could actually do?*

Amber's story began like so many others with cystic fibrosis. Right after birth, she was rushed into emergency surgery because of meconium ileus. A sweat test later confirmed the diagnosis. At the time, the life expectancy of someone with CF was only twenty. "We were devastated," says Amber's mom, Lisa Dalziel. "But we got to work."

Lisa began giving Amber digestive enzymes when she was only three weeks old by putting small granules into apple sauce. "Amber's digestive issues impacted her more than her respiratory ones," says

Lisa. "But we continued to be dedicated and consistent with her breathing treatments. As she got older, I would play video games with her while she did her vest and nebulizer."

"The games and the extra time with my mom made nightly breathing treatments a little more tolerable and even made me somewhat excited to do them," says Amber, who notes she had few hospital stays as a kid.

Still, Amber's parents worked hard to keep their grave concerns about her future at bay and prayed constantly for their daughter's health. They found unexpected hope when, at one of Amber's juvenile CF clinic appointments, "my mom saw two teenage sisters in the CF clinic waiting room," says Amber, "and by all appearances, they looked very healthy. Mom says the image of them sitting there together, happy, gave her hope that someday I'd follow in their footsteps, defying life-expectancy odds while living an active and healthy life."

Amber was encouraged to try new things and kept busy with a wide range of physically demanding activities: gymnastics, cheerleading, martial arts, and diving, to name a few. It wasn't until she was a teenager that the realities of CF presented themselves. "That's when I began to deal with a recurring lung infection caused by pseudomonas and needed a PICC line," she says. "I did ninety minutes of IV transfusions in the morning, ninety minutes at night, and of course, had the PICC line itself in my arm at all times. It was a constant reminder of CF at school and at all of my other activities."

The sudden challenge impacted her as much mentally as it did physically. "I remember thinking how just one bad lung infection could potentially cause irreversible damage," she says. "My lung function eventually got better, but it definitely made me consider my future more seriously."

At sixteen, Amber started reading more about CF on online forums written by people living with CF. What caught her attention were the firsthand accounts of twenty-somethings being abruptly assumed by parents and turned into third-person memorials because they'd lost their battles. "I was scared and confused," says Amber. "How could I have the same disease they did? Would my health suddenly take a sharp turn? Would I be following in their footsteps one day?" Amber started thinking more about the future uncertainties that come with a CF diagnosis, but she leaned on prayer and her faith in God when worry crept up.

It was in middle school when Amber's parents had the family switch churches to a larger congregation at the Overland Park Church of Christ. "My mom told me later it was because they hoped I would date boys from church," says Amber. "Well, their plan was a raging success, and I dated several of the boys I met there. I spent a lot of time with my youth group in high school: I was involved in the teen visitor's committee, weekly small group, and a prayer group. Eventually, I joined the church staff as the Children's Ministry intern."

Church group is where she met Travis, and for four years, they built a close friendship. "Travis was also highly involved in the youth group and was one of my closest male friends," says Amber. "He was loud and crazy, always the life of the party, and we spent a lot of time together."

Amber completed her high school degree in three years. "I was a bit of an overachiever," she says. She won academic and character awards every year and held many leadership positions starting in elementary school. Academically, she was a straight-A student all the way through school, earning her first B her freshman year of college in an English class (something Amber admits crushed her because it went on her "skipped" senior-year transcript, ending her all-As streak). Amber also admits that she was very social and had friends in many different circles. "Personality tests as an adult have pegged me as ninety-three percent extroverted," says Amber, "and I make friends easily." Her last year of junior high, she was elected student council president. She was also cocaptain of the cheerleading squad, and on the yearbook committee that year. In high school, she went on to cheer with the JV squad and joined the diving team.

After her junior and final year, she was offered and accepted the Presidential Scholarship from Lipscomb University in Nashville. Armed with the impressive accomplishment of her accelerated graduation and scholarship, she was heading off to an out-of-state college. "Suddenly, the routine maintenance that was so easy to adhere to at home was all on my shoulders," says Amber. "A diagnosis of cystic fibrosis–related diabetes during my freshman year made it even harder to adjust to managing this full-time disease on my own. After checking myself into the ER, sick and alone, I experienced my first hospital stay without my parents at my side. During my admission, it seemed like everything that could go wrong went wrong. But I became more independent through the process and emerged a different kind of CF patient with a different level of determination and responsibility. I realized I needed to step up and manage this on my own instead of relying on others to help me."

Amber did not go alone to Lipscomb. Travis also attended the school. "We quickly realized our four years of close friendship was evolving into something more," she says. "The beginning of our relationship felt different than most because we'd been so close for so long already. There wasn't much in terms of 'wading into the shallow end' of this new aspect of our relationship—we were diving in deep from the beginning and we knew it.

"Travis proposed in a gazebo on the boardwalk in New Orleans the summer after our freshman year, and we planned the wedding for the summer after our sophomore year. I remember sitting in my car together in the dorm parking lot, discussing CF and future children. Having our own biological children was important to us, and we decided we'd have Travis genetically tested. We knew we wanted to get married regardless of the results of his test, but we wanted to know if he was a carrier. Thankfully, he wasn't. As an adult, I've looked back on our early engagement and wondered if my decision to marry young was subconsciously related to CF."

"The joy of being young," says Travis, "is that it's easy to look past or minimize larger issues such as the impact of CF on your future spouse's longevity. I was well aware of Amber's medical history as we had known each other through our early teenage years; however, it wasn't necessarily a concern that was top of mind during our relationship and eventual marriage. We were young and, for the most part, quite healthy (all things considered), with the routine treatments and doctors' appointments mostly positive, and things just felt like any normal relationship (save for the medicines, appointments, and treatments). In reality, Amber's CF was simply just part of her life and therefore part of mine. It was just my new norm, and we'd take the good or bad in stride."

Amber married Travis the summer after her sophomore year. "The first nine months of marriage was a fairytale," she says. "We moved into our apartment in Nashville, got our first puppy (named Pancake), and spent time on camping trips and hosting our friends for small group 'house church' meetings—similar to the ones we'd grown up with in our youth group."

In the spring of 2005, things took a turn for Amber as her father was in a serious car wreck which had him life flighted, suffering life-threatening injuries including a broken neck, hip, and knee. "He had a brain contusion," says Amber, "and was placed in a medical coma for six weeks before moving to a rehab facility. His mental health was never the same after the accident. My dad was bipolar, and unfortunately, his worsening episodes eventually led to his suicide in 2009. Losing him was devastating, and I think of him often when I'm at my CF clinic appointments. He was usually the one to take me to appointments, and we passed the time waiting for labs and X-rays by playing games like Twenty Questions and I Spy. He never missed an opportunity to remind me of how proud he was of me."

During the time of her dad's hospitalizations, Amber was notified that the state insurance program she was on in Tennessee was going bankrupt and they were purging their list of insured clients. Amber's group was deemed healthy enough to cut. "The irony of that statement was infuriating," she says. "I was only 'healthy' because of the intense and expensive medical treatments I was receiving. I remember hearing Travis on the phone, calling insurance companies. No one would insure me. We were heading into our senior year of college the next summer, and Travis couldn't get insurance for me through his part-time job. I already knew I wanted to be a teacher and wanted to continue as a full-time student, but Travis was wavering on his plans of becoming a youth and family minister, so we made the hard decision to leave our school, friends, and apartment in Nashville and move back to Kansas. We had more family connections there to help Travis find a job that would provide insurance for me, and it put us closer to my family while they were still reeling from my dad's accident."

Amber later wrote a letter to President Obama that was shared with the Obama-Biden Health Care Policy Transition Team in late December 2008 where they were discussing plans for the Affordable Care Act. "In it, I wrote that the fact that two college seniors had to abandon their scholastic and life plans due to medical-insurance needs was unacceptable," Amber says. "Preexisting conditions had to go. His team obviously listened."

In 2005, Travis got a job at his brother's law firm, working the overnight help desk in the IT department, and Amber transferred to MidAmerica Nazarene University, a private Christian university in her hometown of Olathe, Kansas, to finish her education degree. "Unfortunately, they don't give large scholarships to incoming seniors," says Amber, "and I'd had to leave that incredible Presidential Scholarship behind at Lipscomb, so we applied for a lot of student loans. Travis worked his way up to project management in information technology, and after my graduation, I was selected as an early hire to teach in the same school district I grew up in, alongside some of my former teachers."

After college, Amber unexpectedly found one of her great passions when she was modeling for fashion shows at a local convention center. "One of my agencies required that we update my comp card using the in-house photographer," says Amber, "and my mom and I were not impressed with the photos. We felt like we could do better, so my mom researched and purchased a beginner-level camera and we played around with it, learning what we could online and through books, until we knew enough for her to take new photos of me for my comp card. In the learning process, I realized that I liked being on the other side of the camera even better, and I started taking pictures regularly for my own personal use."

Amber began student teaching in fall 2007 before graduating in December 2007. She was an early hire and therefore guaranteed a job but didn't get her own classroom until fall 2008 at an elementary school where she taught sixth grade. She was there for two years until sixth grade moved up to the middle school level and Amber went with them to teach sixth-grade world history in 2010.

Among the first students assigned to her class was Katie, who also had CF. Because of the risk of bacterial cross-contamination, Katie was moved to a different class, but the assignment was fortuitous as Katie found a kindred spirit in Amber. After school, she would go into Amber's classroom and sit way on the other side so the two could chat about CF.

"We talked about breathing treatments and PFTs and all the things CF patients can bond over," says Amber. "I remember her telling me that it felt good to talk to someone who understood exactly how she felt and what she was going through. She was like my little CF sister."

The two talked throughout middle school and they kept in touch when Katie went to high school as well. Amber, who began moonlighting as a photographer, updating headshots, taking family photos, and creating marketing imagery for small businesses after college, even took Katie's senior pictures and, with those pictures, the two created a montage tribute to CF. Amber and Katie have stayed in touch ever since.

"Having Amber be able to visually bring CF to life in such a beautiful and memorable way," says Katie, "is something that will mean so much to me for the rest of my life. Knowing that CF meant as much to me in those photos as it did for Amber makes them all the more special. For a few of the photos, Amber drew on a 'Just Breathe' tattoo with a sharpie that I actually ended up getting tattooed in the same spot on my arm a few years later. Amber has been such a huge part of my life and my CF journey for over ten years, and I will always be so thankful for the friendship we have.

"She continues to inspire me and motivate me to never let CF define me, and every time I look at my senior pictures, which is probably more often than most, I am reminded how lucky I am to be where I am today. [She has] been the image for what I aspire to be as an adult. I am so thankful that I insisted on sitting in [her] classroom and just talking to [her]. I love [her] and can't wait to continue to watch [her] accomplish [her] dreams."

Married to Travis and professional passion in tow, Amber turned her attention to one of the biggest challenges of living with CF:

having children. "We decided shortly after my dad's death," says Amber, "that we were ready to have children."

Travis says that cystic fibrosis also played a role. "When CF became a legitimate concern and something I began to consider," says Travis, "was when we began to discuss having a child together. While Amber was healthy, and the doctors said things would be fine, it was difficult to avoid thinking about what life could be like as a single father if things didn't go to plan."

Soon, the two tried to have children. "After years of crying over negative pregnancy tests, I was losing hope," says Amber. "Finally, I sought fertility treatments, and after two rounds of IUI [intrauterine insemination], I got pregnant in 2012. Nine months later, in January 2013, Oliver was born, surprising us all with his spiky red hair—a perfect tribute to my dad, who was a redhead himself.

"Without a doubt, being a mother was my calling. I think that, sometimes, when women are faced with the possibility of not being able to carry their own children, and we go down that painful and scary road of fertility treatments, we approach motherhood a little differently. We hold on a little tighter to this miracle that we almost didn't get. We fear missing even a moment of this precious time we've been given. This is me, to a fault. I documented so much of Oliver's first year in the form of letters written to his future self that I almost pursued publishing it as a book. He is, not surprisingly, also the most photographed child in existence."

When he was a toddler, Amber taught Oliver about her treatments. Amber takes over 180 pills each week and is connected to two medical devices to monitor her CFRD. "He helps me refill and reconnect my pump now," she says in a story she wrote in November 2015 for the Kansas City Mom Collective (a chapter of a national network of moms providing blogs, local resources, and events for other moms). "He holds the (unopened) infusion sets and watches for drops of insulin as I prime the tubing. He even sings to me to help me be brave when I change insertion sites. Any way that you can involve your children, do! It's both a learning and bonding experience."

Being a CF mother made the search for a cure even more important to Amber. "My family became involved with Great Strides in 2005," says Amber, "and a few years later, Travis's family started hosting an annual barbecue as part of our fundraising efforts to benefit the Cystic Fibrosis Foundation. Over the years, the barbecue became a competitive event, where teams of four register to compete in lawn games. As the size of the event grew to about 150 participants, we started involving a local caterer who actually met and married a woman with CF through his connection to the barbeque.

All in all, we've raised just over one hundred and eighty six thousand dollars!"

Amber left her teaching job in April 2016 to pursue a full-time career in photography. "I love photography because every day, and every job, is so unique. You never know what you're going to walk into," says Amber. "It was just a hobby for many years, something I loved doing with my mom, and I didn't consider doing it as a career until shortly after Oliver was born. Even then, I didn't think it was possible. Then I landed a job taking pictures for a boutique in 2016, and the income was going to be consistent enough that it gave me the confidence to take the leap! I resigned from the school district, joined a networking group, and hit the ground running.

"Being a full-time photographer has been such a blessing to my health and has given me extra time with my family. I especially love that it's something my mom and I do together. She and I are very close, and I cherish that extra time and connection with her. And I love the freedom that photography has given me, to be so involved in Oliver's childhood. I volunteer at school parties, chaperone field trips, etc. We also have a tradition of taking a weekend vacation alone together each year."

While Amber was finding passion in her new full-time career, another part of her life was changing. After twelve years of marriage, Amber and Travis divorced in 2017. "Marriages rarely end because of one problem," says Amber. "Marrying young meant that Travis and I had a lot of growing to do in our twenties, and there was plenty of time for our paths to diverge as we entered into our careers and discovered more about our beliefs, preferences, and passions. Those twelve years threw a lot at us too. The need for Travis to drop out of college to provide health insurance; my dad's accident, mental health instabilities, and suicide; difficulties getting pregnant and fertility treatments; and financial struggles due to student loans. It's a daunting list, even, for more experienced couples, but we were young and not very far into our relationship. He worked his way up in his career, eventually taking on a traveling component and grueling hours that kept him away often. And I dove into motherhood with all that I had. We didn't leave enough time and energy for each other. We didn't leave enough room to accommodate for how we'd grown and changed."

Amber says marrying and divorcing Travis were both important parts of her life. "I will always be grateful for Travis and the relationship we had," she says. "I'm thankful for the priceless memories we made together, for the way it shaped me and helped me grow, and for the people it brought into my life. I love my former in-laws dearly and am still really close with them. Above all, it also blessed us with Oliver. I told Oliver that a part of me will always love his dad because of that."

And yet Amber says, despite the hardships, "2017 was a new beginning, one filled with adventure." Over the next three years, on top of being a single mom, "I expanded my role writing for the Kansas City Mom Collective. I also sought new experiences: I traveled, I went skydiving, I joined a kickboxing gym, and I learned country swing dance."

This veritable Peter Parker (who is also a photographer) has a Spider-Man side too. "It was during these three years that I found the sport of ninja."

While on the Kansas City set of *American Ninja Warrior*, Amber asked around and discovered that there was a ninja gym she could train at, close to home. So, she joined the Apex ninja gym and worked with Alex, a ninja coach. "When I first started training, it was still with the mindset of testing the course one day. But Alex told me that I shouldn't just be training to test the course, but rather to compete," says Amber. "It was encouraging to hear, and it gave me the confidence I needed to really dive in." That's where her training began.

"Training for *Ninja* with cystic fibrosis was tough," says Amber. "Every pulmonary exacerbation resulted in a three- to four-week-long break from training. It was discouraging, but I pushed on. I remember walking in some nights, feeling like I didn't have the physical or mental energy to train. But the smell of the chalk dust and the welcoming smiles of my ninja friends motivated me every time."

Amber says the most impactful outcome of her ninja experience was happening on the sidelines. While training, she met Jerry, who was also training and applying for the show. Amber remembers, "We had more in common than I thought possible, right down to having the same birthday." A couple of years down the road, Jerry would get down on one knee in front of the Warped Wall (a *Ninja Warrior* staple course obstacle) at a *Ninja* competition and ask her to marry him.

"I'm incredibly grateful for the man Jerry is," says Amber. "He supports me, respects me, and loves me completely. I'm so excited for the lifetime of adventures that await us. Swimming with sea turtles, jumping off waterfalls, and sandboarding the Great Dunes were just the beginning."

In March 2020, they married in a little pandemic-friendly wedding, and Amber gained four stepchildren in the process. "I always wanted more children," she says. "I'm very close with my own brother and sister, and it warms my heart to see Oliver building sibling re-lationships. I was nervous about becoming a stepmom—especially with all the cultural stereotypes that paint those relationships in such a negative light. But I have four incredible stepchildren, and I love the relationships I have with each one."

"I have always felt that Amber is the strongest, most courageous woman I've ever met," says Jerry. "I believe that through her lifelong battle with CF, she has developed a personality that not only has a zest for life and a desire to never waste a moment but also a strength to adapt and move through adversity. This is what drew me to her. We happened to have ninja in common when we met. Ninja was simply the expression of each of us taking control of our lives—doing some-thing incredible and new every day."

Amber and Jerry continued to train ninja and rock climb togeth-er, competing at local and even national levels in the National Ninja League (NNL). Amber qualified for and competed in the NNL's National Championship in 2018 and 2019. "I certainly never thought I would get the attention of the show itself, though," she says. "I knew I wasn't likely to attain a level of athleticism like the athletes we see dominating the course on TV, but I was eager to see where this adven-ture might take me! And in 2020, in the middle of the pandemic, I got 'the call.' The one every ninja hopes for. I was asked to compete on season 12 of *American Ninja Warrior*."

Amber officially adopted her ninja nickname, "The CF Warrior Ninja," and did all she could to prepare for filming in St. Louis in just a few short weeks. However, after months of quarantine, Amber wasn't as physically prepared as she wanted to be and didn't do as well as she wanted on the course.

"But I was seven months in on Trikafta," says Amber, "and my lungs were at a record high: 107 percent! The pride I felt taking my airway clearance vest off and throwing it down on the starting plat-form with the cameras on me and lights sparkling all around was a win. And getting to spend the week with athletes from all over the country, representing the best of the sport, was unforgettable. I made memories and friendships I'll never forget, and I'm hoping it's only the beginning of my journey with the show!"

After Amber's appearance on *American Ninja Warrior*, her ninja story was covered by multiple news stations and magazines. She has since been asked to present at a virtual education day to local families and children with CF; has been interviewed by the Piper's Angels Foundation for *The Epic Love Show*; told her story for the end-of-year campaign for the Cystic Fibrosis Foundation Heart of America chapter; and most recently, was selected for the Kansas

347

City CF Star Award. The articles and interviews sharing her story were seen by CF families throughout the nation, many of whom contacted her to tell her they were inspired by her health and accomplishments.

"Knowing that other CF patients, and even parents of newly diagnosed babies, are finding hope in my story brings me to tears," says Amber. "My platform on the show has opened up more opportunities to spread hope, and I finally got to do for others what the girls in the waiting room did for my mom," says Amber.

Amber continues to work hard in the gym while building her photography business and says she lives by legendary poet Maya Angelou's quote: "Life is not measured by the number of breaths we take, but by the moments that take our breath away."

ROB LAW

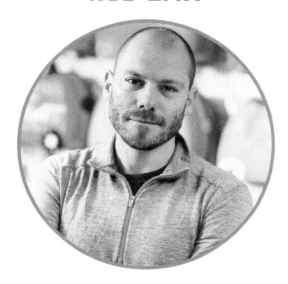

Age: 44
Resides: Bristol, England, United Kingdom
Age at Diagnosis: 3 months

FROM TRUNKI TO TRIATHLONS: ENTREPRENEUR DEFIES HIS DOUBTERS

In 2006, in the wake of being told his business was "worthless" live on BBC's *Dragons' Den* (a show like *Shark Tank* in the United States), Rob Law successfully pioneered the Trunki, the brand behind the colorful ride-on suitcase for kids. Since its launch in May 2006, the company has sold over four million suitcases in over one hundred countries and has won over 120 awards, including the Small and Medium Enterprises (SME) National Business Awards of the Year.

Rob, who is also the author of *65 Roses and a Trunki*—a life-affirming book that tells of Rob's entrepreneurial success while battling cystic fibrosis—has not just played the underdog role in business. Rob's story began in the late 1970s when, just three months after birth, he and his twin sister, Kate, were diagnosed with cystic fibrosis. The two were born prematurely on their mom's thirtieth birthday and both children had the familiar CF symptom of failing to thrive. But despite the later diagnosis, doctors kept them in the hospital for four months before coming home for the first time.

Rob says his stature caused him torment growing up. "Due to my small size," says Rob, "I was bullied at school, everyone knew I had CF and I felt like I was treated differently." Rob stayed active as a youngster by running eight hundred meters in athletics, riding his mountain bike in local forests, swimming, and joining the Scouts.

"My family was very supportive but did not allow us to use CF as a crutch," says Rob. "Mum never let us feel self-pity. She would say, 'There are always people worse off than you.' Dad was very supportive with exercise." And yet, despite his penchant for athletics, what Rob loved most as a kid was creating things. "Especially playing with Legos," he says. Rob's dad ran an interior-design business, and when Rob was fourteen, his dad helped him gain work experience with a product-design company. "Soon after, product design is all I wanted to do!"

Rob didn't talk much about CF growing up, but he had many experiences fighting the disease that doctors believed would take his life in his twenties. "Everyone at my small school knew about my CF," he says, "but I hated the label along with being small for my age. I am dyslexic so I really struggled and even ended up in a class at high school called 'special needs.' I was also probably in the hospital ten times as a kid. I was probably in the hospital more as a kid since the treatments got better as I grew up."

Rob says that at ten, he and Kate were "thrilled" to be gifted an enzyme called Creon that they could take before meals so that they could eat a full-fat diet, which allowed them to gain weight. The twins took enzymes and used inhalers as kids, with their mother doing most of their postural drainage, with the support of a weekly visit from a therapist. "Eventually, I did my own postural drainage until the flutter device allowed me to gain more independence in my twenties," says Rob. Kate's experience was more challenging.

"We were very close as young kids," Rob says about he and Kate. "Like many twins we talked our own language first. We grew apart as teenagers with different gender social groups in school. She got ill when she was around four with stomach problems and the CF really took hold. She was always fighting pseudomonas and in the hospital—miraculously, I never caught it, despite sharing the same tipping frame and stuff. She ended up on the heart and lung transplant list and got a new lease of life when she finally received the operation at fifteen."

A year later, during a family holiday in Canada to celebrate, Kate started getting ill and her body rejected the new organs. Rob was on a school engineering trip when he got a call from his dad that his sister's life was in jeopardy and that she had been hospitalized in London. "My teacher drove me to London," says Rob, "but by the time I arrived, it was too late." Kate was taken off life support and passed away shortly after Christmas at Great Ormond Street Hospital.

"I knew several young people with CF who died growing up," says Rob, "but when my twin sister passed away [from] CF at fifteen, that was the [scariest]. [Seeing her pass away] was a horrendous experience and Mum's devastation was overwhelming. I realized life was short and that I would make a promise to myself that Mum would never lose me."

Rob was ready for a new beginning. "So, when I left to go to [university]," says Rob, "I had a fresh start and kept CF under wraps to only my closest friends. At school (when I was younger), everyone called me 'Robert.' At college, I introduced myself as 'Rob.' Rob was normal, a highly motivated product-design student who was living his life to the fullest, working hard and playing hard."

When Rob met his partner Kathryn in a bar fifteen years ago, he was reluctant to tell her about his CF. "But Kathryn became curious when she saw a bottle of my pills and researched what they were for," he says. "She realized I had CF before I could even tell her." Kathryn was not fazed by his condition, and in fact, when she and Rob discussed having children, Kathryn enlightened Rob to possibilities even he hadn't entertained. "I didn't think I could father kids for most of my adult life," says Rob, "but Kathryn researched IVF and the doctor said ICSI (intracytoplasmic sperm injection) can be successful for people like me. That was a big moment. A few months later, we started treatment and Kathryn got pregnant. We were very excited and let our emotions run away."

Kathryn miscarried before twelve weeks. Six months later, after a second round, Kathryn became pregnant again, and, sadly, experienced a second miscarriage. "A third attempt resulted in a healthy daughter, Ida, now eight," says Rob. Two sons would follow after a subsequent two rounds: Rafe, five at the time of this story's publication, and Kip, now two and a half.

"My children inspired me to make my latest range of folding balance bikes and scooters complete with Trunki tow straps," he says. "It hit me a few years ago, shortly before I turned forty. I was wheeling my daughter on her Trunki (then eighteen months and the first time she could actually probably ride it) through Edinburgh airport. It occurred to me that I was on a journey I was never supposed to make

351

with a child I was told I could never have, on a product I was told was worthless. That was a very proud moment."

Rob is now a Cystic Fibrosis Trust Patron for the Sixty-Five Roses Club, a trustee for the CF Trust, and an inspiration to many people living with life-threatening illnesses.

Applying his business approach to living with CF, he says, "We all have the mental strength to fight our demons and overcome challenges in life and in business. What seems like an insurmountable problem can be overcome, the storm will pass but it will be exhausting, and you need all your mental energy to overcome it. So, use that energy wisely, stay focused on the things you can control, and ignore the rest. You need an open mind to see the opportunities you have and to make the most of them. That may take you away from your initial direction, so be open to change. There are no right or wrong ways, just ways that work and ways that don't. Remember, success is just a hiatus in a series of defeats."

To this day, Rob rarely tells people about his CF. "Not because I'm embarrassed that I have it," he says, "but rather because I don't want pity. I prefer to defy the odds that were presented to me growing up." Yet he adds that, during the pandemic, he has opened up more with his neighbors to explain why he was much less likely to engage.

When not working on his company, Rob enjoys spending time with his young family and is an amateur triathlete, often found cycling around his adopted home of Bristol. He has already competed in twenty triathlons and stays active daily, running two 10Ks per week, swimming two 3Ks per week, and riding one 40K and one 20K on his mountain bike per week. He says that he enjoys pushing his lungs to the limit and relishes every opportunity to cross each finish line in his pursuit of a "normal life."

Rob started a European drug trial in November 2019 for Trikafta but didn't notice much change. "Turns out I was on the placebo, which was Orkambi," he says. "I managed to shake off colds quickly but that was about it. Six months later, in June 2020, I started Trikafta as the second part of the trial, and within a day or two, I really struggled with my physio. I just could not cough anything up and haven't for the last ten months." Rob calls his struggle with his physio a good thing, meaning that he barely has to cough since starting Trikafta. His lung function went from 78 percent to 90 percent. He said the biggest changes for him is that he rarely needs physiotherapy anymore and has now been off antibiotics for the first time after forty-three long years. Rob calls the drug a "game changer."

Rob is a UWE (University of the West of England) Advisory Board member at Faculty of Business and Management, where he was also awarded an honorary degree of Doctor of Business Administration in 2018; he's an ACID (anti-copying in design) ambassador, and a Prince's Trust ambassador and recipient of support in 2002, which is Prince Charles's charity to support young, disadvantaged kids to help them start their own businesses. He has also received an MBE (Member of the Most Excellent Order of the British Empire) from the Queen of England for Services to Business and an honorary degree of Doctor of Engineering from Bath University in 2015.

"All those fancy distinctions just give me the opportunity to be in front of large audiences of future entrepreneurs and offer some guidance by way of creating the most professionally and personally rewarding enterprises," he says. "I was passionate about design from a young age, and the medium provided an outlet for me to create my own business, give back, and, simply, live my best life."

10

FITNESS FIBROSIS:
THE BENEFIT OF EXERCISE

AVERY FLATFORD

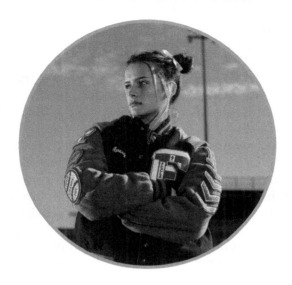

Age: 18
Resides: Knoxville, Tennessee
Age at diagnosis: 18 months

AWESOME AVERY: SOFTBALL STAR STRIKES OUT CF

"**A**t the age of nine, I decided to be a pitcher and never stopped!" says eighteen-year-old all-star softball player Avery Flatford of Knoxville, Tennessee. "Her goal was to be the first kid with CF to play Division I softball," says her father, Chuck.

Avery—who lives with Chuck, her mom, Lynsey, her brother, Rhett (who does not have CF but is a carrier) and their two golden retrievers, Majors and Moose—was diagnosed with CF when she was eighteen months old, just a few weeks after Rhett was born, because of a failure to thrive. Today, she navigates not only a flourishing softball career, but her strict treatment schedule and the occasional annual tune-up.

"My mom is always in the hospital with me when I'm admitted," she says. "She works a full-time job as a teacher, has a small business she does from home, and spends hours upon hours a month on the phone with insurance companies to make sure I have the medicines I need.

My dad spends countless hours in the yard on a bucket, driving me to practices and lessons. He also gives me advice about life and faith."

Today, Avery is five feet, six inches and 125 pounds, so let's just say thriving is no longer an issue. "Ever since I was little, my parents said I have always been self-motivated," she says. "I've always strived to be the best in everything I did: school, art, friendly competitions, and sports. I've never let CF stop me from being the best that I can be. Not too many people in the softball world know I have CF, but I use the disease and the struggles as motivation to be the first college pitcher with cystic fibrosis."

Avery is highly aware of how important it is to make her fitness a priority. "I exercise to make sure I'm staying ahead of CF," she says "but I also exercise for my team. I have to make sure I'm at my best health." Avery has had approximately fifteen tune-ups in her life but only missed two games during her softball career due to CF-related hospital stays.

"Most of my friends and teammates do not know a lot about my CF. It just isn't a part of the normal conversations I have with them. I want them to hold me accountable and not let me slide because I have CF. I'm fortunate that my passion for pitching helps me with strength and endurance, and that practice helps me to play at a high level against some of the best teams in the nation."

Lynsey says that softball is one of many things that motivates her daughter. "Avery is competitive in everything she does," says Lynsey. "She is now doing PFTs without parents and she always comes back with a look of pride on her face when they are up.

"Avery was diagnosed as failure to thrive at eighteen months by her pediatrician, despite all our efforts she was not growing or gaining weight," says Lynsey. "We were sent to a gastroenterologist, and he tested Avery for CF and a few other things. We were numb when the CF diagnosis came back positive. CF did not run in our family. How could she have inherited a genetic disease we weren't even aware of? Chuck and I felt emotionally alone but [we were] strong for everyone around us because we still had this special little girl and newborn son [Rhett]. We felt it was God's timing for us to [find out she had CF]. Had we found out when she was born, we might not have had more children. We immediately became as knowledgeable about the disease as possible, joined the Cystic Fibrosis Foundation, and began attending quarterly CF clinic appointments."

"My parents always told me my CF was a part of my life," says Avery. "I took extra medicine, did daily treatments but otherwise I lived a normal life." Avery's routine has not changed since she was a young kid. "I always completed my chest physiotherapy and breathing treatments twice per day," says Avery. "Having CF has made me tough. I tolerate pain well. The treatments and meds have taught me to understand that hard work pays off. I take those lessons with me on the field."

"I treat Avery like a normal sister," says sixteen-year-old Rhett who often brags about his sister's accomplishments and puts her on a pedestal. "I try to be the best brother I can."

"Chuck and I have always split the caretaking duties," says Lynsey. "I take care of ordering supplies, going to appointments, and staying in the hospital. Chuck organizes treatments and the pill box."

Chuck is also the one who works with Avery in the field. "I played baseball growing up and was fortunate to play in college," says Chuck. "I never got to experience what Avery has been able to do in regard to playing travel and exposure tournaments. I only played softball for a brief time when the kids were younger. I enjoy watching both of them play the sports they love [Rhett is an outstanding lacrosse player] and being a dad. I've had a front row seat to watching Avery grow as a pitcher from the tough years of starting to now. Because of the hours and thousands of pitches I have caught for Avery over the years, I'm able to see things almost before they happen. When she and I work together it is just the little things, not just pitches but the defensive side and mental side of the game. We talk about certain hitters to see how to approach and what pitches to attack with. She is a better player than I ever was."

Avery isn't just passionate about the game; she's very good at it. "Avery first picked up a softball at the age of four," says Lynsey. "She was playing for our local rec league and her dad was her coach. Avery started out as an average to even below-average player. We wanted her to have fun and learn something new. She has played every fall and spring season since then."

At nine years old, Avery decided she wanted to pitch and started in the yard with her dad. "She showed some promise, so she started lessons soon after," says Lynsey.

"My favorite player is former pitcher Matty Moss of the University of Tennessee because of her positive attitude," says Avery. "I modeled my game after Odicci Alexander of James Madison because of her size [she's just an inch taller than Avery at five feet, seven inches] and being underestimated [most Division I pitchers are closer to six feet]."

At ten, Avery had her first travel ball season and her pitching skills grew from there. "We knew she would be a great softball pitcher at the age of fifteen when she had a stellar travel ball season and was a big part of her high school making it to the sub-state game for the first time in ten-plus years," says Lynsey. "She got a lot of time in the circle that year playing varsity. This is also when she started getting some attention from college coaches. With great excitement, Avery verbally committed to play Division I softball at Tennessee Tech University fall of her junior year and officially signed with the Golden Eagles her senior year."

Still, it was her junior season that Avery turned the softball world upside down in the state of Tennessee, but not before a major setback. "Avery tore her shoulder labrum during the fall of her sophomore year in 2019 during travel ball," says Lynsey. "We do not know exactly when she tore it. She started having some dull pain and her pitching was off but not bad. It took us a few months to take her in. She had surgery to repair the labrum in December of her sophomore year and completed six months of physical therapy. Going into the surgery, we told her that she would come back stronger and not to worry." Avery indeed came back stronger. "I wore my arm in a sling and completed physical therapy a few times per week," says Avery. "I always knew I would come back strong, and my pitching career wouldn't be over." Her first game coming back was during the fall of her junior year during travel ball, where Avery threw a no-hitter with fifteen strikeouts. "In another game where she was not feeling her best due to a hip flexor injury," says Lynsey, "she captured the Farragut High single game record of nineteen strikeouts in a seven-inning game. In the spring of 2021, she threw a one-hit shutout with sixteen strikeouts in the sub-state game and this time it took Farragut to the state tournament in Murfreesboro. Over the years, she has thrown multiple no-hitters in travel and high school ball. She is currently the all-time season leader at Farragut with three no-hitters in one season."

Still, Avery and her Farragut team had a goal to win a championship, which they'd come so agonizingly close in both 2018 and 2019, losing to the eventual state champions each by one run and each in extra innings. After the 2020 season was shut down due to the pandemic, Avery was focused on her goal in the 2021 state playoffs. She pitched twenty-nine innings, going 4–0, striking out thirty-nine batters and allowing only four earned runs in the state playoffs, culminating in their first state championship in thirty-nine years. Avery's 2021 postseason awards include Tennessee Miss Softball AAA, All-State, All-District Team, All-District Pitcher of the Year, All-Tournament Team, All-Tournament MVP, 5Star Preps Pitcher of the Year, 5Star Preps 1-Team Pitcher, and a total of twenty-two wins in the circle. And in 2022, she had another tremendous year on the mound with a 23-1 record, finishing her career at Farragut with a remarkable three-year record of 55-3, including 691 strikeouts and a 1.14 ERA (earned run average) . . . culminating with a ten-strikeout, complete-game-shutout performance in the championship game, which led to a second consecutive Tennessee

AAA state title. Following the 2022 season, she received the Courage Award at the Knoxville High School Sports Awards.

"Avery goes about her business on the mound," says her high school coach Nick Green who has been coaching her at some level since the sixth grade when she first attended Admiral softball camp. "She is supportive of her teammates. She works hard to perfect her skills as a pitcher, attending private pitching lessons and countless hours throwing with her dad.

"To look at her, you wouldn't see anything intimidating. She's not six-plus feet tall, she's not going to light up the radar gun throwing sixty-five-plus miles per hour. What people see when she takes the mound is a scrawny, non-athletic-looking girl with a space buns hairstyle. But that's not the impression that they leave with after Avery has made their team look silly. Really good hitters who will be playing in college walk back to the dugout after striking out wondering, *Why did I swing at that pitch, one second I was about to hit the ball and the next I was missing it by a foot*, or *I'm not going to swing at that pitch yet, I just swung and missed it . . .* why? Her ability to spin the ball and make it move is her special physical ability on the mound. Her nonphysical special abilities are most likely a product of her life with CF: determination and perseverance."

"Our goal for Avery is, and has always been, to be healthy and happy," says Lynsey. "The great thing about softball is, it has helped in both areas. She plays softball to be healthy and she stays healthy to play softball. We hope that her college ball experience will encourage other CF patients to stay active in a hobby or play a sport."

When Avery is not on the field, she and her family have spent more than a decade raising money for the Great Strides walk and other fundraisers that benefit the East Tennessee Chapter of the CF Foundation. Chuck was a member of the CF Foundation Board for five years. Avery was named Team Boomer CF Workout Warrior of the Month by the Boomer Esiason Foundation (BEF) in January 2017. She was soon named Team Boomer Co-athlete of the Year (along with fellow CF warrior Michael Caruso Davis) by the BEF in 2017, becoming both the first Tennessean and the first softball player recognized by the foundation. She would compete in Boomer Esiason's Run to Breathe four-mile race in New York City that same year. Lynsey also raises money for the East Tennessee Children's Hospital by leading various fundraisers and volunteering at the Fantasy of Trees event each year since 2010.

Along with playing for Farragut High School, Avery competed for the Force Elite Champions 03 out of Dalton, Georgia, during the 2017–2018 season, the Firecrackers-TJ out of Southern California for a couple of tournaments in Summer 2019, and has been competing for the Frost Falcons 18U out of Chattanooga, Tennessee, for the last three seasons, during the fall and summer.

"I'm known for my softball ability as a strong lefty pitcher with a calm demeanor on the mound," she says. "I love being inside the pitching circle, the one-on-one battle between me and hitter, the pressure, getting a strikeout or ground ball out when the game is on the line or close!"

But Avery is still just an eighteen-year-old high school senior, and while she has accomplished one of her biggest dreams—to play college softball—she admits that she leaves room for her *many* dreams. "I've wanted to be a marine biologist, racecar driver, real estate agent, and an interior designer," she says. "Most of all, I want to have my own family."

BREANA SCHROEDER

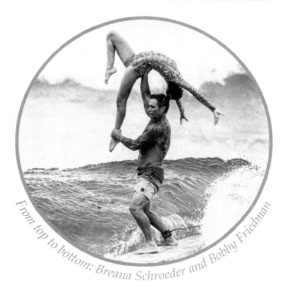

From top to bottom: Breana Schroeder and Bobby Friedman

Age: 21
Resides: Long Beach, California
Age at diagnosis: 6

BREATHE BREANA: THE EVOLUTION OF A TANDEM-SURFING STAR

Breana Schroeder was nine the first time she stepped onto a surfboard. And fell off. She got back on. And she fell off. The cycle repeated itself, but Breana just kept at it and, in the process, fell in love with the sport.

"'She's so good at this, she needs to pursue it,'" Caryn, Breana's mom, remembers many surfers who observed Breana's efforts saying this. But then there were parents who openly impugned Caryn's parenting: "'She has *cystic fibrosis*,' they would say emphatically, like I didn't know. 'She shouldn't be out there.' And I'd just reply, 'She's living her life and having fun.'"

Breana got the opportunity to try out the sport that would become her calling through the Mauli Ola Foundation, which recruits professional surfers to volunteer their time to teach people with cystic fibrosis how to surf. Caryn learned about Mauli Ola through

Breana's CF clinic social worker, who said studies had shown that saltwater can benefit those with CF by thinning the mucus in their lungs. "The ocean is kind of like a breathing treatment," says Breana. "I could breathe better after surfing and breathing in the salt water."

When Breana was a toddler, Caryn observed that when she ate— "which was three times as much as me!" says Caryn—she would develop a big bulge in her stomach. Not long after each meal, she would defecate, and the bulge went away. Caryn recalls that Breana had an insatiable craving for salty foods.

Three years later, at the age of six, Caryn expressed concern to Breana's pediatrician that while Breana had been an apparently robust forty pounds at three years old (the CDC puts the average weight of a healthy three-year-old girl at twenty-six to thirty-eight pounds), she hadn't gained weight since then. "'She probably just has a very high metabolism and will always be very thin,'" Caryn says was the pediatrician's response, but she wasn't convinced. Caryn demanded to see a pediatric gastroenterologist who looked at Breana's symptoms, including clubbing of the fingers, which indicates a lack of oxygen to the blood, and on observation alone, deduced that Breana had cystic fibrosis. A sweat test confirmed the diagnosis. "I was devastated," says Caryn. "I was crying at work. I felt mad and alone."

Caryn was not going to sit back and let cystic fibrosis win. "I didn't want to deter her motivation to do anything she desires." Caryn, a single mom, went all in to do whatever it took to not only help Breana but motivate her daughter to help herself. Caryn says Breana's social worker at the hospital was very helpful and taught them new concepts each time they were in the hospital and, on learning that Caryn had been a competitive swimmer for thirty years and had Breana in the water at just two weeks old, reinforced sports as an important aid to keeping Breana healthy. The physical activity, sure, but also the discipline, since the doctor prescribed physiotherapy twice a day. "We get up an hour earlier than everybody else," says Caryn proudly, "and we go to bed an hour later than everybody else."

While consistent growth continued to be an issue, Breana seemed to be following in Caryn's footsteps, becoming a competitive swimmer and, at age eight, finishing third in both the butterfly and freestyle at the Orange County Swimming Conference which featured the top-ten swimmers in Southern California. Then Breana found gymnastics and was no less successful, finishing first in bar at the SoCal South State Championships. When she hurt her knee in gymnastics, she ditched the mats and took on diving, qualifying for the Junior Olympic team!

And yet, despite her accomplishments, the sport that brought her the most personal satisfaction was surfing.

Breana was appearing at every Mauli Ola event and, at age nine, met Bobby Friedman, a world championship tandem surfer in the eighties and nineties who would come out and do tricks for the kids. Tandem surfing is a discipline in which two opposite-sex partners ride on one board at the same time. It combines gymnastics and acrobatics with the man hoisting the woman into a series of lifts and poses. Breana came up to Bobby and asked, "Will you take me surfing?" Breana had a blast.

A month later, Breana was back and asked Bobby to take her tandem surfing. The sport quickly captured her imagination and she implored Bobby, then in his mid-fifties, to train her. Bobby obliged, coming out of retirement to surf with Breana.

Bobby came to deeply care for Breana, seeing himself as a father figure. Though Breana had competitive aspirations, Bobby was just keen to see her healthy. He'd carefully notify lifeguards before they went out because he didn't want her underwater for too long and he wanted them on full alert. Determined to keep her motivated while they were surfing together, he'd visit her each of the few times she was in the hospital when she was sick and be ready to hit the waves when she was recovered. "He was amazed at Breana's bravery," says Caryn. "Not only did she take five hundred pills a week, she surfed with a feeding tube!"

At the age of thirteen, Breana received a G-tube to help her gain weight. Ingrained with her mom's discipline, each night Breana would prepare her G-Tube so she was ready to ingest 1,500 calories while she was asleep. After three hours, she would unhook the device and go back to sleep. The result was that she gained twenty-two pounds and four and a half inches in just a year and a half!

In 2015, after having success at a handful of competitions, Breana and Bobby entered the Oceanside WTTQ Championship, which they won, and qualified for the Tandem Surfing World Championship in Oahu, Hawaii, on the west side at Makaha Beach, making Breana one of the youngest to ever qualify and compete in the event, and after which, Bobby finally retired from competition. Breana no longer competes because she said that Bobby is difficult to replace, but she stayed active after her competitive career was over, surfing at various Mauli Ola events with other CF kids, teaching and, more importantly, inspiring them.

Breana's story is featured in Duke Addelman's award-winning documentary *Breathe Breana*, which can be found on Google Play, YouTube, Tubi TV, and Apple TV, among other platforms. The film details her journey with cystic fibrosis and her introduction to and success in tandem surfing. *Breathe Breana* has won Best Documentary at the Five Continents International Film Festival, the Golden Era Humanitarian Award at the Idyllwild International Festival of Cinema, and the Award of Merit from the Accolade Global Film Competition.

Breana kept her CF a secret from a majority of her classmates during her career because, "my family and especially my friends had, to that point, helped me lead a normal life," says Breana. "I didn't want my peers to show me any special treatment, which helped me not feel controlled by cystic fibrosis or have it make me believe I'm different from anyone else."

Eventually, though, her achievements could not be ignored. Most notably when her picture was painted onto buses and used in newspaper ad campaigns to promote the Miller Children's & Women's Hospital Long Beach. On the heels of her athletic success, she was named Hill Middle School's "Most Inspiring Student." The following year, as a freshman at Wilson High School, she immediately established herself as a straight-A student and a standout junior-varsity cheerleader, earning a coveted spot on the varsity team her sophomore year.

Breana eventually made the difficult decision to stop surfing toward the end of high school to focus on her academics. "I feel that surfing, at times, distracted me in school because I only wanted to focus on the sport because it was so fun." While Breana admits to missing her days on the waves, her sacrifice has paid off in other ways, as she earned three As and two Bs her most recent semester at Cal State University, Long Beach.

While in college, Breana's interests have evolved to include painting and drawing. She wakes up every morning at 5:30 a.m., clears her airways by using her vest, inhales various medications while using her nebulizer, followed by an inhaler and a nasal treatment. She follows the same routine at night. She still takes five hundred plus pills a week, mostly composed of enzymes to help her maintain her weight, and, in March 2021, started Trikafta, which dramatically improved her lung function from 94 to 114 percentile. And, not surprisingly, she remains highly focused. "I want to graduate college and get my master's degree in psychology and then move on to build a career for myself," says Breana. "I want to be able to have a stable income and never worry about not affording medication or good health care. Once I am steady on my own feet, I want to possibly start a family."

Breana also recently finished emergency medical technician (EMT) school, as she has taken a job as an EMT for PRN Ambulance, and plans to get into nursing when the pandemic is over. Breana says she wants to be an inspiration to those outside of the surfing world too. "I feel like people can still look up to me just for something more academically centered. I think some people can feel discouraged when going into the medical field, but I want people to know there are safety precautions in place so that we can do whatever we can handle."

As far as returning to tandem surfing, Breana says that she's likely done competing; however, she would eventually like to return to Mauli Ola, with which she still follows closely on social media, and help other young people see what surfing can do for them.

SHANIA MURPHY

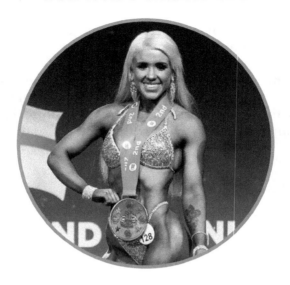

Age: 22
Resides: Dublin, Ireland
Age at Diagnosis: Birth

SHOWING HER MUSCLES:
SHANIA'S BODYBUILDING TRANSFORMATION

Inspired by American bodybuilding legends Jay Cutler and Ronnie Coleman, Shania Murphy began researching everything there was to know about bodybuilding on YouTube when she eventually found the bikini division. "The girls were gorgeous," says Shania, "a mixture of perfect hair and makeup with amazing bodies and a perfect amount of muscle. I wanted to look like a bikini competitor." Suddenly, she had found her life's purpose.

Shania's CF journey started at birth when she was rushed into emergency surgery because of a blockage in the intestine. "I had meconium ileus, and during the procedure, a large amount of my bowel and small intestine was removed," says Shania. Shortly after the procedure, along with a later surgery for a bowel obstruction that left a scar to her stomach, she was diagnosed with cystic fibrosis.

"We were extremely scared, confused and couldn't even conceive of a future for her at the time," says Shania's mother, Iris. "Shania was ill from the moment she was born. She received an emergency, lifesaving operation within her first twenty-four hours and spent the first month of her life in [the] hospital. It was difficult to think beyond the day-to-day care of Shania for many years. Her world revolved around drugs, physiotherapy, and hospital appointments."

Shania says she kept healthy in the early years by staying active. "First off, my family and I work on a sheep farm in Ireland, which requires a lot of energy," she says. "I also got involved in many sports and physical activities. I took dance lessons—ballet, tap, and jazz—did gymnastics and swimming also. I also did physiotherapy treatments for my lungs twice a day, even though it was a struggle fitting it in between school and extra activities." Then she was diagnosed with distal intestinal obstruction syndrome (DIOS), which she says manifested as excruciatingly painful stomach episodes for which she'd have to go into the hospital for treatment. In her teens, she was admitted nearly two to three times a year.

Things got more difficult for Shania in 2012, just as she was making the big transition to secondary school. "I was diagnosed with cystic fibrosis–related diabetes," she says. "This was extremely scary for me as I suffered from hypoglycemia on a number of occasions. Also, I was encouraged to eat lots of food throughout the day, which isn't easy when you're on the bus at eight a.m. and not home until five p.m. from school. So, I had no choice but to carry crisps and sandwiches and things of that nature, which in turn caused me to gain weight." Shania was also diagnosed with CF-related arthritis, which resulted in painful flare-ups. "I would miss school for days because I was too sore to carry out normal daily activities like showering, getting dressed, or walking up stairs," she says. "[CF is] a hard life . . . especially when you're younger and you want nothing else but to be like everyone else."

And despite the weight gain, which, along with the scar on her stomach and CF issues, gave rise to body insecurity, she was further confused by the fact that doctors and dietitians would be concerned about her weight in the other direction—telling her she was "too skinny." Then, in 2014, after trying it with a friend, Shania discovered boxing.

"The thrill of getting into the ring was like no other," she says. "I enjoyed the training because it was so intense. It felt amazing after completing a session, and I always felt great after landing a few punches."

"She announced one day that she wanted to be a boxer and immediately started [working] toward this goal," says Iris. "Getting doctors to sign off on her boxing [became an issue because of] the ever-present worry of her getting a 'hypo' [low blood sugar] before, after, or during a boxing bout, but Shania persevered and worked extremely hard in her boxing career."

In 2016, competing in the forty-six-kilogram, under-eighteen division, she won her first fight, which was part of an international tournament called the Monkstown International Box Cup, in Dublin. She competed in several amateur bouts between 2016 and 2017, winning most of her matches. She eventually stopped because her CF-related arthritis in her wrists and hands would be extremely sore after boxing. Then, in 2018, she discovered bodybuilding.

"I love all aspects of bodybuilding," says Shania, "from the bulking phase in the offseason [putting on as much lean mass as possible] to the cutting before a competition [getting as lean as possible while maintaining as much muscle as possible] to the show day itself where I am able to get dolled up because I am quite girly to the aspect of competing."

Shania registered for her first-ever bodybuilding competition in 2018, which took place right after completing her final secondary school exams. "I prepped for fourteen weeks," says Shania, "and training was intense. Leading up to the competition, I would get up at five a.m. and do an hour or more of cardio before school, go to school, then go to the gym for two hours of weightlifting, and then get home at around half-past seven to do some studying. And then there were my physiotherapy treatments, which I had to do before bed." The result: she took home three first-place trophies and one second-place trophy.

"When I first started bodybuilding," says Shania, "it was a lot harder because I was still in school. So, after very long days, I would have to go train and remember being extremely tired. I would also have to go to posing lessons on the weekend before my competitions, so I was very busy. Now, I enjoy my bodybuilding a lot more because I have lots more time to train and to rest. Rest is extremely important for muscle growth and preventing injuries. Also, because of Kaftrio [which Shania started taking in March 2021], I have a lot more energy and it has really helped my digestive problems that I suffered."

Shania competed in two Northern Ireland Fitness Model Association (NIFMA) competitions in 2019 and, combined, took home six trophies. She also won an overall bikini title at one of the NIFMA competitions where a competitor is judged on a mixture of things such as muscularity, tone, symmetry, shape, and stage presence. "That title was, to that point, my ultimate dream fulfilled!"

Shania's healthful approach to her sport also dramatically improved her CF symptoms. "[The year] 2019 was the first year I didn't have to be admitted to the hospital since I was a teenager!" she says.

"She has taken to bodybuilding with great enthusiasm and has embraced all that goes with it," says Iris. "She still has to make time for appointments, doing nebulizers, and medicines but she powers through, and we feel like she has finally found her niche."

Concurrent with her bodybuilding successes, Shania became a qualified personal trainer, nutritionist, and gym instructor and eventually started her own business, Girly Gains Fitness. She now teaches fitness classes and does online personal training. In the summer of 2019, she also became a licensed security officer and works security all over Ireland.

She also serves as an ambassador for Cystic Fibrosis Ireland, raising funds and awareness through sponsored events, media appearances, and even church-gate collections.

"She has been through so much and has great empathy not only for other people with cystic fibrosis but for everyone," says Iris. "I think she is a beacon of light for younger CF sufferers to see that they, too, can live life to the fullest and do amazing things despite everything CF might throw at them."

Since starting Kaftrio, she says she can eat a lot more without being sick the next day. She hopes that's just the beginning of health improvements.

In 2021, Shania moved to Dublin, which was a goal of hers because she loves the city. In September 2021, she competed in an International Federation of Bodybuilding (IFBB) competition in Tampere, Finland, and placed second in junior bikini. The following month, she competed in the amateur division of the prestigious Arnold's Sports Festival UK in Birmingham, England, and received first call outs (which means the competitor was one of the top choices for that category), which Shania says is "amazing" at such a big event. She is now working as a fitness instructor and personal trainer in Dublin while also working as an online coach.

Shania continues to prep for future competitions including a 2022 IFBB Pro Qualifier Amateur Olympia event in Tokyo, Japan, where she hopes to place. She has also set goals of receiving her pro card, becoming a professional bikini competitor, and competing all over the world. In order to earn her pro card, she must win an IFBB Pro Qualifier competition where the winners win prize money. If she gets her pro card, the next goal would be to qualify and compete in Mr.

Olympia, the biggest bodybuilding competition in the world. In the meantime, Shania continues to grow her personal trainer business and has even started a YouTube channel documenting her workout routines and detailing her journey to the bodybuilding stage.

"When I think back to the time she was born," says Iris, "and the worry at seeing her attached to ventilator tubes after her operation and losing weight rapidly, and to see her now as a beautiful confident woman both in life and on stage during her bodybuilding competitions, just makes me the proudest mother in the world."

CHELSEA SPRUANCE STAHL

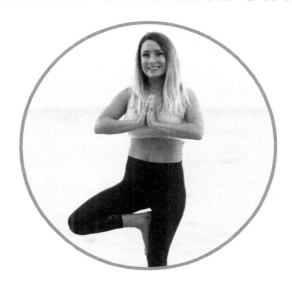

Age: 28
Resides: St. Thomas, Virgin Islands
Age at Diagnosis: 4 months

ONE BREATH AT A TIME: BECOMING A CF YOGI

After graduating cum laude from the University of Tampa at the age of twenty-two with a BA in psychology, despite multiple hospital admissions and setbacks, Chelsea Spruance Stahl chose to go to the one place she thought would be conducive with being active, eating healthy, and self-care: San Diego, California.

"When I moved to San Diego it was clear that health was not only my main priority but it was within the culture. From outdoor activities to healthy food options, it was clear that I was not the only one focusing on and understanding the importance of my health." Among her ambitions was to take up yoga. "The first class I did was horrible," says Chelsea, "but something in me told me to stick with it. Because of this I was able to gain lung function and strength back, far past the amount the doctors told me was possible."

Chelsea was born in her parents' home state of Delaware, though her parents, Tom and Linda, were living in St. Thomas in the US Virgin Islands, where Tom had set up his business. During her first four months, while she and her parents were traveling, she was not gaining much weight. "At four months, I weighed just eight pounds," says Chelsea.

Tom and Linda sought care from several doctors in Delaware, but it was a doctor in St. Thomas who recognized the symptoms as being "genetically wrong. But we do not have the resources to diagnose her here," he said. Upon returning to Delaware, Chelsea was admitted to Alfred I. duPont Hospital for Children and remained there for four months before she was diagnosed with CF.

"My treatment regimen as a child was pretty basic," says Chelsea who spent her first eight years living in St. Thomas. "I had a feeding tube that was put in when I was an infant, because at four months, I still only weighed eight pounds and was diagnosed with 'failure to thrive.' But, after diagnosis, things were very smooth overall." Chelsea was active and healthy and only did a few treatments a day—Albuterol and Pulmozyme—in addition to her vest or CPT and had enzymes. "One beautiful memory my father and I have," says Chelsea, "is that when I was too young for the vest, we would walk up and down the mountain we lived on, and that I now live on again. He would 'tap' my back as we looked up at the stars, where I would always point and say, 'Mr. Moon!'"

"Treatments became a normal daily event," says Tom, "which I tried to use as a time to be closer to Chelsea."

"But I in no way grew up in a bubble," says Chelsea. "I could do what every other child my age was doing. My parents always instilled in me that though CF is a big deal, it is just a part of who I am, like my hair and eye color. There wasn't anything I was going to do to change or hide it because it is simply me. This helped cultivate such confidence in who I was as a person and took remembering when I was feeling less confident."

Chelsea says the treatments were just part of the family's daily regimen, that there was always time for the stuff of "normal" families. "We always did what we planned to do regardless of CF, whether that be traveling," she says, "going out to have fun, school, meeting friends. All in all I felt normal with an added element of nebulizers and pills."

Chelsea says that CF wasn't a common subject of conversation in her earliest years, but that when it came up, she was happy to talk about it. "I wasn't ashamed or anything like that. I think growing up on St. Thomas, in addition to having CF, helped shape me into the person who I am," says Chelsea, "which is very personable, always wanting to help someone else—in addition to someone who tries to seize the moment every chance she has."

Chelsea says that, early on, CF did not concern her when it came to her life aspirations. "Ever since I was a little girl, I wanted to become a mother. My childhood clinic was amazing at allowing me to dream, imagine, and plan as if I had as normal a future as anyone else. There was never someone who told me I could not be a mother, but my parents and doctors were almost too encouraging of any of my future plans and conveniently avoidant to any more-pressing future questions I had."

Yet, while Chelsea says she grew up relatively healthy with no real signs of CF aside from her daily regimen of medications, an increase in treatments and a more serious tone to the CF conversation created a greater awareness of her condition. "I think many [CF patients] see, as they age, the natural progression of CF slowly taking over," says Chelsea. "I was put on Pulmozyme twice a day at around ten to twelve years old, then started adding in inhaled TOBI, and started to more frequently have to be [adding] oral antibiotics. It was when I was twelve that I vividly remember thinking there was something my parents weren't telling me about CF. So I went to Google and typed in 'cystic fibrosis life expectancy.' In bold numbers, I saw the age twenty-six glaring back at me, and my world crumbled. All my future goals and ambitions vanished before my eyes."

As Chelsea got older, CF became more of a mental burden than it was physical. "Thankfully, CF did not impede my life at all [during middle school and high school], aside from daily treatments," says Chelsea. "Looking back now, I know I was very lucky to not have had any issues with my heath before the age of eighteen. But even with a lack of outward CF issues, I was still dealing internally with what CF meant for my future. Following the discovery of CF life expectancy, I became depressed and defiant for a short time. I stopped doing treatments, thinking, *Well, I'm going to die, so why bother?* This was around the time I began dabbling with dating and I started having to think about how to explain my uncertain future to someone else. This stayed an undercurrent for a few years.

"I think a lot of the mental anguish and depression within CF (for me at least) comes from a lack of control. There are so many things in life that no one can control, but for most people, their health is not one of them. For most people, they don't even think about their health until they absolutely have to. It would be ignorant to talk about CF without talking about the mental stress it puts on someone.

"Most of this stress for me occurred in my teenage years. These were the years where most friends were becoming independent, figuring out who they are and what they want in their future. Whereas I was figuring out what my illness means to me, my future, and how different my life truly was. I remember the first feelings of truly knowing how different my life was and will be when going to sleepovers. I could not just pop over to a friend's house after school for a spur of the moment sleepover. My life did not allow me the luxury. I would have to go home and do treatments, pack pills, pack morning treatments, and then be able to do what most children did without thinking. It was truly challenging trying to become an independent person while knowing there is a huge part of my life that I will never be independent from."

Chelsea continues, "CF is who I am, it will always be there, and it was a challenge no one could necessarily help me with. I had to learn on my own how to cope with the feelings of being different and knowing how different my life was. It was through support of friends and family that I was able to see CF as a part of me rather than a hinderance to me. Trying to navigate it alone was terrifying. And even though friends didn't have or fully understand CF did not mean they could not be there for me when I needed support. It was hard, but I had to look at the big picture. How CF had shaped me into such a determined person. I also had to accept and feel those feelings of sorrow, to mourn the life I see others living, that I will never live—a life free of CF. I tried to begin to look at my sadness as a human emotion rather than something to avoid and push away.

"But there came a point that my mindset began to shift. It shifted from giving up and letting CF 'do what it's going to do,' to fighting it. It didn't happen overnight. But slowly I realized that giving up meant letting CF win and letting it take control of my life. I still had dreams and a future I imagined for myself, and I had a choice. Let the life expectancy win and become true, or to fight and not let CF win. I decided to fight. I am eternally grateful for that because once I became sick at eighteen, it wasn't like what I had seen happen to other [CF patients] where they are sick for two weeks and then not again for a year or two. At eighteen, my health took a complete turn, and it was then where my fight really began.

"When I got to college, I added in hypertonic saline. This was also the time that started the ball rolling with recurring need for IV antibiotics, which I had never needed until the age of nineteen. It was only when I moved to Tampa, Florida, and went to college that CF began to truly show how powerful it is. In a matter of three years, I went from a healthy, vibrant eighteen-year-old with eighty-six-percent lung function to a twenty-one-year-old who could barely shower without getting out of breath at twenty-six-percent lung function. My lungs took a beating those years."

Chelsea says her CF center at the time did not have a good

treatment plan and she believes it cost her physically. "It is apparent in CF care," says Chelsea, "that patient advocating is one of the most important things in the treatment of one's health. This is the ability to know what is going on in our body and to be a contributing factor to our treatment plan based on our knowledge of our own disease and body. Many clinics see this as an integral portion of care because you are not just treating the disease, but the patient. In my eyes, this constitutes a good care center—a CF care center being an area of a hospital that is devoted to the care and treatment of CF patients. A good care team, and thankfully one that I have found with my team at Johns Hopkins, involves the patient as a specialist, because they are a specialist of their own body. They prescribe medications while factoring in what that means for the patient day in and day out. The patient is involved in each and every decision. Unfortunately, the care team I was with in college in Tampa did not share that same idea."

At twenty-one, Chelsea received a port to access IV antibiotics easier since she was getting them so frequently. She eventually ended up in a hospital bed unable to walk up a flight of stairs. "I found myself depressed, thinking thoughts like 'I don't want to live if this is my life now.'"

Around that same time, Chelsea began making more friends online as she was looking for answers to help her health and also to learn about what may be in store for her future. "Some of [these people I met online with CF] had children already and spoke about the challenges, the lung function requirements for a safe pregnancy, and the worries both they and their care teams had. This was before any modular therapy for CF and around the first time in history there were more adult patients than pediatric. Up to this point, pregnancy wasn't an item most clinics discussed or even thought about because of the average life expectancy. Knowing where my health was at that time, I knew pregnancy would not be advised, and also at that time I was unsure if I would ever get healthier. This continued to reinforce the idea that my dream of a family was a fantasy."

Chelsea continues, "When I was at my sickest moment, I was twenty-one years old and in a hospital with a care team I did not trust, 1,500 miles away from my family and my home center. There were plans to transfer me to my home center in Baltimore, Maryland, at Johns Hopkins in the coming weeks, but I was still in the hospital near college. This left certain doctors tense at the thought they were treating 'someone else's patient,' and I could sense the distaste for how involved and in control of my care I was. With this already uneasiness in the air, one morning a doctor from the team (and my least favorite doctor) came in at seven a.m., woke me up, and, in my groggy state, he sat down and, in a sarcastic manner, said, 'Well, it looks like you should start planning to head up north to get new lungs.'

"I don't know what it was, but something in me said that this wasn't my time," says Chelsea. "I was eighty-nine pounds with twenty-six-percent lung function and on oxygen, and still, I thought, *It isn't time for new lungs.* I never missed my meds, even in college; I did everything that was 'prescribed' to me but . . . I believed I could do more. This was when I started truly listening to my body, what it needed, what it was telling me, and put my heath at the very top of any priority list. My dream became to regain my physical strength."

In a Hail Mary attempt, Chelsea's father drove her up to Johns Hopkins. "Thankfully, after six weeks in the hospital," says Chelsea, "I was released, but I was released nowhere [near] where I wanted to be. I was only around ninety-two pounds and my doctors, with the help of medications, were only able to get my lungs back up to forty percent. This is outside the window of lung transplant, but not by much."

Once out of the hospital, Chelsea began her quest by drinking three weight-gain shakes a day—"I would have coughing fits and occasionally spit some of the drinks out!"—and doing pulmonary rehab. "This new regimen was not necessarily prescribed but suggested," says Chelsea, "and I knew in my body it was time to put the pedal to the metal and get my health back where I wanted it: in my control. The pulmonary rehab was a suggestion from my team at Johns Hopkins that I jumped on, but once the three months were up, I knew that was not the end for me. I needed to push myself. I could no longer use the negative narrative that 'I can't' because I did not have a choice if I wanted to live a life I wanted. A life as unrestricted by CF as possible. This took a choice every single day to not only do what had been prescribed by doctors, by doing my medications and hour-long treatments, but also by recommitting to my body, choosing to do the things that I needed to, even though it was hard.

"Working out three to four times a week, even though it was hard to walk around the block; eating over three thousand calories a day, even though I wasn't hungry; pushing my body to do more each day instead of feeling sorry for myself. It was like taking on a full-time job in addition to taking a full course load in college and graduating on time despite all the medical setbacks and time away. The first thing I thought about each morning and the last thing I thought about each night was what more I could be doing to help my body recover. It was my job to help my body now, to give it all the resources it needed to become stronger, and I needed to start working with my body and not against it. I had to stop hating its inabilities and accept where it was that day and work with that.

"It was a constant battle," says Chelsea, "to not compare myself to other twenty-one-year-olds and only compare myself to who I was yesterday to see my progress. This was my fight to fight, and no one could do it for me. I had to ask myself in the hardest moments how much I wanted to live. I let myself cry when I needed to, be upset when I needed to, but I couldn't stay in that moment. I had to keep pushing because I was not done living yet—far from it. I slowly started to make my climb out of the hole I was in. It took a lot of determination and personal strength, but through changing centers and devoting my time to my health, I began my long climb back to normalcy. I was told this may be my new normal and I could not accept that. It took years [to get stronger]."

Chelsea's dream has come true as she is now much healthier. She is now a yoga teacher with 55-percent lung function and weighs 125 pounds, more than double her lung function in her early twenties, and nearly forty pounds heavier. She primarily works with people dealing with cystic fibrosis to help them improve their lung function. "Soon after becoming a yoga teacher," says Chelsea, "I started teaching for CF Yogi, a nonprofit directly formed to bring yoga to [people with CF] from people in the CF community."

Yoga turned out to be the perfect recipe to make Chelsea healthy again. "I wanted to find out what more I could do for my body," says Chelsea, "and through pulmonary rehab and exercise, I stumbled upon yoga. When I found a yoga class that fit me and my body at that moment in time it was transformative. It helped me reconnect to my body. I slowly started looking at it as strong and beautiful instead of damaged and faulty. The physical elements of yoga and its benefits for CF is apparent—focus on the breath and strength gaining, but rarely is the emotional and mental element spoken about. This was a multi-year journey that brought me back to myself, to loving myself, and because of this I wanted to help other people from the same dark place I was.

"We all know how important exercise and mental health is within any disease, specifically the CF world, but when I was starting my yoga journey, there was no one like me. There was no teacher who understood what having a coughing fit in the middle of a class felt like, no one who understood how breathless I could be, no one who understood how I felt. So, I wanted to be that teacher to people. I wanted to be the teacher who has CF and can honestly tell students, 'I get it,' 'It's okay to cough,' and every other statement I wished someone would tell me."

Chelsea later joined Beam, another company focused on fitness in the CF world, as a CF yogi instructor. "CF Yogi to me is a place where other people just 'get it,'" she says. "It is a place where we all know how hard it can be to exercise, try something that challenges us, and push our body when we don't feel well. It is not coming from a physical therapist who has not lived it; it is a place where the teachers and students alike know what it is like to have a coughing attack mid deep breath."

Yoga continues to teach Chelsea valuable lessons. "Yoga helped me understand that what we resist persists," says Chelsea. "So, by allowing those deeper emotions room to be felt, I released their control over me rather than bottling them inside to fester. These deep and depressing thoughts still exist today but I have acquired so many methods of coping and dealing with those thoughts in a healthy way that I did not have in my teens. Like anything, it is a growing experience, and I am thankful for my teen years because it was the beginning of my journey with my mental health. It helped me work through hard times, and by worrying through them, I slowly began acquiring tools that work for me."

Since starting Trikafta, Chelsea's world has continued to change. "Though I did not gain any lung function, my day-to-day life improved to the point I was able to begin working full time and still had energy to explore more hobbies than ever before," she says. "A life with CF is one full of so many rollercoasters, but when you learn to see each opportunity as a change for growth and learning, they all become a little easier to bear."

Chelsea has cochaired both BreatheCon and FamilyCon for the Cystic Fibrosis Foundation, a keynote speaker at CF Foundation events, and a guest on podcasts, speaking on behalf of the Boomer Esiason Foundation. Her family is also hugely involved directly to the Johns Hopkins CF adult center and have done fundraisers with them for many years while helping get the transplant initiative from Johns Hopkins Hospital to hospitals across the country. Chelsea also attends Johns Hopkins regardless of where she is living. To this day, her dad, at the age of seventy-four, still attends clinic visits with her.

"Clinics provide the opportunity to personally learn about Chelsea's progress and the challenges that confront her," says Tom. "I always want Chelsea to realize that this is a team effort."

Chelsea's view on life is reflected in "how much life I can squeeze out of this one. I have been cage diving with great white sharks, moved across the country, alone, three times, solo traveled for forty days throughout seven countries in Europe with all my medications, and seen so much of the world—Thailand, Guatemala, Costa Rica—I've been to so many more places than I could've dreamed of!"

After a move to Atlanta at the age of twenty-four, Chelsea eventually found herself back in St. Thomas, where she currently resides, while aspiring to one more goal. "My ultimate dream is to be a mother," says Chelsea, who calls her husband, Connor, whom she married in summer 2022, her biggest supporter. "I remember reading at a young age that it would never happen because of my CF. This alone has been a driving factor of why I wake up and do my medications each and every day. I put in the work now to spend time with my future children, who mean enough to me now that they push me to keep myself healthy. And at this past year's clinic, I brought up potential family planning and was given the medical green light to embark down the path of becoming a mother whenever I want."

In the meantime, Chelsea and Connor opened a two-part business in January 2022, in which Chelsea runs her own yoga studio while Connor, a free-dive instructor among other professions, runs his own free-diving school.

And yet, Chelsea admits she'd one day climb Kilimanjaro. "And travel the world by sailboat," she says. "Overall, I want to live to be old enough that my obituary says that I died *with* CF, not *from* CF."

MEGAN DiBENEDETTO

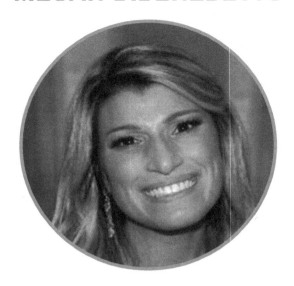

Age: 29
Resides: Brooklyn, New York
Age at Diagnosis: 9 months

MEDICAL ATTENTION: NURSE WITH CF WORKS DURING PANDEMIC

Megan DiBenedetto admits the last few years have not been easy but, in her case, as a registered nurse, it has been even more difficult, with regard to having CF and trying to avoid COVID-19. "I never thought about quitting and I never will," says Megan, "because every patient needs a nurse to take care of them, and nursing is my career."

Megan was born on September 24, 1992, to Madeline and Carmelo DiBenedetto. From two weeks of age, Megan had symptoms of bronchitis, but her doctor ensured Madeline that was all it was. At nine months old, with symptoms still prevalent, Madeline took Megan to get a sweat test. The diagnosis was confirmed. Megan had cystic fibrosis.

"Devastated, shocked, and in denial," Madeline said on receiving the news, "but I made up my mind: I would never let this affect Megan. She will never see the weakness I had initially. I became strong for her and me." Yet, as much as Megan's parents wanted her to feel "normal," there were tough moments.

"I don't remember how old I was, maybe about seven or eight years old," says Megan, "my mom was reading me a book called *Stevie's Secret*. It was about a girl with CF, and I remember asking my mom if I was going to die. I was still very young at the time so I couldn't fully grasp the concept of CF, but it was a feeling of uncertainty and confusion because I didn't understand what my life was going to be like. Mom said, 'That's not going to happen. We are going to do everything to keep you healthy.' My parents raised me to power through. I went to school every day, and there were no excuses unless I really did not feel well. Growing up, my brother treated me as if CF wasn't even a thing. My family shows me no pity."

Megan says her parents were especially disciplined when it came to sports. "They signed me up for practically every sport," she says, "and the one that stuck was swimming." Megan started swimming competitively around the age of five and competed in roughly two to three meets per week for the next sixteen years. "In high school, I won almost every meet I was in," says Megan. "I had meets every weekend, and sometimes twice a weekend."

Megan walked on at Wagner College, a Division I school in Staten Island, New York, and won some races which culminated in an Northeast Conference (NEC) team championship in 2014.

As good a swimmer as Megan was, she still believes she could have been better. "I still got out of breath [because of CF] when I swam," says Megan. "I had over 110-percent lung capacity [in college], but swimming still got me winded, and when your body lacks oxygen, it slows down. During practice, I would have to stop periodically to catch my breath or to cough sometimes. I even ran outside to get fresh air and then I would jump back in the pool and finish the set. It was like second nature."

Megan attended Wagner to get her bachelor of science in nursing (BSN) degree. During her senior year at Wagner, she started going to therapy because the stress and change of life was a lot to handle. "I started going to therapy because after college starts adult life," says Megan. "I had to figure out how to balance 'adult life' with CF and start my career as a nurse."

Megan finished her college career at the top of her class, with her BSN, in 2014. She became a hematology/oncology/bone marrow transplant–registered nurse through NYU. Megan has since received her oncology nurse certification in 2016, became an adjunct clinical professor, received her bone marrow certification and an master of science in nursing (MSN) from Wagner College in 2018, and received the highest promotion in the clinical ladder at NYU Langone Health in 2019. "I decided to go back for grad school in nursing education," says Megan, "because I figured if I was ever too sick to do bedside nursing, at least I could teach."

She again went to therapy because "bone marrow transplant sometimes can be mentally exhausting," says Megan. "But mental illness does play a specific role in CF. CF is mentally challenging, it's stressful, it's scary at times, and there are a lot of feelings you want to say to the people around you but can't because they will never truly know. A therapist not living with CF won't ever truly know either but having that person to talk to and confide in plays a big role in keeping a positive mindset." Megan says that aside from going to therapy, working out also helps clear her head. She also finds mental solace in snowboarding, hiking, and trips to the beach.

When Megan was living the lifestyle of an elite athlete, her lung function was frequently over 100 percent, which fell off as she transitioned to post-college life and the demands of her chosen path. "It suddenly became a challenge to, after work, do my medications and work out when all I wanted to do was sleep," she says. "When I got sick, my lung function would drop into the high eighties, which in comparison to most is not bad, but as a former Division I athlete, I considered that low."

At twenty-seven, Megan was diagnosed with CFRD and got an infection so bad she thought the only reasonable answer was to throw in the towel. "I was exhausted, and was on antibiotics at least five times every month, and virtually never slept," says Megan. "I was a walking zombie. I was on so many antibiotics that they stopped working, and if they didn't stop working then I was getting allergic reactions. Nothing was helping so I thought to myself, *What is the point if I'm doing everything right and everything by the book, and after all the hard work I put in over the years, nothing is helping?* But my doctors said one more time, one more try, and my parents too.

"Every doctor's appointment, my parents had a look of hope. I told everyone how exhausted I was and how sick I felt after everything was thrown at me. I got sinus surgery in 2018 (I could smell for the first time in my life for about three days), had a PICC line [inserted] in 2019, and was trying antibiotic after antibiotic. I had every right to be tired. But how can you look at your parents and your family when their hope is so high and tell them you are done? You can't."

So, with her family's support, and her resolve to serve her patients, Megan plowed ahead with another round of medications and antibiotics. Little did she know that her life would change a few months later when Trikafta was approved by the FDA in October 2019.

384

Megan started soon after and noticed changes immediately. "The first week into Trikafta, I was coughing up a lot," she says, "but after that first week, I coughed maybe once a day. Right after starting Trikafta, I went snowboarding in Utah, and when we were on the chairlift going up the mountain, I turned to my parents and said I could take a deep breath for the first time in twenty-seven years. I could feel the cold air at the bottom of my lungs, and it tickled, and I had never felt that before. I remember having so much air flow I didn't know what to do with myself."

"I had tears in my eyes. I cried when I was alone," says Madeline. "We were so happy and then to hear no more coughing we were like, *Is she okay?* My husband, with a big smile, asked her, 'How does it feel to take a deep breath?' Megan replied, with a big smile, 'I feel my lungs and chest expand. It feels awesome.'"

Since starting Trikafta, Megan has been able to stop all antibiotics. "My first PFT after Trikafta, my lung function was back to 115 percent," says Megan. "It was a number I never thought I would see again." Megan says she can tell a difference at work too. "I'm a nurse so I feel like I will be chronically tired, but it's different. I'm not chronically tired from work and coughing nonstop, I'm just tired from work. I can *finally* sleep through the night without an annoying nasal drip or waking up gasping for air. I can finally work out until my body is tired and not my lungs. I felt like an athlete again because, for the first time since my college swimming days, I was able to run three miles and not be tired. I was not even out of breath. I had energy like I had never had energy before and no cough, all while still working two nursing jobs. It's a feeling that is very hard to describe."

Trikafta also led to more goals for Megan. She will be graduating with her family nurse practitioner degree in December 2022. "My first masters I did," says Megan, "was because I figured, one day, I would be too sick to be a nurse. Then Trikafta happened, and my teachers did a good job twisting my arm, so I figured, let me go back and finish another degree."

Then, the pandemic hit. "Working during the pandemic was extremely difficult, not because I have CF but because we had no choice but to go to work and take care of people," says Megan. "COVID or not, nursing is a hard profession. Hospitals are filled with extremely sick people. Now add a global pandemic to the mix, and it makes it that much harder. Nurses became burnt out, but we had no choice. We couldn't work from home—we had to go to work. Everyone is scared to go to work because everything was still unknown. Things changed every day, and we had to take it one day at a time. And yet, though I have a lung disease, I was more worried for my parents! I made sure I did everything safely so I wouldn't come home and get my parents sick."

Megan says her hospital family was looking out for her. "My co-workers and management knew I had CF and made sure we all stayed safe," she says. "It was known I could not work with COVID-positive patients, so if I had to, my coworkers would do it for me. My coworkers also tried to make sure my assignment was safe for my condition but there is only so much one can do. I personally could not care for COVID patients given my condition so I would take care of the patients who were negative on my floor, but that was also a gamble because, at one point, there were a lot of COVID patients."

Megan—who has helped raise approximately $30,000 for the Cystic Fibrosis Foundation over the past ten years, with the support of her friends and family, who assemble as part of her Great Strides team, Megan's Mob—continues to eat well and stay active. She works out most days, runs, walks every night after dinner to make sure her blood sugar stays within the normal range, and rides a Peloton during the rough winter days. And, of course, she does her therapy every night before going to sleep.

"And having a good support system is crucial," she says. "My parents, my brother, Vincent, and my fiancé, Patrick, work as a team when things are hard. They are there when I need to laugh, to cry, or just to be told it's going to be okay. They are there when I need a long hug, a shoulder to lean on, or a hand to hold. They make fighting this battle a little easier."

Megan knows what it is like to consider letting CF win, so her advice for those in the same situation is, "Hang in there. Find someone else that has CF you can vent to, because that struggle needs to be spoken about and the only people who would understand [are those] going through it. So, vent, sulk, cry, do whatever you have to do. And when you're done, look yourself in the mirror, wash your face, and push through, because tomorrow is a new day."

ROSS CRAIG

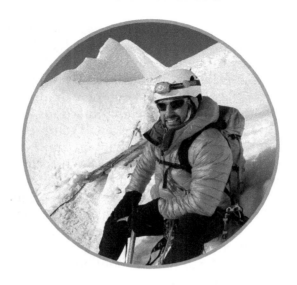

Age: 38
Resides: Richland, Washington
Age at Diagnosis: 3 months

THE CF MOUNTAINEER: CLIMBING TO NEW HEIGHTS

Super-athlete, outdoorsman, and CF warrior Ross Craig, with his wife, CJ, have explored multiple corners of the globe. With their hiking boots and backpacks, Ross and CJ have taken to descending river valleys and summiting mountains, reaching their highest altitude in 2012 when, over a four-day span, they hiked the Inca Trail to Machu Picchu, which boasts an elevation of fourteen thousand feet. And when he's not in rarefied air, embarking on strenuous multi-day hikes or running marathons, Ross is a passionate physical therapist, sharing with his patients his greatest love: healthy living.

"Exercise is my medicine," says Ross. "It has allowed me to pursue a lifestyle that hasn't been dictated by my diagnosis."

Ross was born and raised in Brookfield, Connecticut. He had meconium ileus at birth which indicated to doctors that he could have CF.

A sweat test, after various other tests, finally confirmed the diagnosis when Ross was three months old.

Ross says his parents, Sue and Bill Craig, were instrumental in not letting him pity himself because of his disease. "My parents helped me lead an active lifestyle despite my diagnosis, which has been the cornerstone of my successful fight against CF," says Ross. "They started me out on the right track, enrolling me in sports from a young age."

"Some [parents with CF children] kept their children quite isolated from normal activities in fear of catching infections," says Sue. "Not that we were not worried but [Ross] wanted to do everything other boys [his] age were doing, so we went with our gut instinct and, with some precautions, let [him] be as normal as we possibly could."

Ross says growing up outside the bubble was a blessing. "[My parents] encouraged activity, came to all my games—grandparents and family too—and I excelled. I may not be the biggest one out there, but I certainly tried my hardest. And I was never the 'CF kid.' In fact, I didn't tell my close friends [about CF] until later in my teenage years. It just wasn't something I had to talk about because it didn't rule me. Most kids and families growing up didn't know I had CF and that helped on the field because I wasn't treated any differently. I was held to the same standard, I ran the same number of laps as everyone, I swam in the fast lane to make myself better, and I played hard. Yes, my sweat is a little saltier and I housed the halftime snacks and Gatorades, but I excelled."

Ross is a middle child, with older sister, Jennifer, and younger sister, Kimmy. While neither sister has CF, Kimmy has been working for the CF Foundation for the past four and a half years, for the Connecticut Chapter, and helps provide necessary funds for the amazing research that is happening within the CF world.

"Growing up, my family has been involved with the CFF," says Ross. "We grew up doing ski rallies in Vermont, Great Strides in Connecticut, my father organized a golf tournament for nearly twenty years, and various dinners/balls, and other events when they came up. I remember as a child going door to door in my neighborhood asking for donations from friends and neighbors pre-internet days and having to collect checks and whatnot."

And, like most folks who live and thrive with CF, Ross arrived at a point where he had no choice but to face the mental challenges of realizing the statistical realities of the disease. "When I was a young child, maybe eight to ten years old," says Ross, "we were at a CF event, a ski-a-thon in Vermont. The evening after the event there was a large dinner and auction/raffle with guest speakers and CFF staff giving speeches. For many years, my parents would escort me away during these speeches, but for whatever reason I got to stay for this one, and the honesty behind the disease hit me.

"I never had to deal with severe illness or sickness up to that point, and even into my late teens, but here was somebody telling a large crowd who may not know much about CF why we hold events to raise money. It was because I was going to die. Apparently, the black and white of it was because people with CF die. And they often die young. How did I not know this? I mean, I felt fine. I didn't understand, but the honesty was difficult to wrap my ten-year-old brain around. This was a hard realization for me at that age. This is pre-internet time frame and access to information about CF generally only occurred at MD appointments up until this time for me, so, until then, I wasn't at all preoccupied by outcome statistics."

Ross grew up enjoying skiing, soccer, and swimming. "From the age of nine," says Ross, "I had participated in a summer swim club at our local lake. For six weeks during the summer, I swam at Candlewood Lake, in my hometown, for the Muskrats."

When he was a teenager, Ross discovered competitive swimming, which captured his imagination. "Between trying to figure out how to swim, to avoiding the seaweed coming up from the lake's bottom, to trying not to freeze in the cold lake temps," says Ross, "I slowly learned how to swim freestyle and, after a couple summers, butterfly. This prepared me for the high school swim team my freshman year. My longtime coach and childhood mentor for the Muskrats, Doug, was also the high school swim team coach, and I couldn't wait! I wasn't the biggest or the fastest out there, but for a freshman, I could hold my own.

"At practice I was put into the same lane as the juniors and seniors, and it really pushed me to advance my training. I quickly had to get used to the workouts which were much different than summer-league practices. But sure enough, my times started to drop, and I was entering high school events trying to take valuable first, second, and third place points depending on the events. I was put on the A relays with my older teammates, and we were winning. We had some great talent thanks to our coach, who really pushed us to achieving something our team never had.

"Doug really thought I could do even better and urged me to consider joining a local YMCA National Team, the Wilton Wahoos," says Ross. "I had a few other teammates already on the team who were excellent swimmers, and I knew the caliber of athletes that trained there went on to become very successful swimmers in college. Part of this meant I had to really decide whether or not I wanted to up my game. Into my junior year, I was still playing soccer and enjoyed other sports such as skiing and snowboarding in the winter. I had to commit to joining a year-long swim team and leaving my other sports behind. Joining the Wilton Wahoos in Connecticut my junior year was a huge decision for me and probably one of the best ones I could have made. It certainly helped pave the way to become a collegiate athlete, but I truly feel it helped keep my lungs so incredibly strong and healthy."

Ross continues, "But it was hard. Everybody on Wilton was good. I thought practicing at the high school level was hard enough. This was only the next level in difficulty. Over the next couple of months, after being broken down with some of the hardest workouts I had ever done at the time, I started to see changes. I was getting faster. Practice was getting easier. I was switching lanes at practice and working out with faster swimmers. I was leading some of the workouts at times. I was starting to do really well in swim meets, winning my heats at times and scoring points for the team.

"Something else started to happen. I was watching my times get closer and closer to National Cuts for championships. The work was paying off. Not only that, I was contributing more on our high school team and really started to succeed in butterfly." Ross eventually helped his high school swim team win the Connecticut Class S State Championship his senior year for the first time in the school's history. His participation became an opportunity to bring attention to the disease with which he lived.

When Ross was eighteen years old, as his high school senior project, he organized his first CF fundraiser for the CF Foundation—a swim-a-thon that raised approximately $22,000. Ross's athletic success and activism garnered him the Hero's Award in 2002 as the Connecticut CF Athlete of the Year, presented by ESPN's Chris Berman and Joe Tessitore along with the NFL's Steve Young and many other star athletes, broadcasters, and CFF supporters at the Sportscasters Super Ball at the Oakdale Theatre in Wallingford, Connecticut.

Ross went on to swim at Springfield College in Springfield, Massachusetts, where he participated in the one-hundred- and two-hundred-yard butterfly and the two hundred and four hundred individual medleys. "I was always in the middle of the pack in college," says Ross. "I was never the fastest, but I was always striving to get third place to score [more] points for our team. We had some pretty incredible butterfliers on our team and depending on the meet, I would be the B or C person in the event for our team. I never achieved an NCAA National Cut, unfortunately, and never got to go to NCAA Nationals, but I was able to contribute during our regular season and postseason regional championships that included competition against MIT and Coast Guard Academy, which were our main competition."

Ross dealt with a few pulmonary issues throughout high school and college, including three sinus surgeries and a PICC line at the age of eighteen for a pseudomonas infection. He also had some GI complications during his college years. Ross's ascending colon was removed due to an intussusception when he was twenty-one and his appendix and gallbladder have also come out due to CF complications and mucus build up in his GI tract. But he doesn't harp on these medical interventions and instead focuses on the fact that he was able to "get away with" only doing his nebulizers approximately two to three times per week because of his swimming regimen, which he calls his "medicine."

In 2006, Ross received his bachelor's degree in physical therapy and in 2007 his master's in the same discipline. "While in PT school, I was in cardiopulmonary class," Ross recalls. "CF was on the agenda that day and the 'textbook' version of CF was presented to the class, and it wasn't pretty. Most of my peers knew I had CF at this point in my life, at age twenty-one. Here I was sitting in a class of thirty-four of my peers being taught what the book said about CF and how I was going to die at a young age. I felt really small at that moment, like everybody was staring at me and pitying me."

During his last semester of graduate school, the National PT Conference happened to be in Boston, less than two hours from where he was studying in Springfield, so he was required to attend some of the presentations. "As part of the conference, there was also a huge job fair," says Ross. "My best friend was looking to move out west with his then girlfriend (now wife) to start their PT jobs. One company out of Puyallup, Washington (near Tacoma, Washington, south of Seattle), was offering to pay for travel for in-person interviews and had sign-on bonus opportunities. My buddy and I took the opportunity to fly out at their expense and interview at multiple different clinics within the company. We were offered jobs the next day and that was that."

Ross passed his state board certification in orthopedic physical therapy in 2011, but in Washington he found so much more. Practically upon arrival, Ross found a passion for exploring the mountains in Washington. "It was pretty incredible when I went out for my job interview," says Ross. "As you fly in, on a clear day, you get to see Mt. Rainier, Mt. Adams, Mt. Hood, Mt. Baker, and the whole Cascade Mountain range depending on what side of the plane you are sitting on. It was stunning. And from there, all I wanted to do was explore. Here is where I started to really enjoy the Pacific Northwest outdoors and continued my commitment to remaining active and living a life without CF boundaries."

In June 2011, while supporting mutual friends who were competing in an Ironman Coeur d'Alene in Idaho, Ross met CJ. "I was immediately smitten," says Ross. "I told her early on about cystic fibrosis and being a PT—she was not fazed by it." In April 2013, ten yards before the finish line of his first marathon, the Wenatchee Marathon in central Washington, running alongside CJ, Ross got on one knee and proposed.

"When I first met Ross on the streets of Coeur d'Alene during our best friends' Ironman," says CJ, "I was immediately captivated; he was unlike anyone I had ever met. He had this dynamic energy and endless positivity. Within ten hours of roving the streets while our friends competed, I knew he was someone very special. I had no idea he had CF. I was just magnetically attracted to him, and I wanted to know more about him. Essentially, I wanted more of him, all of him. From day one, I never had any doubts about Ross, and I never looked back.

"When I did find out that Ross had CF, I was ignorant. I honestly had no idea what it was, really. I played it off, that it was no big deal, but immediately got off the phone to Google it. *Oh, this isn't good.* And that's about as far as I got with those thoughts. I was undeniably head-over-heels in love with this guy and the fact that I just found out he had a terminal illness did not seem to pose a threat; it was not a deal breaker. The way Ross made me feel; the way he treated everyone with kindness; his patience, his intelligence, and success as a physical therapist; his steadfast existence that was softened with compassion and empathy; his very way of being, was all that seemed to matter to me. Even if I only get ten years with this guy, they will be the best ten years of my life . . . I'd figure out the rest later. We cannot predict the future, and I was determined to live in the now, with Ross, for as long as I could have him."

"My dad was on the bridge with the ring in his pocket," says Ross, reminiscing of the moment he proposed to CJ, "and without CJ noticing, he gave me a high five and handed the ring off to me while in stride to the finish line just a short two hundred yards away." They were married in October 2014 and spent their twenty-one-day honeymoon hiking all over New Zealand.

"On June 26, 2011, on the streets of Coeur d'Alene, I met a man," says CJ. "Two and a half years later, I married that man. He has always been the perfect man for me, even before I knew about CF. Ross lives life bigger than anyone I know. He works hard, speaks soft, laughs often, and loves deeply. All I knew on that day, was that I wanted a life with him, all of him, CF included."

In 2016, Ross and CJ completed the Tour du Mont Blanc over nine days, hiking through France, Italy, and Switzerland. In November of 2017, they spent eight days hiking the O-Circuit in Patagonia, Chile. In September 2018, they completed the GR20 on the island of Corsica, hiking 140 miles over fourteen days and forty-eight-thousand-foot elevation gain/loss (elevation gain is the total amount you will climb in a day, and elevation loss is the total amount you will descend in a day).

In July 2017, Ross completed his second marathon, the Jack and Jill Marathon in North Bend, Washington, with CJ in a personal record time of three hours, forty-nine minutes. After that they then began switching their focus to checking mountain summits off their Pacific Northwest bucket lists, with successful summit attempts of Mt. Rainier (14,411 feet), Mt. Hood (11,275 feet), and Mt. Adams (12,275 feet) unguided. Ross found a mountaineering company based out of Seattle where he learned about and studied basic mountaineering for their first attempt of summitting Mt. Rainier in 2018. Unfortunately, weather got the best of their group that night and kept them from a summit attempt.

This was right before they embarked on their first IVF journey to start a family. "Undertaking IVF seemed like something I had known about as a young adult," says Ross. "I had heard the chances of males having children without IVF were very slim. I did not know until I approached the subject with my CF doc that only two percent of males with CF have an intact vas deferens. A quick test showed I was one of the ninety-eight percent without an intact vas deferens.

"CJ and I did a lot of international traveling prior to starting the discussion to have a family. We didn't want to jump right into a family. We were young and healthy and wanted to see some of the world. We wanted to grow our relationship through experiences. I think we did a pretty good job at that. When we were ready, we met with an amazing fertility doctor out of Seattle, Washington, who did monthly visits to eastern Washington with the hospital system we both work with. After meeting with him and going over his recommended plan of IVF, we didn't think it was going to be too difficult to conceive. We couldn't have been further from the truth. We met with our doctor in April of 2018. We did our first stimulation cycle to harvest CJ's eggs in January of 2019. We suffered through two miscarriages in the first half of 2019. Then my wife was diagnosed with stage II-B colon cancer and had emergency surgery to remove the tumor blocking her intestine. As lucky as we were catching it early, her life changed dramatically."

After everything they dealt with trying to conceive children, things got even tougher for Ross and CJ. In November 2019, Ross suffered his scariest CF moment. "I went into respiratory failure and required a life flight from my home in Richland, Washington, to Seattle, where my CF team is based," he says. "My wife took control of all my medical decisions, and I had to fight harder than I ever had in my life. I have never gotten so sick, so quick, and I have never not bounced back quickly. This was certainly new territory for me, and it was a struggle. All I could do was attack it like I had previously and listen to my medical team. I had to be intubated for a temporary time while my lungs calmed down and I was given high-dose IV antibiotics and steroids. While at the University of Washington Medical Center, my MRSA pneumonia was treated, and it was identified I also had a severe allergic reaction due to a fungal infection from ABPA [*allergic bronchopulmonary aspergillosis*]." At his clinic appointment just a few weeks earlier, his FEV1 was 82 percent, and after, at the time of discharge from the ICU, his FEV1 had plummeted to 59 percent, the lowest lung function he had experienced in his life.

Ross has worked hard to return to his previous baselines and get back out running and hiking with CJ and dog Kepler, a Pomsky (half Siberian Husky and half Pomeranian), as well as their new puppy, a sixty-pound Siberian Husky they rescued in Montana that they named Kafta after Trikafta, which Ross would start in mid-December 2019.

"Hiking with CF certainly has its challenges," says Ross. "I feel like I have hiking 'pre-Trikafta' and now 'with Trikafta.' Pre-Trikafta I was constantly making sure I had enough food, water, and electrolytes. I learned quickly that I need, like, twice the amount of water than most people, so my pack was always heavier than everybody else's. I often would see if others could carry a little extra for me. I also was always exploring electrolyte replacements. This was especially difficult on our trips abroad. How was I going to keep my nebulizer meds cold? And how was I going to use my nebulizer overseas? I found out through trial and a lot of error that the best way is generally finding a portable nebulizer or aerosolizer that is run on batteries. Electricity isn't as consistent in some areas of the world we've traveled in, making rechargeable batteries difficult to depend on.

"I also worked with my doctors to try ways of not needing my Pulmozyme for a two-week period and would test this a few months in advance at home by doing Albuterol and hypertonic saline twice a day instead. This was a big stress relief that I wouldn't have to travel with Pulmozyme, trying to keep it cold for twelve to twenty-four hours of travel and keeping it on your person for one to two weeks in the mountains. I always travel and hike with prophylactic meds too . . . usually Bactrim, prednisone, and Cipro, but [hiking] with Trikafta I seriously feel like a mountain goat. I feel so strong. I don't get winded. I don't need as much hydration anymore. I don't have raccoon sweat stains around my eyes anymore. I don't need as many electrolytes anymore to supplement my salt loss from sweat. I feel . . . 'normal.' I have so much energy overall it is amazing. My wife and I did quite a few backpacking trips within a three-hour drive of our home during the COVID-19 lockdowns and carrying a forty-pound backpack was easy compared to previous years. Ten-to-fifteen-mile days really didn't seem daunting to me. I never see myself, my wife, and my dogs ever stopping hiking. It is just what we do. It gives us our peace."

Ross says Trikafta has helped him come to terms with, "something that I wasn't sure I would even experience—aging! When I hit my thirties, I realized that I am much more dependent on my daily treatments. When I started my nine-to-five job as a physical therapist and my time was dedicated to my career, I realized the need to do my nebulizers regularly was much more. I couldn't just dismiss them as time better spent elsewhere. When I got married and my wife and I were planning international hiking trips, I became more and more anxious and scared about traveling abroad for fear of not getting my treatments in and for fear of getting ill while abroad. Generally, my troubles lie in trying to live a normal adult life and maintaining my health as best as possible, and Trikafta helps me immensely with that." Since starting Trikafta in late 2019, Ross has been hospital-free.

Ross continues raising funds and awareness for the Cystic Fibrosis Foundation as he did with swim-a-thons when he was younger. "I've been involved with the Washington CF Chapter and regularly participate in the CF Cycle for Life, wine and brewery events, CF Stair Climb in Seattle, and golf tournaments," says Ross, who, in the fall of 2019, traveled with CJ to Virginia to participate in the Virginia Xtreme Hike with family from Charlottesville, and completed 13.1 miles with his mother and aunt, "while my wife completed the full marathon with my other aunt."

Ross and CJ continued to try and have children in 2020 when COVID struck. "We continued with another stimulation cycle to get more eggs," says Ross, "when CJ was feeling better [after her bout with colon cancer]. Unfortunately, she developed OHSS [ovarian hyperstimulation syndrome], and we had to hold off on doing any live embryo transfers. We were exhausted. We never thought it was going to be this hard. We had a third miscarriage in early 2021 and that started getting doctors really concerned and working us both up with more genetic tests, autoimmune syndromes for CJ, clotting syndromes for CJ, and much more. All negative. *Phew.*"

Their therapy was simple after another devastating setback. "We hiked three days in a row," says Ross. "We watched our dogs run wild. We got our daily dose of exercise in with some vitamin D. We talked through our pain and struggles. And hiking is truly our mental therapy to be able to move on and cope with our loss. We will always hike. I never want to think about a day that I couldn't."

Things finally took a turn for the couple. "Luckily, we had quite a few embryos left in the bank," says Ross. "And now, I can faithfully say my wonderful wife is pregnant with our future child and doing great. It certainly is not the road we thought we were undertaking. We have had more sadness, and tears, and heartbreak with IVF than anybody should ever experience. But looking back at all we went through and how strong we were to keep moving, I know my wife and I can tackle anything together. And I know that child is going to be loved so much."

And there is Ross's profession as a physical therapist, which he says has complemented and enhanced his physical pursuits. "I feel grateful to have been working full time as a physical therapist for more than fifteen years," he says. "I've only had to take a minimal amount of time off due to my disease and therefore have been able to help others get back to the things they enjoy doing through my work. I am thankful that I have been able to give back to others what my medical staff has been able to provide to me."

Ross's next goal is to run the Boston Marathon for charity to raise money for the Cystic Fibrosis Foundation, but most of all, he says he's dedicated to taking care of himself. "Exercise is my medicine and I'm fortunate that my wife and I share that common passion," says Ross. "My wife and dogs are my cheer squad every day and my medicine! We truly enjoy the great outdoors and often spend our weekends driving to trail heads for a day hike or an overnight. Participating in trail runs and supporting local community groups and charities are generally how we also enjoy more formal events, but there isn't a time that I'm outside with [them] that I don't constantly smile and laugh."

And Ross recently gained a new member of the pack—a daughter, Shane Lawrence Craig, born two months earlier than expected on December 12, 2021. The unexpected is par for the course for Ross and CJ, as CJ had an emergency C-section and Shane, who weighed three pounds, fourteen ounces at birth, spent seventeen days in the NICU and was discharged in time to celebrate New Year's Eve with her parents.

"The birth of my child happened so fast," says Ross. "One minute my wife was resting comfortably on the birthing floor. The next, a full code team was in the room and running my wife down to the operating room for an emergency C-section. Less than six minutes later, I heard my daughter crying and my fear turned to pure joy after learning they were both going to be okay. The love I have for these two ladies cannot be put into words."

Ross now gets to experience something he never thought he could. "I am beyond excited to be a father," he says. "With my CF, I never knew it would be possible to have a family. With all the medical advances to treat CF over the course of my life—and now with the ultimate drug, Trikafta—I look forward to being able to be a part of Shane's life. And nothing makes me more excited than to think about my wife packing our child up a mountain with our dogs running wild."

MARTEN DeVLIEGER

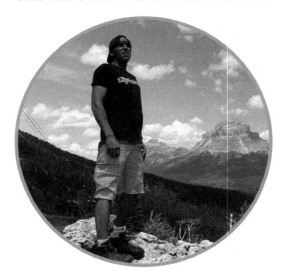

Age: 40
Resides: Crow Nest Pass, Alberta, Canada
Age at Diagnosis: 3 weeks

NO TIME TO REST: THE ADVENTURER'S LIFE

"**W**hen a man is faced with the need to survive, his natural instincts are to create an event to survive," says Marten DeVlieger. "The longing for freedom, family, and adventure comes from within."

Marten (@cf_adventurelife on social media) and his family moved from Holland to Canada, where CF outcomes were better. And it wasn't just Marten who suffered from CF—so did his sister, Karen, who was four years younger.

"We loved each other very much," says Marten, "but we were very different. Karen was more of the stay-at-home type, the patient one. I was the adventurer. Growing up with a sister with cystic fibrosis was a good thing because we could relate to each other and help each other through hard times, because we were both going through the same thing. On the other hand, it was very tough on me because it was my little sister, and she was very sick. I often struggled with the fact that she was not doing as well as I was and was not involved in exercise and sports like I was, and I think that would've helped her."

Growing up on a farm, one of Marten's chores was to shell peas. For him it required long hours of being kept from the "adventurous" things he wanted to be doing, so he instead invented a machine he hoped would shell the peas faster. The machine worked . . . sort of. "It did shell peas," says Marten, "but much too fast as it shot them all over the yard and the result was a bunch of inedible shells."

Despite suffering from CF liver disease and CF-related diabetes, Marten is sponsored as a mountain biker, kiteboarder, and snowmobiler. He also has run two marathons, including the Boston Marathon in 2005. He learned as a teenager the simple truism that exercise contributes to better health. "I was always very active in my life playing hockey and sports and all kinds of other activities," says Marten, "but as my disease progressed and things got harder and I started to take less care of myself, I started to look up to a lot of athletes. When I was in junior high, I would look up to people in my windsurfing and kiteboarding group, and seeing how fit the older people were and how healthy they were staying, it motivated me to push myself, and I thought I could make myself feel better. I really started to think about my future. It really made me understand that every day is precious."

Marten says that running helped him feel better and feel some sort of freedom from the disease that so frequently kept him out of the game. "After changing my lifestyle," says Marten, "I really started to see the benefits, and I never stopped."

But Marten hasn't just fought cystic fibrosis with an adventurous lifestyle. Marten also has done it by way of invention (refer to previously mentioned makeshift pea-sheller!). At age seventeen, Marten used the welding skills he'd learned on the farm growing up. He was sick of doing his physiotherapy while feeling paralyzed on a couch. He wanted something that was strong enough to make him cough and get his mucus out but, at the same time, would also allow him to continue his adventures without having to waste more than two hours a day doing therapy.

With his parents' support, he began scouring a nearby garbage dump for parts and began playing with sewing machine motors, off-centered weights, and electrical currents and vibration. Marten spent many hours in his laboratory—the family car garage—and the result was the "Iron Maiden"—a vest-like device that would allow him to continue his adventurous lifestyle while still staying healthy by doing his treatments.

The initial problems with the vest were not only that it was too abrasive—the heavy steel bruised him—the power was overwhelming. Simply turning on the Iron Maiden caused him to be knocked off his feet. So, Marten got in touch with a company called StarFish Medical in Victoria, British Columbia, and inquired about improving the vest. The company noted Marten's ingenuity and agreed to work with him. The resulting new-and-improved vest was made of aluminum and had pods to beat certain areas of the chest, sides, and back, allowing individual patients to ultimately determine what they needed. It was also gender-friendly to allow comfort and effectiveness for all genders. Marten said the new vest was like his mother having eight hands and doing his postural drainage. Soon he developed a technology known as the ChestMaster high-frequency chest wall oscillation (HFCWO) system and the Iron Maiden was renamed the ChestMaster 5000.

Eventually, he sold the technology to Hill-Rom to create the Monarch Vest, which has now been distributed all over North America to help CF patients do their chest PT while still getting exercise and remaining active. Marten says that he considers seeing a CF patient put on the Monarch for the first time as his greatest achievement.

"At first, I was surprised at how strong [Marten] was and how positive he was about his CF," says Marten's wife, Janine, whom he met by chance at a bar in 2004. "He could still accomplish anything, but I see him struggling every day and fighting for his life behind the scenes."

In keeping with his sense of adventure, Marten worked as a commercial helicopter pilot in the oil industry for seven years. Two days prior to what would be his last flight, at age twenty-six, he had his scariest experience with CF.

"I was running on the treadmill at a remote camp up north, as I was training for the Boston Marathon," says Marten. "I started to feel heartburn after that. I left the next day on crew change. That was my last flight. I was due for days off. When I got home, I went to Janine's house (this was prior to the us getting married) and that's when I started to really feel sick and had really bad heartburn, or so it felt like. I got up, walked to the sink, and started vomiting blood."

His soon-to-be father-in-law rushed him to the hospital, where the doctors had to band his veins to stop the bleeding, as Marten was hemorrhaging from his CF liver disease. "I spent over a week in the hospital," says Marten, "with several different banding sessions to get rid of all the bad varicose veins."

Marten stopped flying helicopters commercially because, after the incident, the government took away his commercial medical insurance, so he had no choice but to retire from flying for a living.

"Janine and my family were quite worried because we did not really know what was going on at the time," says Marten. "And it was definitely life threatening. With a lot of prayer, everything worked out." Now, Marten says that he has to have his liver checked more frequently.

Times got tougher for Marten as Karen needed a transplant. "She did very well until she needed a transplant. The transplant went very well." Unfortunately, five years later, Karen, who was married and the mother of twins, lost her life at the age of thirty-three. Marten was thirty-seven.

"She contracted West Nile disease and went into a coma," says Marten. "At that point, I was very angry at cystic fibrosis, not for myself but for her life. I was shocked and angry toward the disease and wished I could fight for her, so she didn't have to go through the pain she did. It just did not seem fair that she had a second chance—and she was doing so well and [she had] her two kids—to be all taken away from her in one second. It was a lesson for myself, that we need to take every day and make the best of it and not take anything for granted, because it might not be there tomorrow. She and I often talked about that and that we would be going to heaven, and we would be in a safe place away from cystic fibrosis. It is sad that she's gone, and she would be sad to leave everybody behind, but I know she's in a better place."

Marten continues, "Once I got over the initial grief, I started to look forward to using it as a strength to guide me to fight even harder for the family I had. I never look back. None of us in life knows when our number's up. Neither do I. So, I'm not going to let some number or statistics slow me down in life. I am just going to make my situation push me even harder to accomplish things that I've always dreamed of and to push me out of my comfort zone to make big achievements in my life that the world did not think was possible. [Karen] was very strong and had great faith and was not scared to die. That taught me a lot and that's how I live my life as well. I will do the best while I'm here and be the kindest person I can, but when I leave this earth, I will be in a better place and at peace from cystic fibrosis."

Marten and Janine, who were married in 2006, have two children through a sperm donor: a son, Noah, who is eleven, and a daughter, Kabrina, who is eight. Both his children have taken on Marten's adventurous life with biking, skiing, snowmobiling, hiking, fishing, camping, traveling, and kiteboarding. The family rides what Marten calls an "adventure bus," which they use to seek their next adventure. "Even as his disease progressed and got worse and worse, he still managed to be an excellent father, husband and friend," says Janine, "always putting everyone else ahead of him as much as he could."

Marten does a lot of work for CF Canada, where he helps children with cystic fibrosis by encouraging them and their families. He also spends time advocating for new treatments and new drugs being brought into Canada "so all people with cystic fibrosis have access to the best care and medication, as it's been a real struggle in Canada." He also is a big advocate for lung transplant and organ donation because that was something Karen supported.

He uses his YouTube channel to advocate for those four-thousand-plus Canadian patients with cystic fibrosis and does his part in getting breakthrough drugs accessed in Canada. "I try to motivate on YouTube and promote positivity and encourage that cystic fibrosis is not a life sentence," says Marten. "I'm also very involved in all the sports activities I do on social media, such as I am a sponsored mountain biker and a sponsored snowmobiler in the winter. I like to encourage people with cystic fibrosis that activity, sports, and adventure can help you live a long, active life. Life can be short, and I want to live life to the fullest, and I want everybody to be able to do that and understand that we are here for a good time, not a long time." And in keeping with his social entrepreneurial spirit, he works with a promotional company in Holland called yoursurprise, which helped him create his CF Adventurer Life apparel line, which donates 50 percent of all sales to cystic fibrosis research in Canada, Europe, and the United States.

"My adventure exploits have not only given me opportunities, they also provide me with a mental break from cystic fibrosis," he says. "I'm kind of blessed to have CF and I'm kind of not blessed to have CF. One thing I have learned: don't do things tomorrow."

DR. CRAIG D. REID

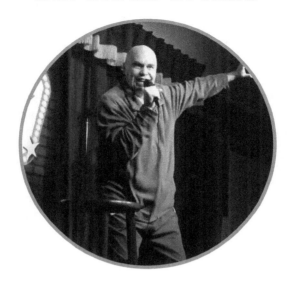

Age: 66
Resides: San Diego, California
Age at diagnosis: 2

THE CHI GONG MASTER:
HOW BRUCE LEE SAVED A CF WARRIOR'S LIFE

Craig Reid—who was born in Reading, England, before immigrating to Endicott, New York, with his family in 1967—says his mother told him that before being diagnosed with cystic fibrosis at age two, he ate all day and had diarrhea every few hours.

"I wasn't gaining weight," says Craig, "but had a large swollen belly from malnutrition. I always violently coughed and had extreme difficulty breathing. Whenever I cried, it wasn't loud or for long, not enough wind."

Post diagnosis, Craig shared that in the late '50s in England, they used *pats*, a daily two-hour postural drainage therapy (without vibration) on twelve parts of his thorax. "I was raised to never complain," he says. "Soon thereafter, I'd be in hospitals sleeping in oxygen tents and, at four, was aware of the creepiness of nurses and doctors looking at me through the distorted plastic like I was a dying puppy."

England started socialized medicine in 1948 so, fortunately, all of Craig's medical costs were covered by the British government from ages two to eleven. When the US government recruited his father to work in America, his parents had to cover Craig's medical bills, which in 1967, drug treatments alone cost $25,000 per year. They couldn't afford it. "The only way to get free medication was to be a test subject," says Craig, "of which I did almost every six months for twelve years. Though losing count of how many test drugs I was on, I've prevented many CF folks from the physical, mental, and emotional grief and anguish by not having them use drugs that don't work, and thus eliminated the psychological hope of getting better that would never have happened. I've also saved CF people from having to experience the horrid side effects I went through [while] using drugs they'll never use."

And yet, "we never complained about our predicament inside or outside the house," says Craig. "Beyond family members, no one else knew I had CF and even when they did, they didn't know what it was. CF was never a topic of conversation inside the house or during meals, and thus I wasn't constantly reminded about being sick. My dad was a professional soccer player in Scotland, so he made me play soccer. Though I couldn't run much due to exhaustion, he'd never be, 'Come on, Craig, you can do it'; it was, 'Keep kicking the ball, lad.' Being raised in a traditional British family, we don't cry, complain, or whine about anything. I was never treated like I was going to die, and thankfully my two older brothers treated me like I was normal—pushing me around like any pesky younger brother would be treated."

In 1973, at age sixteen, Craig was taking thirty pills per day (enzymes, steroids, antibiotics, decongestants, multivitamins, and the unknown "Pill X"), enduring daily painful chest therapy, and in the hospital every three months. "I was enduring explosive diarrhea fifteen times per day while lung-deforming mucus made me often violently cough throughout the day," he says. "Once I started coughing, it would last for five minutes. I'd barely have time to inhale before the next uncontrollable hacks began." These episodes included him sweating profusely, his face turning bright red, his neck veins bulging, and his lungs straining for air. The suffocating gasps created rib-breaking pain and incessant dry heaves. The breathing distress and elevated heart rate caused his enlarged heart to beat so loudly that he couldn't sleep at night.

Craig remembers his doctor saying he'd be dead in five years due to CF and there was nothing Craig or his family could do about it. "To this day, [that] is the scariest piece of news in my life," says Craig. "I never, ever feared for my life until the doctor told me I'd be dead in five years. When we're in pain (physical, emotional, mental, spiritual), it makes us think, and with thought comes wisdom, and isn't wisdom partly about not knowing? I didn't want my parents to have to watch me slowly waste away, I quickly decided that I'd commit suicide by not taking my medication because I knew that would kill me within two weeks."

Ironically, it was when Craig heard this horrific news that he turned to humor. "I was back at school and forgot about my two-minute speech that I had to do in American History class," says Craig. "On the spot, I made up a two-minute speech crazier than a Monty Python sketch that stunned the teacher and students into utter silence. During that crucial moment in my life, the realization of humor helped me laugh and, for a brief moment, forget about death." Craig enjoyed comedy and the escape from reality that it provided so much that he performed routines in talent shows throughout high school and college.

Moments away from dying and still just a teenager, Craig's brothers fulfilled one of his dreams: taking him to a drive-in movie theater. The second film was *Fists of Fury*, starring the little-known Bruce Lee. "While my brothers were making out with their girlfriends," says Craig, "I was squished in the back seat not caring about anything. Then a thug lunged at Lee with a knife. When Lee threw the two fastest kicks in kickdom history, hitting the knife then the ruffian's face, I howled like a banshee, which scared the crap out of my brothers. In that split second, I went from being depressed and waiting to die to wanting to live and learn what Lee was doing. A life purpose had found me, and I wanted to breathe again." Craig swore that if he survived, he'd pay homage to Lee like no other.

Craig began to read martial arts magazines. The first one he read was about Bruce Lee's training techniques. "The centerfold of the magazine detailed how sickly kids were often left on the steps of Shaolin temples where monks would take them in and nurse them back to health using kung fu and chi gong and they'd become Chinese kung fu heroes." Yet there were no training methods or explanations. He says, "I'd never heard of chi gong and there were only pictures of Bruce doing kung fu, so I decided to teach myself kung fu using his pictures."

While at SUNY Cobleskill (a public college in Cobleskill, New York), from 1974 to 1976, Craig diligently practiced martial arts eight hours a day, copying the moves he saw in Lee's films and sparred with any martial artists on campus he could find. In 1976, upon transferring to Cornell University in Ithaca, New York, Craig says his martial arts knowledge and skills broadened. "Most of my friends at Cornell were Chinese, many of which were exceptional martial artists and we ended up sparring and sharing techniques," he says. "I joined the Chinese Student Association to see if I could learn more about martial arts and took such an active role that I was nominated for president . . . and won!"

During his first year at Cornell in 1976, Craig worked at dining halls and, in January of 1977, joined an Okinawan Goju Ryu karate school where he practiced karate two hours per day, four days per week. During the summer of 1978, to continue the training, Craig had a summer job on campus cleaning apartments. "We did some insane training," says Craig. "During winter we'd jog around Ithaca barefoot in the cold winter weather in our gis [karate uniforms], the first time there was three feet of snow on the ground. After each jog in the freezing temperatures, I'd catch a horrible cold, doubled my antibiotics, then struggled for weeks to restore my health."

As a senior, he walked to his job at a grocery store where he did the night shift—nine p.m. to seven a.m.—and walked two miles back to school to make his eight a.m. class, five days a week. Yet Craig's resolve was stronger than ever, as he was saving money for a very important trip.

In 1979, after graduating from Cornell—"the first [CF patient] to graduate from an Ivy League school," says Craig—Craig's search for chi gong, a style of breathing said to benefit the lungs, led him to National Taiwan University to pursue a master's degree in entomology.

Craig arrived with no scholarship to aid his tuition and still unable to speak Chinese. "I slept in a room with a bed made of plywood and my pillow was a brick covered by a towel," says Craig. "That was the least of my dorm issues: rats in the bathroom, no hot water, crouched over hole-toilets with no partitions, 110-degree heat, 100 percent humidity. Meals were pig ears, chicken feet, and meat bits. I'm amazed I survived the dorms. Plus, many folks hated me, the only American in the dorm. It was tough, nerve-racking, I'd question myself, 'Why the hell am I here?' Yet I always knew why I was there. I was dying and believed I had no other options."

When he met grad student Silvia, a weekend volunteer at a leper colony, it was love at first sight, and they were engaged months later. When he told Silvia he might die soon from CF, she cried, "Little time with you, better no time with you."

Craig initially picked up Chinese from watching Chinese kung fu films then later took classes at National Taiwan Normal University. While teaching English, via one of his students, a TV personality in Taiwan, he became an actor and stuntman and appeared in several

Taiwanese TV shows and movies, including *Little Sister-in-law* and *The Flying Tigers and the Kung Fu Kids,* with such roles as an American airman, an assassin, and an opium dealer.

During a TV show, Craig met an ascetic chi master who, during the monsoons, subjected him to a perilous thirty-day test of perseverance, endurance, and worthiness on Monsoon Mountain. Over the previous five years, Craig learned that by disciplining the mind, body, and spirit, one could build a strong moral character with patience, confidence, and tough training. These martial lessons and his love for Silvia gave him the physical, mental, and emotional strength to pass the test.

Five months after learning chi, "strange things happened," says Craig. "One of the many that occurred was that my digestive system began functioning better. Over the next month, I went from a lifetime of going to the bathroom fifteen times a day to three times a day, without the runs. Yet what happened in the summer of 1981, literally blew me away."

During a major typhoon in Taipei, with eighty-miles-per-hour winds, after being chased by a pack of cat-sized rats through waist deep, sewage-inundated, toxic flood waters, Craig challenged himself by practicing chi in the heavy rain at a construction site riff with flying debris. Days later, he says, "I developed a serious lung infection, quickly followed by a 105-degree Fahrenheit body temperature." Prior to learning chi, a similar illness would require Craig to double his antibiotics, have a long hospital stay, and would take months to fully recover. But this time, he recovered in three days. "I don't claim to be cured, yet I feel much stronger since mastering chi," says Craig, who, in 1981, became the first non-Asian to earn an MS from National Taiwan University's Agricultural School and defended his thesis while utilizing two years of Chinese language experience.

Five years after learning chi, Dr. Warren Warwick from the University of Minnesota's CF center wanted to better understand Craig's chi breathing skills. "Dr. Warwick [who passed away in 1996] conjectured that the chi gong motions loosened mucus by decreasing its viscosity [making it liquify] thus making expectoration easier and aiding digestion," says Craig. "With that revelation, he was inspired to invent The Vest that, three years later, hit the market. Without realizing it, I had given back to the CF community and am honored to be part of his inspiration behind that important CF therapeutical device."

In 1986, to demonstrate that his vast health improvement was for real, with both lungs 30 percent deteriorated by CF, as ascertained by Dr. Warwick's tests, Craig walked three thousand miles across America (a marathon per day for 115 days) from Ithaca to Seattle, Washington, to pay his respect to Bruce Lee's grave. The achievement garnered national attention as he received a letter of support from the Queen of England, a letter of bravery from President Ronald Reagan, a MADD Humanitarian of the Year Award, and an invitation to the Washington Press Club to address senators, congressmen, and dignitaries about CF.

The walk was a way to teach children, teens, and adults with CF, or those who know someone with CF, that in Craig's case, martial arts, chi gong, exercise, falling in love, having an aim in life, and a positive mental attitude were important therapies in his fight against CF. Dr. Warwick told the *Chicago Tribune* in 1985 that chi gong would be useful for people with CF and any folks afflicted with other lung diseases.

From 1983 to 1991, while at the University of Illinois, Craig was a twelve-time award-winning teacher of eight science courses, including pre-med biology, medical entomology, and microbiology, and in 1989, he became the first person with CF to earn a PhD at the university. Craig was still performing planned comedy routines and extemporaneous routines around everything he did when talking to an audience (including, he says, when he curated and spoke at film festivals, spoke at Yale School of Drama, and even when he defended his PhD thesis) and says one of the reasons he was considered a top teacher was that kids wanted to be in his class to experience his humor and presentations.

In 1992, he turned his professional ambitions toward writing and — in addition to having published more than 1,800 magazine articles, being a former reporter for Reuters of Asia and a Reuters Los Angeles bureau correspondent, and a medical writer—Craig was also a fight choreographer in Hollywood, wrote screenplays (*End Game* (an uncredited rewrite) and the short *Lost Time: The Movie* presented in *Red Trouser: The Life of the Hong Kong Stuntmen* documentary), and has written a five-hundred-thousand-word book titled, *The Ultimate Guide to Martial Arts Movies of the 1970s.*

On his sixtieth birthday, he performed his first comedy routine in a comedy club "just to see if I could pull it off as a profession." Craig was successful and after the routine, he did a handful of other clubs, open mics, and was even invited to the Entomological Society of America annual convention to do a routine but then, alas, COVID hit. Craig has also written his share of humorous speeches for others, which has ranged from presenters at the United Nations to TEDx Talk lecturers. "Comedy is a major part of my life," he says.

Apart from becoming a stand-up comedian, Craig was also a post-production writer for the short film *Shadow Glass*, which won the best psychological film award at the 2021 Cannes Film Festival.

Yet Craig has never forgotten the path that is linked to saving his life and now, at age sixty-six, Craig and his wife of forty-one years, Silvia, are chi therapy vanguards, using their knowledge of related techniques to help others live healthier lives. "Since 1987, we have volunteered our time working with Olympians from seven countries and helped various US Armed Forces special ops/special forces and ranking officers to improve their breathing and well-being issues," says Craig, "which helped them become physically stronger, mentally sharper, and emotionally healthier." Craig realizes the irony that a CF patient is teaching "normal" people how to breathe better. He says that he and Silvia have helped over eight-thousand-plus people over the years.

"Martial arts made me mentally and physically tough," says Craig. "Chi gong taught me how to connect with my emotions, understand the importance of emotional toughness, and I've always said that martial arts is about training not to fight and to heal rather than hurt. I have learned to control CF and not have it control me and firmly believe that one is only limited by what they think they can't do."

11

THE POWER OF ADVOCACY: FINDING WAYS TO MAKE A DIFFERENCE

CASSIDY EVANS

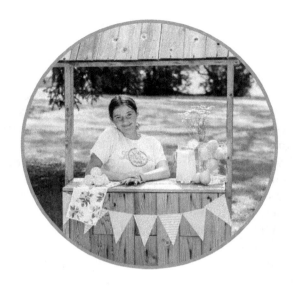

Age: 13
Resides: Saskatoon, Saskatchewan, Canada
Age at Diagnosis: 4

WHEN LIFE GIVES YOU LEMONS: CASSIDY'S LEMONADE STAND

I n May 2013, just a few months after her cystic fibrosis diagnosis, then five-year-old Cassidy Evans decided to turn lemons into lemonade. Despite it being a very cold day, she set up a stand in her driveway in Saskatoon, Saskatchewan, and waited for customers. "I wanted to help raise awareness and funds to find a cure for CF," says Cassidy, now thirteen. "That's what inspired me to start Cassidy's Lemonade Stand." By the end of the day, she had raised $100 and was delighted.

A year later, in 2014, she did it again, this time raising $300. In 2015, though her family had moved to Moose Jaw, Saskatchewan, she ingratiated herself to her new community by handing out flyers to her Grade 1 class and to her younger sister Lucia's preschool class for her third annual lemonade stand. As she prepared the lemonade with her mom and some friends, she looked out the window to see 150 people standing on the driveway, waiting for her shop to open. Cassidy's Lemonade Stand was official, and since then, along with selling lemonade, Cassidy and her family host charity events and sell merchandise through an online boutique. All told, Cassidy's Lemonade Stand has raised over $100,000 for cystic fibrosis research and advocacy for Cystic Fibrosis Canada.

"We knew this was the start of something very special," says Cassidy's mom, Kimberly.

Saskatchewan did not yet have newborn screening for cystic fibrosis when Cassidy was born, so her family was without a diagnosis for four long years. "The lead up to her diagnosis was years of us trying to figure out what her digestive problems were," says Kimberly. "Cassidy always had a very distended abdomen and, from birth, went to the bathroom fifteen to twenty times a day. She was hard to settle as a baby and, as she got older, she was able to tell us that her stomach was sore. We went through a variety of tests, food allergies, and other digestive tests when the doctor decided to try to rule out a few things and suggested that we get Cassidy sweat-tested."

After repeating the sweat test on Cassidy, Kimberly and Jesse, Cassidy's dad, sat in a sterile office only slightly offset by colorful butterflies painted on the walls, as one after the other, the cystic fibrosis specialists were sent in. Results had confirmed that the heart-wrenching diagnosis was true. "Amid the streaming tears, we tried to put on a happy face for Cassidy so that she knew everything was going to be okay," says Kimberly, "but in that moment, life had instantly changed as we knew it."

And yet, Cassidy soldiered on. Despite a treatment routine that consisted of medication through her nebulizer, respiratory physiotherapy with her PEP and vest, lots of medications, enzymes before every snack and meal, nasal saline rinses, and getting in as much exercise as possible, which in the winter, where she lives in Canada can be quite tricky when it is so cold, Cassidy maintained and continues to maintain a positive attitude.

"Cassidy has always been a spirited girl with a zest for life," says Kimberly. "She loves to sing and uses that as therapy for breathing! She has the ability to enjoy life and live in the moment, and even though days can sometimes be really hard, she doesn't dwell on her diagnosis."

"My mom has been a big positive influence in my life in showing me, through her words and actions, how to be brave and to stand up for what I believe in," says Cassidy. "Because [my mom] is an entrepreneur, she has helped me grow Cassidy's Lemonade Stand and is always ready to run with all my big ideas."

In 2017, the lemonade stand expanded with a mobile lemonade

truck that attends events across Saskatchewan, allowing Cassidy to not only raise funds but share her story and information about the disease in the hope of gaining support for awareness and access to advanced, lifesaving treatments. "When I was eight years old, a lady came to one of my lemonade stands and started talking to me about how she lost her child to cystic fibrosis," says Cassidy. Though her parents overheard the conversation and stepped in to help manage the emotional exchange, "I couldn't stop thinking about it. Later that night, I asked my mom if I was going to die from cystic fibrosis."

"I told her that every single person in the world has numbered days and none of us know what they are," says Kimberly, recalling that hard conversation. "That all we know is that we need to make each day count. Whether you have CF or whether something unexpected comes up in life, we all get to choose how we spend our days and if we sit at home worrying about what might happen tomorrow, we will miss out on all of the amazing things in between."

Cassidy, who somehow finds time to enjoy swimming, aerial silks classes, and jumping on her trampoline, has spoken at the Saskatchewan Legislature with the Premier of Saskatchewan and sung the national anthem at a Canadian Western Hockey League game in front of thousands in order to bring awareness to cystic fibrosis. She mostly loves to speak in front of her peers to not only share her story but inspire others to take dark circumstances in their own [lives] and turn them into something positive. "Never stop believing in *hope*, because miracles happen every day," says Cassidy. "No matter what is happening in your life, there is always something great just around the corner, even if it's just the little things."

Cassidy has won the Community Builder Award for the city of Moose Jaw and received the National Mila Mulroney Award from Cystic Fibrosis Canada, which honors a family impacted by cystic fibrosis that has made significant ongoing contributions to the foundation. She sung with country music artist and cystic fibrosis advocate Tenille Arts at the family's SOAR for Cystic Fibrosis Gala, a travel-themed event held in an airport hangar. Cassidy has even met the cast of the TV show *Fuller House* through the Make-A-Wish Foundation, which her family also supports. But she mostly has lemonade on the brain.

"I want to grow Cassidy's Lemonade Stand and open lemonade/bakery shops all over the world," says Cassidy, who dreams of traveling to space as well.

"First, I'm looking forward to being old enough to be able to drive my own lemonade truck!"

ELLA BALASA

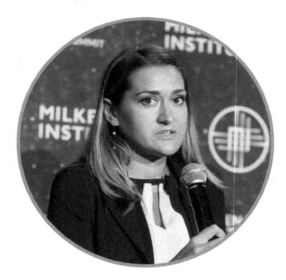

Age: 30
Resides: Richmond, Virginia
Age at Diagnosis: 18 months

BECAUSE I LIVE AND BREATHE:
THE JOURNEY INTO THE WORLD OF CF RESEARCH

"**B**ecause I live and breathe . . . *fill in the blank*," says Ella Balasa. "I believe having dreams and feeling fulfillment comes from motivation. Motivation to do and to be better for whatever parameters you set for yourself. My motivation for life comes in the most innate form, which is the will to live the fullest life I can in the time I am given to live it."

Ella is a writer, a patient advocate, and a health care consultant. Having a science education and having worked as a microbiology lab manager, she finds the connection between the bacteria that live in the lungs of those affected by CF fascinating as well as the way these same organisms thrive in the environment. She now utilizes her knowledge and health experiences to serve on various research committees and advisory boards with health care companies providing the patient perspective to advance research and health care strategies.

"The happiest day of my life was watching Ella graduate from Virginia Commonwealth University with a degree in biology," says Ella's dad, John.

"I assume that's because he never thought I would live long enough to accomplish it," says Ella.

Ella, now thirty years old, was born and raised in Richmond, Virginia. She was diagnosed with cystic fibrosis at eighteen months old. "My sister was born four days before my eighteenth birthday," says Ella's sister, Erica, "and I recall commenting that when I kissed her sweet little head it was salty. After returning home from college the following summer I noticed that she was still tiny, very petite in size for her age. It was that summer that she was diagnosed with cystic fibrosis."

"Having never heard of CF when Ella was diagnosed, when I researched it I began to cry because her future looked so bleak" says Ella's mom, Agnes. "Once a few weeks passed and she came home from her first hospitalization, we got our heads and hearts in sync and began to focus on the quality of life and not the quantity."

"It was during a time prior to life without the World Wide Web and the information was limited," says Erica, "especially about this genetic disease. The only words that I recall hearing were 'failure to thrive,' 'no cure,' and 'fatal.' It was an overwhelming feeling of hopelessness, helplessness, and complete despair in the family. Reflecting back, I believe I distanced myself from the reality of my sister's disease as a defense mechanism. Our mother was consumed with Ella's care and fighting for her youngest child's next breath."

Growing up, Ella's parents always wanted her to do everything that every other kid did, and they never tried to stop or shield her. "I played sports as much as I could," says Ella. "They also fed me with lots of whole foods and treated me with holistic care, which I think only complemented my normal CF treatment routines. Even when I was very thin as a child, they really advocated for me when I didn't want a feeding tube and cooked the kinds of foods I wanted and needed to get the optimal nutrition."

Ella made a concerted effort to stay active, like a majority of friends, by scootering and playing soccer. But unlike her friends, she was required to go to the nurse's office before lunch to administer an inhaled breathing treatment, drink a weight-gain supplement, and take her enzymes. As she got older, it did not get any easier.

"In the third grade, I had four separate hospital stays," say Ella, "each two to three weeks long, during which I received IV antibiotics to treat lung infections."

She says it was around this time that she learned about the severity of her disease. "I was probably like ten years old, and I secretly read my mom's diary where she wrote about my disease and how my life would progress," says Ella. "I distinctly remember reading the word 'inevitable' and knowing exactly what it meant. I was traumatized, and I would think about it sometimes when I was sick growing up."

Since she was a child, Ella has had countless hospitalizations to receive intravenous antibiotics to treat the intractable lung infections. Despite these hardships and the physical exercise limitations she has, along with a 25-percent lung function, she has never let CF be her excuse. "Ella has had many highs and lows over the years," says Agnes, "but we get through them because we believe in a brighter tomorrow. Ella always says, 'Don't worry, Mom, I'll get through it.' She has a very deep well that she can draw from to surmount the struggles and setbacks of CF. It amazes me!"

A few years back, while still at Virginia Commonwealth University, Ella's lung infections became more severe. She had four lung collapses, each requiring surgery to reinflate the lung. "I missed five weeks of calculus my freshman year because of hospitalizations," says Ella. "Throughout my college years, when I wanted to be as carefree as my peers, I very often had to consider the repercussions of my actions on my health. I had to rest more, I had to go home earlier sometimes, I had to skip events for my treatment schedule. There were many times, too, that I ignored what I knew I needed to do to maintain my health, and I did pay the price, but finding that balance is vital. Living life with care and regard helps someone like me with CF live longer, but a life of exciting and wonderful memories, although perhaps for a shorter time, is equally fulfilling.

"I graduated a semester late from college from taking a smaller load of classes to assure I could complete all requirements. Walking across the stage at graduation certainly felt like an accomplishment. It's a milestone that too many of my fellow CF peers never got to do. I had lived long enough to complete one more monumental step."

Over the past few years, as the progressive symptoms of lung infections and lung-function decline have required her to work less and spend about four hours a day taking care of her health, doing breathing treatments and airway clearance, Ella has become increasingly involved in the CF community. "It was Ella's curiosity and science degree that triggered her involvement with advocating for herself and fellow CF friends about new therapies and improving existing protocols," says Agnes. "This has taken her to lead patient advocacy groups and even speaking at the FDA. All of these activities add up to improvements in the CF community and provide her fulfillment of a life cursed with disease yet blessed with love and hope."

"I had decided to turn down my first 'big girl' job a year after college," says Ella. "Having cystic fibrosis, my life had other plans in store, and keeping up, in that sense, wasn't in the plan. At the time, already only having thirty-percent lung function, realistically, I wouldn't be able to maintain eight-plus-hour workdays and take care of my health to keep infections away and stay out of the hospital.

"In our society, so much emphasis is placed on the origin of our success through our careers, and I felt this pressure too, despite being aware that I was someone with a chronic illness who didn't know what even a few months might bring. Whenever we meet a stranger, one of the first questions we ask is, 'What do you do?' It was one of the hardest decisions in my life—feeling like I was giving up a part of my identity."

Ella continues, "I vowed to find my success in other ways. I began working part time in a microbiology lab with a focus on the public health outcomes of antibiotic resistance in municipal water. I became interested in how the public is educated on health matters and then more specifically how patients uptake health information and the value of this in self-advocacy.

"Not only this but some of the microbiology work that I did had intersection with CF too, as common infections in CF lungs and antibiotic resistances they acquire are also commonly found in the environment. With this combined knowledge, I became interested in how I can utilize my voice as a patient and explore my involvement in CF research. I began working with the CF Foundation, participating in various research-related advisory committees tasked in providing patient perspectives on research questions as well as working with researchers and professionals and helping them and the general public communicate and relate to each other.

"This expanded to opportunities speaking at conferences about my health care journey, the value of the patient voice in research, and how we as patients can harness this raw understanding of the health care system to work with researchers and industry to advance health care together. Since my lab closed for a while during [the pandemic], I decided to focus even more on my patient-advocacy work, and I have most recently established myself as a patient-advocacy/engagement consultant, building my website and brand and having more opportunities to work with health care companies in patient-advisory roles and giving input on advisory boards, committees, and panels.

"Along with this interest, I have developed a passion for writing," says Ella. "Through writing, I have been able to provide a scientific voice and encourage empowerment to the CF community by occasionally writing about past research experiences as well as introspectively sharing on my *Cystic Fibrosis News Today* column called 'This Lung Life' about the increasing hardship yet countless triumphs that come along with living a life with a chronic disease that significantly affects day-to-day life."

Outside of the science world, Ella has also been named both the 2019 and 2020 CF Ambassador for the Virginia Chapter where she fundraises for the annual Brewers Ball and speaks there to tell her story and raise awareness. Her role as an ambassador has helped to raise over $100,000 toward advancing research through sharing her story and giving her time to meet with community members and businesses to help the cause. She is also on the committee for the CFF young professionals network Tomorrow's Leaders, for which she plans events and participates in engaging the young professional community in Richmond to be active in philanthropic efforts, specifically for the CF Foundation.

In late 2018, Ella's disease gradually became more visible, as she began to require the use of supplemental oxygen with any kind of physical activity. "The reliance on supplemental oxygen feels like a leash," says Ella. "It's so difficult to accept that my disease changes from the invisible to a visible illness. It makes me embarrassed, fearful of judgement, fearful of pity. Perhaps the pity is the most bothersome. It's hard to accept that I have no control over my health, in that I can't just double up on treatments that day and I'm going to be breathing fine—it isn't nearly as easy."

As her lungs weakened, Ella wanted to try phage therapy, which she'd heard about from another cystic fibrosis patient. Phage therapy is where viruses are inhaled into the lungs to fight certain strains of bacteria because these infections have become antibiotic resistant. Ella's treatment was performed at Yale University in January 2019 and lasted seven days, during which she inhaled billions of phages and was covered by both the *Associated Press* (AP) and the *Huffington Post* (for whom Ella wrote the article) to explain more about the novel therapy. Phage therapy is not FDA approved and only a few research institutions have the resources to attempt it. Ella was only the eighth patient at Yale University to try this approach.

"I'd been preparing for a double-lung transplant," says Ella. "During the peak of my sickness, my body was a shell of an existence—at eighteen-percent lung capacity, supplemental oxygen was constantly filling my nostrils. But after trying an experimental therapy, my body started to clear that infection, and I knew it was time to begin the transplant process before another infection might tip the scale into lung failure—the lungs' inability to provide me enough oxygen to sustain my life."

Ella coughed out fewer bacteria soon after the treatment, began feeling better a few weeks later, and was eventually able to quit her antibiotics. Following phage treatment, she was referred to Duke University for a double-lung transplant in February 2019. Then, some exciting news arrived. She was granted the opportunity to use Trikafta on compassionate use in September 2019 weeks before it was even FDA approved.

"In the months leading up to getting compassionate use for Trikafta, I wanted to be hopeful but cautiously optimistic, so that if it came, truly, too late in the game for me, I would be at peace with knowing I tried everything I could," says Ella, "meaning if I didn't experience any benefit, I [would] know I did everything before I went down the road to transplant. I also wasn't sure I would even be able to hold out long enough with my native lungs to be able to take the drug since my lungs were so weak.

"In the moment, I was thrilled that I was able to get it. And I was hopeful that my life would be prolonged to some extent by this medication. That may translate into one year or five before I will need a transplant, but any length of time is enough for me to be thankful to have lived long enough to benefit to some capacity."

Still, while Ella was excited to try the new drug, she did not want to display that to her family and peers as she was very nervous that the results would not change her status as needing a lung transplant. "Once I shared the news that I'd been able to start the drug, the cheers and questions and elation from loved ones, fellow CF friends, and acquaintances on social media came flooding in. Accordingly, I found myself overinflating my response, trying to match my enthusiasm to theirs," says Ella.

"It's not that I wasn't excited about the drug's possibilities, but I still felt the need to keep my expectations in check. It's difficult to articulate the nuanced changes the medication has brought: My results have been gradual and moderate in comparison to other patients. Day to day, for example, mucus reduction has been slight, but over the course of a few weeks, I've found relief for a few more hours between breathing treatments. I am thin, but I've gained a few extra pounds. The volume of my breaths has increased by five percent (from twenty-five to thirty percent)—as good as my highest lung function in the last three years, albeit a small overall change."

In October 2019, about a month after starting Trikafta, Ella was strong enough to travel to Washington, DC, to speak at the Milken Institute Future of Health Summit, sharing her experience as a patient who had received experimental phage therapy to fight a drug-resistant bacterial infection and to advocate for the development of novel therapies. Ella was one of only a handful of people in the country to attempt this type of procedure to specifically combat pseudomonas. While she seems to notice some success with it, she is proudest of the fact that her efforts have made a difference.

"I think I have paved the way for more patients to be treated and for the rapid advancement of this treatment into clinical trials." The ability to travel to DC and from there fly to Nashville for the NACFC [North American CF Conference] was an important triumph for Ella. "It was a hectic week, but I was already feeling somewhat stronger and wanted to push my body to do things I used to be able to do—like travel with relative ease," says Ella. "It's one of the biggest markers of health and quality of life for me because I like to travel as much as I can. By the time I was starting Trikafta, and the months leading up to it, there was no way I was able to anymore."

Ella realizes her lungs are still not in the best shape and that a transplant is probably her best hope at regaining strength. "I am not against transplant," says Ella. "It's an incredible research advancement. I hope to successfully receive [a double-lung transplant] one day when my lungs can no longer breathe for my body to sustain life. I've been very close to that cusp but now am walking that fine line, stabilized enough that I can wait a bit longer before I need it."

Ella says, now, instead of listening to music while riding her bike, she listens to the clearer, fuller breaths that fill her lungs. She has concluded that Trikafta will extend her life and delay her need for a double-lung transplant. Her siblings, who don't have CF, are amazed at how Ella has continued to fight the disease. "My sister Ella is the strongest person I know," says her brother, Jonathan. "The physical and mental challenges she has overcome and the continued fight and determination she possesses is inspirational to me, her family, and all those around her. She is a true warrior behind that beautiful smile!"

Erica agrees. "The struggles and limitations my sister faced and continues to face are incomprehensible for most," she says, "yet she continues to fight for her next breath and selflessly advocates for the CF Foundation. As adults, my sister and I share a special sisterly bond. We both believe that living each day with purpose, passion, and positivity is a choice. Ella chooses to wake up every day ready to fight the daily challenges of her life with CF while she advocates for the entire CF community and serves as an amazing resource to those who are feeling helpless and hopeless. Through her inspirational writings, which can be found on several health-related websites, including her own column at *Cystic Fibrosis News Today*, and with her voice, she connects with people who are directly and indirectly affected by CF sharing her research and medical trials."

Ella exercises consistently, enjoys cooking, drawing, spending time with friends, and traveling as much as she can. Her biggest motivation, though, is using her passions for science, writing, and personal health to assist others with CF to rise above old statistics and pessimistic thinking. "Although it limits my life tremendously, it has shaped me to be the person I am—tenacious, fulfilled, and grateful," says Ella, who was part of a 2021 BBC documentary discussing how she combats antibiotic resistance. "The CF community has provided me with so much joy from both gaining and giving support to others with CF who face similar challenges with this disease. I have created many friendships from connecting with others through social media and serving as a director for the US Adult CF Association, as well as fostering meaningful connections with others with CF in person."

CF has not stopped Ella from dreaming of a bright future. She still wants to travel, get married, and continue to be a patient advocate. "There is light at the end of the tunnel," says Ella. "Everything in life is impermanent. Your situation will change; just keep persevering through with a strong will!"

DR. JACOB WITTEN

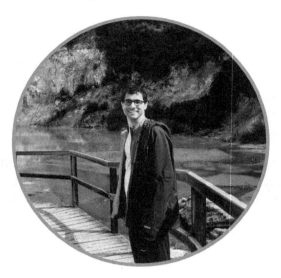

Age: 29
Resides: Cambridge, Massachusetts
Age at Diagnosis: 2 months

LIFE SCIENCE: CURING HIS DISEASE

Twenty-nine-year-old Jacob Witten does not just want CF to be cured, "I want to be the one to cure it!"

Jacob was born in upstate New York and lived in Saratoga Springs. Doctors were not comfortable with his pace of weight gain, so at two months he was given a sweat test. The diagnosis: cystic fibrosis.

"When Jacob was diagnosed at two months old, we were completely devastated," says his mom, Nancy. "We read in *What to Expect When You're Expecting*, our main pre-internet source of information, that the predicted age of survival was eighteen and that his childhood would be full of constant illness and hospitalization. Honestly, my first thought was to run away to Hawaii, to live as well and long as possible in perfect serenity and denial. But when we met the CF doctor the next day, he said we should ignore everything we'd read— that the prognosis for CF had changed fundamentally and that with the new drugs and treatments, Jacob would grow up, go to college, have a family, and live a good life. We clung to that statement like a life raft."

"When Jacob was diagnosed, I lost whatever faith I ever had that God might exist," says Jacob's father, Matt. "But even though I didn't believe in God, I was angry at Him/the universe for creating a baby with this health issue. For bringing me and my wife together to create a baby with this issue. Life seemed like a cruel joke. I also felt some hope. The doctors and the newspaper articles we read said there was a very good chance that, because the CF gene had recently been identified, CF would be cured by gene therapy within ten years. I knew I had to be as strong as I could for my wife, Jacob, and my other son, and it wouldn't do anyone any good if I gave way to despair."

"Growing up, I didn't have any symptoms," says Jacob, "and while I had to spend an hour a day on my treatments, it was usually a minor imposition as I could just read or watch sports during the treatments." He credits his parents' no-nonsense approach for helping him to have established good habits as an adult and for maintaining an FEV1 in the one hundreds. "I definitely attribute my good health, at least in part, to near-perfect compliance to all my treatments," says Jacob, who has an older brother, Zack, who does not have CF. "My parents made air quality a priority in where they chose to live, which could not have hurt. I moved to Los Angeles near Santa Monica in the second grade, and I think the ocean breeze was good for [me], at least relative to other urban areas."

Jacob says he is grateful for his parents masking the scariness that CF brought to their family. "I'm in awe of how good my parents were at keeping their anxiety about CF from affecting me," says Jacob. "I never got any scary or stressful messages from them about CF, and I grew up blissfully unaware that there was any kind of risk of something bad happening to me. I didn't understand it at the time, but in retrospect, my parents did an incredible job of making me feel safe and secure."

Jacob remembers his first statistical encounters with CF. "When I was eleven, I was in the library and stumbled onto a sci-fi book where the main character was being manipulated by aliens who held the only treatment for the main character's wife, who was dying of CF in her twenties," he says. "Oddly, it didn't have a huge impact on me. I dismissed the book as having an out-of-date representation of CF even though a glance at the front matter told me the book was only a few years old." Jacob later Googled the life expectancy for CF and confirmed a less-than-forty life expectancy. "My actual understanding of the dangers of CF came more gradually with no real eureka moment. One thing that definitely tracked my awareness is that, growing up, whenever I would talk to a new medical provider, they would ask me if I'd ever been hospitalized. They would always be surprised when I said no. As I got older and more aware, their surprise went from funny to ominous."

Still, the stability in Jacob's health allowed him to turn his attention to doing something special. "I found myself loving every math and science class I took," he says, "and I decided I was going to cure CF when I grew up. That desire to cure CF set the tone for my education and professional development."

Jacob went to Amherst College to study math and biophysics, then to MIT to study computational biology. Now he is doing postdoctoral research at MIT working on gene therapy. "I have definitely been privileged to have a number of excellent teachers and mentors, but I never really needed any encouragement or inspiration to get into math and science," says Jacob. "I've just always been good at it and enjoyed it and I couldn't stop thinking about science if I tried. I've had times where I've woken up at three a.m. suddenly knowing the answer to tricky math problems. My brother is the same way except a little better at math so it's presumably something innate."

Since 2012, Jacob has published twelve scientific articles including extensive work on the properties of lung mucus. "I haven't made any earth-shattering breakthroughs yet," says Jacob, "but there's still time in my scientific career." Jacob is studying how to use gene editing to cure the disease. "CF has continued to have only a minor impact on my health and lifestyle, for reasons that are unclear," he says. "I have a nasty CFTR genotype [W1282X/G542X] associated with severe disease and untreatable by any of the targeted drugs on the market, but my lung function has always been good, and I've never been physically limited."

Jacob attributes his success to treatment compliance, a focus on exercise and a healthy diet, and good ole fashioned luck. "I define 'luck' as having good 'modifier genes' that determine each patient's unique CF phenotype, not happening to catch one of the really nasty infections, and maybe other factors I haven't even considered," he says. "The balance among those three factors—including, of course, the unknowns—is not clear, but regardless, CF's main effect on me thus far has been to channel me into CF therapeutics as a career, as opposed to some other scientific field. Additionally, in some ways, it's a mental health burden, because by having CF I'm vulnerable to catching some new and nasty infection and having my health go downhill quickly, so there's always some added stress and fear related to that. And every time something is different physically, like if I can't run as quickly as I used to or something similar, I wonder if that's CF starting to kick in. Of course, awareness of one's inevitable mortality is pretty much the human condition, not really a CF-specific issue, but I think it's fair to say that CF amplifies that awareness."

Since Jacob hasn't really had major CF symptoms, besides, perhaps, coughing more than people without the disease, he has always been confident he could fight CF. "Specifically my somewhat obsessive exercise and focus on a healthy diet is based on my belief that if I do everything right, I can maintain the level of health I have now," he says. "Whether this confidence is delusional or not, only time will tell."

Jacob's positive mindset with regard to having CF has been especially noticeable to his wife of three years, Lisa, who he met while they attended Amherst College. "From the beginning, I think I just followed Jacob's lead in how to think and act about CF," says Lisa, who also has a background in medicine as she received her PhD in biological and biomedical sciences from Harvard while researching the role of small RNAs in cancer.

"He always treated it like a fact of life," says Lisa, "the way other people might treat a gluten intolerance or a tendency to get occasional migraines. As he became more and more a part of my life, it's impressive how quickly it really became just that for me: the twice daily treatments, not something I had to think consciously to remember to fit into the daily routine, and the fact of his having this rather horrible disease just an unfortunate truth, along with his annoying habit of not wanting to spend time planning a vacation in advance. Sometimes, something will make me step back and see it differently for a moment—how much it has impacted him and his career choice, how scary the statistics are, and how lucky we are with his health. But then we get back to the day and it fades into the background again, a fact of life, and certainly not the most important one."

Jacob wakes up every day around six a.m. and goes for a jog. When he returns home, he does his vest airway clearance. All in all, he runs five days a week, lifts weights twice a week, and does his airway clearance twice a day for a total of approximately two hours. In the last five years he has broken 275 pounds deadlifting, a seven-minute-mile pace for a 5K, and 1:50 for a half-marathon.

"At first, I didn't know what CF was," says Zack, Jacob's brother. "I just knew that my brother had to take some capsules before he ate and had to get thumped on the back a lot. No weirder than the rest of the world. The older I got, and the more I learned, the more impressed I became with Jacob's resiliency and, most of all, his discipline. I sometimes think to myself, if Jacob can do his nebulizing routine twice per day for his whole life, I can make myself do [pretty much anything]. The only thing is, ever since he got faster than me, I wish he were a little less disciplined about running."

Treatment-wise, Jacob inhales hypertonic saline twice per day, Pulmozyme once per day, and an inhaled corticosteroid. He takes his digestive enzymes with meals. He also takes CF-specific vitamins and alternates Tobramycin and Aztreonam month to month. And regarding his work, he's sure to make his colleagues aware about his condition when it's relevant for safety reasons. "So I can make sure not to be in labs where people work with nasty CF pathogens," he says.

Jacob is doing non-clinical research, so anything he discovers is at least a decade away from FDA approval. "But without going into the gory details, I'm making some cool progress," he says. "The idea is to either do CFTR gene delivery or gene editing of the native CFTR gene (CRISPR Therapeutics is working on this kind of thing)."

Jacob currently has a fellowship from the CF Foundation and is incredibly grateful for all the support that allows him to do his research. "I also spend time reading and writing," he says, "and I've just completed a manuscript for a futuristic sci-fi thriller called *Immune* that I'm looking to publish!"

Matt says his son's enthusiasm for life has been a pleasant surprise considering his own concern when Jacob was newly diagnosed. "Twenty-eight years later, Jacob seems, to me, like a pretty happy young man with a good life and a lot of joy and zest," says Matt. "I wish I had known twenty-eight years ago this would be the case. I wouldn't have worried so much. Now, I still have fears about the future. I have medical-related fears with everyone in my family, actually, not just Jacob. So, I try to follow the example I perceive Jacob and his wife as setting: live life one day at a time, cherish the moment, don't give in to fears, keep on going. Because the truth is, the next twenty-eight, or fifty-six, or eighty-four years might be as good as the last twenty-eight."

ANNA PAYNE

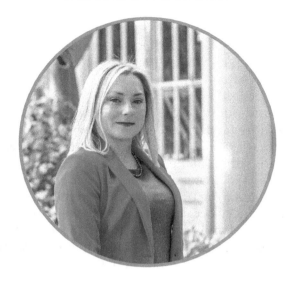

Age: 34
Resides: Middletown Township, Pennsylvania
Age at Diagnosis: Birth

NO "PAYNE," NO GAIN:
POLITICIAN'S FIGHT TO BEAT CF AND COLON CANCER

"**W**hen life puts you in tough situations, don't say, 'Why me?' Just say, 'Try me.'" Those are the immortal words of former professional wrestler and mega star Dwayne "The Rock" Johnson, whose positive attitude has made CF warrior and political up-and-comer, Anna Payne, a super fan.

"I love The Rock," says Anna, "because, growing up, I used to watch WWE and it would be the one show that the hospital would get. The Rock pumped me up and cheered me up. He is and was my hype man. Helping me forget how sick I was."

While Anna loves The Rock, her passion is helping others. "I realized at a young age that the government and politicians have the ability to influence lives and can make laws that help or hurt people," says Anna, an aspiring US presidential candidate. "Growing up with CF and having a different life perspective really helped me understand why it was so important to vote and get involved. I remember when I turned eighteen and how excited I was to vote. I finally felt like I could exercise my right to make my voice heard."

Upon her birth, Anna was rushed into emergency surgery due to meconium ileus, "which was a giveaway that I had CF. A sweat test later confirmed it. After surgery, I was diagnosed with CF and that is how my story began."

"When we found out we were pregnant, we were so very excited, and so was the entire family," says Anna's mom, Kathleen. "Anna was going to be the first grandchild on my side of the family. I remember, after giving birth, sitting alone in the hospital room waiting for the nurse to bring Anna in. Instead, a group of pediatricians came in stating that Anna needed to be transported via ambulance to another hospital to perform surgery because she had a bowel blockage. I stayed in the room, waiting for family to come and visit. They showed up, excited, all with smiles on their faces, and I had to break the news to them that she was en route to another hospital, which would be performing the emergency surgery.

"This is how our life with cystic fibrosis began. When Anna was born, she weighed five pounds, thirteen ounces, and when she came home three months and three major surgeries later, she weighed four pounds. We were determined to follow all the treatment plans, doing postural drainage therapy every day and all medications."

Anna was hospitalized for the first six months of her life. She actually had two colostomy bags at one point. When she finally got to go home, it was a constant battle to support her weight gain. Her parents were very disciplined with her treatment regimen, always making sure she got her enzymes and did her treatments. Still, they were not given much hope.

"When my parents were told of the diagnosis," says Anna, "they were informed I probably wouldn't live long enough to graduate high school. But it turned out that being diagnosed at birth was a blessing, because I could have treatment sooner, could get on the right diet early on, and had time to find the right doctor. I also had a better chance to have different treatment options and participate in drug studies as a young person."

Anna was "relatively lucky health-wise," up to preadolescence. She was only hospitalized a few times, mostly with bowel obstructions, one at age seven and another at age ten. "Bowel obstructions can be super serious," says Anna, "because you could need surgery to get them corrected. I was hospitalized for a couple of weeks but didn't need surgery. To me, surgery is the high mark of severity. My high mark is probably a lot higher than the average person. Some patients are in and out of the hospital all the time for different things, so I consider myself pretty fortunate health-wise."

It was when she was ten that Anna became interested in politics. "I remember watching election returns with my dad and grandparents sometimes in the hospital for the mayor of Philadelphia or the governor [of Pennsylvania]," she says. "Growing up with a rare disease, at a young age, sometimes you need more help, and the government can provide that help to you. So when we would watch the election returns, my dad would explain to me that the mayor can have a positive impact on the city. That kind of sparked my interest in politics.

"The election I really paid attention to was the 2012 election between George W. Bush and Al Gore. I liked Al Gore because he was big into the climate, and as someone who has trouble breathing, air quality is important. Obviously, it had a lot of drama around it as we didn't know who our president was for weeks. We were learning about that election at school. That really solidified my interest in politics. In 2005, during George W. Bush's reelection, and while still in high school, I even made T-shirts asking people to vote because I was still too young to vote but a lot of my friends were old enough."

Anna's lungs had few issues, until she was thirteen. "That was when I contracted mono," says Anna. "I was hospitalized for thirty-one days and home for another two weeks on IVs."

What helped Anna, though, was being open about her condition. "I was sick a lot and did not keep CF a secret," she says. "It has always been important to me to spread awareness and make sure that people understood CF. When my school would do fundraisers, they would always choose the CF Foundation and I feel that was because I was so open about having CF. My openness never showed up for me as much as when I missed school and my great group of teachers helped me keep up with my work and get back on my feet."

It was after this that Anna started to be hospitalized more often, around the age of fourteen. "I was hospitalized when I was in seventh grade for a month and home for IVs for a month, for both winter and fall," says Anna. "This was for a double ear infection, and I had developed Bell's palsy and had to get tubes put in my ears. That cleared out the infection. I was able to relearn how to use my face after a few months. I still can't smile like I used to.

"Meanwhile, I was still hospitalized and out of school for a few more weeks, but I was used to it at that point. Being in the hospital for a few weeks was not a big deal to me. I'd end up missing about half the year during seventh grade. I felt lonely then. I was falling behind and missing the social aspect. My middle school teachers were great. My friends would come visit me in the hospital and at home when I was on the IVs. My teachers even came to see me.

Anna says, "I went for about three years before running into any more issues." Then, when she was sixteen, both of her grandparents died—on the same day. "This broke my spirit," she says. "My grandparents Nancy and Bob [Anna called her grandfather Big Bob] raised me for a while so, to me, it was really hard. They babysat me all the time. I lived with them full time from fourth grade to ninth grade because my parents were divorced and my mom, who had custody, worked two jobs and my dad worked nightshifts. I had to live with someone since I was younger and couldn't be alone. My grandparents would stay with me at the hospital. My grandfather would wake me up for school, and because he had emphysema, we would do treatments together. My grandmother would cook me food and my grandfather would help with my homework. They weren't my parents, but they definitely filled that role. They were like second parents."

Nancy, a diabetic, passed away at seven a.m. on December 29, 2003, after being in the hospital for weeks dealing with heart issues. Big Bob, who had been in the hospital for just a few days, and had been dating Nancy since they were in their twenties, passed away twelve hours after Nancy, at the same hospital but on a different floor, from a torn aorta. Though he'd had a simple procedure and was expected to come home, Anna suspects that maybe there was more to it. "My grandfather never knew of my grandmother's passing. Maybe he knew my grandmother passed away without knowing and died of heartbreak.

"Life hits us all and I'm no exception," says Anna. "I didn't handle things well and my health took a backseat. I was depressed, and I wasn't taking care of myself."

The following year, Anna was hospitalized twice. Once in February and another time in the spring. "I had neglected my health and paid the price," she said. "I was also diagnosed with mycobacterium avium. I was actually out of school for so long they wouldn't let me come back and I had to be homeschooled for the remainder of the year. I lucked out that they didn't hold me back a year. Mr. Murray, my science teacher, volunteered to come to my house to help me out."

On her second visit to the hospital, Anna asked to speak with a psychiatrist. "I needed help dealing with everything from my grandparents to my own mortality," she says. "Asking for help was one of the best decisions I have ever made. The psychiatrist helped me process grief in a healthier way instead of not taking care of myself and helped me pull out of the depression I had sunk into. If you're not taking care of your mental health, you're not taking care of your physical health. The two are definitely connected. By the summer, I was doing better mentally and health-wise. Not being able to go to school stunk, but as I became more present with myself, I recognized the time to rest was important to my overall healing."

Still, Anna had to mentally manage not only the school she missed — by the time she reached high school, she had been hospitalized over a dozen times — but there was also a looming statistical life expectancy of thirty years old. "I recall being eighteen and assuming that time was quickly ticking, and that I wasn't sure what I would be able to do and accomplish," says Anna. However, with cues she developed from her focus on mental health, she got better at managing, whether it was teachers willing to spend extra time with her or friends stepping up to help her academically. "The children's hospital also had a teacher," says Anna. "The school sent the work to the teacher who would help me with the homework while I was doing my IV meds."

Anna decided to go to a community college right after graduating high school where it was closer to home and she had plenty of people she knew in the area who could help her. She ended up going to Bucks County Community College in Newtown, Pennsylvania, and majored in business administration.

"During college, I worked two jobs and managed various hospital-izations in between," says Anna, who was hospitalized every year for a tune-up which prolonged her time in college and she eventually received her associate degree in five years rather than the two years it was supposed to take her. Unfortunately, her lungs hit new lows and her baseline was now at seventy percent. "Looking back on it now," she says, "I wish I had listened and slowed down a little and remembered to take care of myself. Sometimes life gets crazy, but we have to remember we can win if we do our treatments."

By age twenty-three, Anna began working full time as a teller at a local credit union, as she needed the health insurance, and she started raising money and working with the local chapter of the CFF. "I liked the job because I was familiar with it, as I had worked there part time for three or four years. Also, it was close to home. I didn't have futuristic plans to stay with the company forever. I knew I liked politics and doing fundraising and advocacy work."

In 2012, at the age of twenty-five, Anna got more involved in politics. "I got in touch with the Obama reelection campaign and began working for them. I showed up at a person's house. I started making calls, knocked on doors, and found volunteers. This led to a part-time unpaid internship from the summer of 2012 up until election day in November 2012. I met [future president of the United States and current vice president] Joe Biden that same year and even got to drive in his motorcade. I felt like I was making a difference. I can't feel upset about something as long as I did what I could to stop it. I started to realize this is what I wanted to do.

"In 2015, I got into politics for local elections. I got connected with the local political party for my township and my county. I volunteered for local candidates while knowing that I was going to be a delegate in 2016. In December 2015, I had to commit to a candidate to be a delegate. Most people were applying for [presidential candidate and senator] Hillary Clinton. I was applying for a spot to represent [presidential candidate and senator] Bernie Sanders because of his stance on health care and how everyone should have it."

In 2016, Anna became one of only seven elected delegates from her home state to run for a spot at the Democratic National Convention (DNC). "The reason I wanted to be a delegate and get involved in politics was because of growing up with cystic fibrosis and realizing that the government can do a lot to help you or it can do things to hurt you, like taking away the ACA [Affordable Care Act]," says Anna.

Depending on how many votes Sanders received, that's how many elected delegates would be selected. Anna's strategy was to have a lot of volunteers helping her garner more votes than the other Sanders delegates. Each candidate got one delegate for every 15 percent of the vote share. The strategy worked. Since Senator Sanders received approximately 44 percent of the votes, there were only three selected candidates selected to represent Senator Sanders, and Anna was one of them. In fact, once Senator Sanders received 15 percent of the vote, due to a rule of the Democratic National Convention, Anna automatically received a spot at the DNC as the top vote-getting female delegate by approximately eight hundred to nine hundred votes. Her interview at the convention was even televised on the local NBC affiliate.

In 2017, Anna, a democrat, ran for local office and won the election by approximately nine hundred votes to become the township auditor of Middletown Township in Bucks County, Pennsylvania, which Anna calls more of a "placeholder position and a steppingstone, and has very little influence on the township." Two years later, Anna began her climb up the political ranks when she was elected to township supervisor, which holds the ability to influence what happens in the township. "I was surprised that I beat my opponent," says Anna, "but my running mate and opponents were not surprised, as I outworked my opponent and knocked on more than two thousand doors [to secure votes]."

Never losing sight of the cause closest to her heart, in 2018, the year after Anna turned thirty, she raised over $40,000 for the Cystic

Fibrosis Foundation in honor of her thirtieth birthday, breaking her previous fundraising goals. "The challenge was thirty for thirty [raising $30,000 for her thirtieth birthday]," says Anna. "My network had expanded. Getting involved in politics probably didn't hurt. I created an ad book with thirty different people with CF in the area, writing their stories and including their pictures. I had companies sponsor and place ads in the book. I think people really liked the book. People said they were surprised [by] all that the disease entailed and how easy I made it look."

In 2018, Anna became a founding member of the Drexel Cystic Fibrosis Center's Family Advisory Council, which was later renamed the Jefferson Cystic Fibrosis Center's Family Advisory Council.

In 2019, the year that Anna won the KYW (a radio station that serves the Philadelphia area) Rising Star Award for the Delaware Valley, she ran for and won a seat on her local board of supervisors. She was also chosen as one of only two patients to serve on the Pennsylvania Rare Disease Advisory Council, where she uses her voice to advocate for other patients with rare diseases and offers a real-life perspective to the council. "I'm currently vice president [of the Pennsylvania Rare Disease Advisory Council] and it really is my passion to try and make things better for patients across the commonwealth."

To that end, while Anna's love of public office and advocacy are vitalizing, she stresses that her ambition is driven by her desire to help others find the resiliency that's helped her overcome health challenges. Not surprisingly, one of her primary issues is universal healthcare. "My biggest accomplishment is being alive and healthy enough to [run for office and advocate for CF patients]," says Anna, who has done a lot of work during the pandemic trying to get those with cystic fibrosis into Group 1A in Pennsylvania, which helped expedite COVID vaccines for those who share her condition.

Anna also had a little help with her health challenges in November 2019, when she began taking Trikafta. "I was able to stabilize my weight and gained too," says Anna. "I went from 113 to 120 pounds. My lung function improved as my FEV1 went from 1.40 to 1.78. I was able to do [fewer] breathing treatments, and my energy improved too. I was excited. I finally felt like I was going to live, and I could have limitless dreams and that my vacation days might be able to be used for a vacation instead of sick days."

With her newfound energy and improved health, Anna decided to end a yearlong marriage that "just wasn't working" and had hopes of starting her own 501(c)(3) in 2020 called the Bucks County Cystic Fibrosis Alliance, which will have several members of local CF families on the board. "We were supposed to have our first event in 2020," says Anna, "but the pandemic put that on hold. Our first event will now be in 2022. What I hope to be able to accomplish with it is to give money and awareness to the CF Foundation and other CF 501(c)(3) organizations. Long term, I'd like to be able to write grants to CF centers for patients struggling with certain things like food insecurity or missing time at work to take care of themselves—all these things you have to take care of on top of managing their illnesses. If that works out, it will be my biggest accomplishment yet."

Anna is not just an asset to those fighting CF. She inspires those like her physician, Dr. Michael J. Stephen, who she has been seeing at Thomas Jefferson University in Philadelphia since 2011.

"From the moment I met [Anna]," says Dr. Stephen, "I knew I was around somebody special. Anna has a way of bringing out the best in people, making people comfortable while sharing the stories of her illness and journey. Never one to let herself get down, she has risen to the many, and extraordinary, challenges life has presented her. She is a catalyst for getting the word out about CF to the whole community and serves as the de facto patient representative of our center. Where she finds the energy to be there for so many CF patients as well as herself, I will never know.

"She is a true inspiration in every sense of the word. She gives you breath when you feel as if you have run out of your own. She gives people hope when there is a vacuum-like sound in their lives of hope running out. She does this all the while battling her own illness and issues. Anna is a meteor, one that burns brightly, illuminating the troubled sky for those who have any trouble. I have been honored to watch this meteor in flight, every night a beacon of hope for those who are struggling."

While the pandemic has been difficult for many, it has been especially difficult for Anna, even after receiving so much hope in 2019 from Trikafta.

"On July 20, 2021, I found out that I have stage IV colon cancer, which spread outside of the colon," says Anna. "Colon cancer is more common in CF patients, but unfortunately, we don't screen CF patients until the age of forty, which would be six years too late for me. I was never screened for colon cancer, and it wasn't really discussed. A lot of the symptoms with colon cancer are similar to those with CF, with GI issues, so they're often missed or written off."

Going from having her life extended to now being in jeopardy is not something Anna ever expected. "If I had told myself how all of this would go," says Anna, "I wouldn't have believed it. I wouldn't think, at thirty-four, I'd be alive, let alone divorced and facing cancer head-on. I wouldn't think I had been given a second lease on life . . . with new breakthrough medication. Contemplating how I live my best life now that my CF symptoms have improved, I thought, like we all did, that 2021 would be a better year, and so far, it had been.

Anna continues, "Something deep down told me otherwise, and I believed it. I knew something was wrong. I knew it in my bones. I wasn't totally sure what, but I knew something was wrong. When they told me I had stage IV colon cancer, I was devastated. I spent days wishing my premonition was wrong, but I knew. I knew since the biopsy that it wasn't going to be okay.

"Although I was not surprised to hear that I had colon cancer," says Anna, "something had been telling me that something was really wrong for two months. Back in May of 2021, I started having some digestive symptoms, I recall thinking that maybe I should get them checked out. I started asking questions about a colonoscopy, and my team stated they would help me get it after I returned from a trip I took in mid-May.

"By the time I had returned from my trip I had noticed a lump in my groin area. I was immediately concerned even though it was small. I made an appointment to go to the doctor. They performed an ultrasound. Nothing alarming came from that. I was told to see a general surgeon. Over [a few] weeks, the lump had nearly tripled in size. I made an appointment with a general surgeon but had to wait because of summer.

"In the meantime, I felt digestive symptoms again, and went to my CF doctor. He prescribed a colon cleanse as they did an abdominal X-ray and found that I had DIOS. I did two cleanses to clear the blockage. They worked for the most part, but my bigger concern was the symptoms in tandem with the mass. I saw the general surgeon the following Friday. He didn't know what it was either. He said I needed a CT scan.

"That Sunday," says Anna "after the two cleanses and the appointment with the surgeon, I didn't feel well at all. My body was telling me that I couldn't wait another week to get the scan. I contacted my CF team for help. They had me go to the ER to get the CT scan and see where we could go from there. I stayed in the hospital for four days, getting different tests and scans. At no point did anyone think it was cancer, besides me. When day four came around, after a much-awaited MRI, the doctors came into the room and told me they thought the mass was cancer. They couldn't be sure until they biopsied the mass, which I asked for two days prior. My mind and body had prepared for this, but my heart sank into my stomach. I just wanted someone to tell me everything was going to be okay. I was alone when they told me that they suspected cancer. One doctor who read my file told me she knew my journey had been rough and told me it was 'going to get a little more rough.' They were pretty damn sure it was cancer.

Anna continues, "I tried convincing myself it'd be okay while waiting for the biopsy results. I got a call on a Wednesday from my CF doctor who diligently checked for the results so I wouldn't have to wait. I knew when he called me that it wasn't good news. He was insistent that I come down and see him. I drove down with my friend. My mom met me at the office. He came in with a box of tissues. He told me that the mass was colon cancer and had spread outside of my colon. I was mad at myself for being right. Oh, how I wanted to be wrong. I never wanted to be right. I wasn't surprised it was colon cancer. I asked if that was a possibility while in the hospital. Deep down, I just knew. I cried for a half hour straight, just ugly crying.

"I didn't know what the future held," says Anna. "I was scared and anxious. I knew that I was at the beginning of this chapter, and I didn't know how it ended. I didn't even know how to tell most people, let alone how I'd keep my resolve on tough days.

"After a couple days of processing things, I knew I was not going to live in a world where I talked about numbers or percentages. I was going to live in the same world I have for thirty-four years. One day at a time. I'm not just a number on a spreadsheet with medical history and data points. Sure, we can measure and track trends, but I refused to be average. I'm above average. I'm not ever going to fall into that category. I'm starting my own category, my own table in the graph, and my own tab on the sheet. My story won't end average. It will end triumphant, historic, and groundbreaking. Just as it had before. I knew and still know it won't be easy. But I've never backed down. And I'm not going to now."

Anna's advice to others is to listen to your body. "If something is off, believe it," says Anna. "If something doesn't feel right, don't ignore it. Colon cancer is silent. By the time I had symptoms, it spread to other parts of my body. Catching it before it moves elsewhere is key. I think it's super important to tell people with CF that we need to get colonoscopies sooner. If a person has more digestive issues with CF, they should be screened sooner. I'm going to do everything in my power to convince them to change it so people are seen sooner. I have started talking to CF organizations including the CF Foundation."

In December 2021, she took part in a thirty-minute-plus podcast called *Anna Payne's Colon Cancer Crusade* for the Cystic Fibrosis Research Institute (CFRI), raising awareness for colonoscopies and getting screened earlier. "I'll take it to whoever I have to in order to get it changed," says Anna. "Colonoscopies aren't fun but finding out you have stage IV cancer is less fun. That I promise you."

Anna began immunotherapy treatment in mid-August 2021 and had infusions once every three weeks. In late September, she began chemotherapy after the immunotherapy was unsuccessful. "Unfortunately, I'm going to have to figure out how to beat cancer," says Anna. "I was so excited to be on Trikafta. Obviously, this feeling was short-lived, as a pandemic rolled in and now, a cancer diagnosis. This is the biggest thing I've ever faced. I'm facing two dead-weight diseases at the same time. I feel confident but I'm also nervous because this is new," says Anna.

"When you grow up with any chronic illness that's been trying to kill you your whole life, you have that mentality that the grim reaper is always hanging out around the corner. Does the cancer thing make him more apparent? Yeah. Is he easier to ignore when you're on Trikafta and feeling better and not doing as many breathing treatments because you don't need to? Yeah, but at the end of the day, the reality is, whether it's cancer or CF, anything can change with the drop of a dime. For me, I have to be confident going into treatment because I don't know how else to attempt to beat something I've never faced before without being confident."

And yet, Anna continues to stress the turning point of her outlook, when she requested assistance with her mental health so many years ago. "I currently see a therapist twice a month," she says. "It was once a month pre-COVID, but with everything going on in the world over the last year I started going twice a month. I would recommend seeing a therapist if you can. It has been especially helpful over the last year."

Anna also gives her attitude a name. "I call it 'living with an expiration date' syndrome," says Anna. "You never quite know when your time is up. I don't have a lot of fear about things. When I'm given an opportunity, I don't talk myself out of it. Life is short. If you think it's challenging and hard, you're not doing yourself any favors. I don't take life for granted. I don't take experiences for granted. I don't take opportunities for granted. I appreciate birthdays more."

And what does Anna look forward to on her thirty-fifth birthday? "Hopefully, I plan to have kicked cancer's ass by then," says Anna. She is well on her way to accomplishing this feat. As of May 2022, after an unpredictable ten months—which included two rounds of immunotherapy, sixteen rounds of chemotherapy, and news that her cancer was spreading and growing rapidly—her tumors have suddenly begun to shrink and disintegrate.

"I have gone from having ten-plus tumors on my liver to three," says Anna. "I now know that the impossible is possible." While Anna knows her fight is not over, her outlook continues to be positive.

"There is no cure for stage IV colon cancer, but if I can continue to beat it back and handle chemotherapy, that will be a win."

During Anna's fight with colon cancer, someone picked up on her story—Anna's inspiration, Dwayne "The Rock" Johnson, who sent her a three-minute-long video message—which has since gone viral with over three million views—followed by several autographed gifts, a large cut-out of him for her house, and requests to his fans to reach out to support Anna too. Anna's friend Isaac, a newspaper reporter, reached out to The Rock through his production company, and the rest is history. "I was shocked," says Anna. "He is such a positive inspiration for me and so many others."

With The Rock in her corner, Anna has witnessed how big of an inspiration she is. Her goals are to run for congress, run for president and, someday, write a book about it all. "Growing up, I wasn't sure I would live long enough to even get married or buy a house, let alone pursue my dreams," says Anna. "I also never thought I'd be healthy enough to run for public office or be able to handle the stress that comes with it. Now I know that I can do all of these things, and my purpose is to achieve all my dreams while inspiring and helping others to achieve theirs."

STACEY BENE

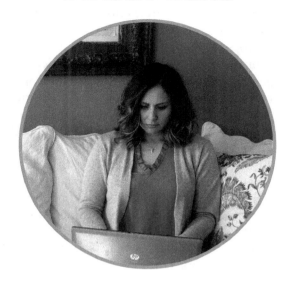

Age: 46
Resides: Medina, Ohio
Age at Diagnosis: 2

THE VACCINE QUEEN: HELPING OTHERS TO STAY SAFE DURING THE PANDEMIC

At the beginning of Ohio's COVID vaccine rollout in January 2021, as she tried to navigate the system for her parents, "Vaccine Queen" Stacey Bene realized that the entirely online registration system was not going to work for many of the senior citizens.

"I know that seniors have lived the past year with the same anxieties and often the same feelings of being unworthy during the pandemic," says Stacey. "They were desperate for the lifeline that the vaccine offered, but most could simply not access it. I knew I could help."

Stacey's story began in January 1978, when she was diagnosed with cystic fibrosis at the age of two at Akron Children's Hospital. She was hospitalized for several months for pneumonia that wouldn't resolve.

"My reaction to the diagnosis was total fear and sadness and some anger. To sit there and watch what her doctor was putting her through hurt me to the core," says her father, Daniel.

"We were told that she had cystic fibrosis, would maybe live until age fourteen and would require intense therapy and medication," says Stacey's mother, Patricia. "Her father and I were devastated, emotionally and spiritually; grief settled in immediately. We pledged to do everything the doctors told us to buy time for our lovely [little] girl."

After several months in the hospital, during which time many invasive tests were performed with no sedation while Daniel and Patricia listened to their child scream, they took Stacey home not knowing what to expect but having an extensive list of things to do for her survival. Once at home, the anger set in. "Anger that we did not know we carried this killer gene," says Patricia, "anger that it took so long to diagnose, and anger that all pre-diagnosis treatments were the opposite of what was needed for cystic fibrosis. Stacey's health seemed to improve once on the proper therapies and medications."

Stacey's childhood was filled with treatments, hospital stays, and medical appointments, along with what she refers to as the "normal" things, like sleepovers, dance classes, and shopping malls. "Growing up, I did nebulizer treatments, combined with therapy where my parents had to clap on different areas of my chest and back twice per day," says Stacey. "I followed up with doctors at least quarterly and in between when sick. My parents did about ninety minutes per day of actual physical labor to keep me well. As I aged, The Vest was developed to take the place of my parents' efforts. I remember how painful my mother's wrist became from the repetitive movements and only as an adult did I begin to appreciate how much she sacrificed for my health. I think my family helped growing up by just treating me like a normal kid. I did normal kid things. I just had to fit treatments into the mix."

"She was so strong playing and doing what we called her exercises [physiotherapy] twice a day without any complaining, no matter where we went," says Daniel. "Whether in a VIP room in the Honolulu airport or a hotel room in Washington, DC, she never complained."

"I knew I was different from my friends," says Stacey, "so only those closest to me really knew about my disease. I always felt conflicted about talking to others about CF. I really wanted to be like everybody else, but sometimes it was difficult to hide. I had a couple of very close friends I shared everything with and who actually learned how to do my treatments so I could go on school trips and to sleepovers."

Stacey made it through school with a few prolonged absences, saying she realized the severity of CF when she was about seven or eight years old when the made-for-TV movie *Alex: The Life of a Child* aired in the 1980s. "It was the first time I even became aware of what others with CF were experiencing and that there was often a tragic ending."

Living with the constant knowledge that people don't often live long lives with CF, Stacey dove right into life after high school, graduating from Cleveland State University with a bachelor of arts in social work in three years and obtaining her master of science in social administration from Case Western Reserve University in Cleveland, Ohio, in one.

"My dream was to help people cope with scary medical diagnoses similar to what my parents received when I was diagnosed," says Stacey. "I wanted to work with those affected by cystic fibrosis, but due to infection control, I knew that could not happen. I, instead, did an internship in the pediatric hematology and oncology unit at Rainbow Babies and Children's Hospital in Cleveland."

During the latter part of that internship, Stacey met a seventeen-year-old Japanese exchange student who had acute myeloid leukemia (AML). She says the student developed a flesh-eating bacterium in her arm that meant she needed to be transferred to the ICU. She did not have a great chance to survive, and the surgeon explained that she would likely lose an arm—which was made even more sad by the fact that she was a violinist. "This was a realization that even if she lived, [the student's] life would never be the same. I hugged [her family]—whose travel to the US I helped coordinate—for a long time. This expression was the only language we shared at the time."

The student lived and was even able to keep her arm, as the medical team was able to contain the infection. Before leaving, the family made hundreds of paper cranes and strung them around the Ronald McDonald House (an organization that helps reduce stress and financial burden for families who travel far for medical attention for their child) across from the hospital as a thank-you and a wish for health for all of the other children fighting illnesses.

"I was twenty-two years old, not even an official master's prepared social worker," says Stacey, "yet I think my empathy transcended the language barrier." Stacey says this story is why she wanted to work with blood cancer patients and would lead to her passion to help those who were in need of her support.

She worked as a medical social worker at the Cleveland Clinic in oncology and spent thirteen years helping blood cancer patients navigate their disease and all that it entailed at the Leukemia & Lymphoma Society. Her experience working with patients in serious need brought her attention back to herself, though Stacey admits that she was doing pretty well, as her CF had been well-managed and she had only been hospitalized once just prior to starting her career. "I felt like I had the energy to support others experiencing a health crisis during this time in my life. I think when I started my career working with cancer patients, I saw so many miracle cases and started to realize that maybe I could be one of those too."

In 2002, Stacey married Matthew, whom she knew in high school but didn't date until several years after. She gained a stepdaughter and then, with Matthew, had a daughter and son by the time she turned thirty. At the time she got married, her health was in good shape, and she tried her best to keep it that way. "I made sure to focus on doing treatments and exercising to keep my health as stable as possible," says Stacey. "I had a family I loved and that counted on me. It was more apparent that my health didn't only impact me anymore."

For years, Stacey's health remained strong despite the concern that those with cystic fibrosis experience more CF-related symptoms as they get older. "My CF didn't steadily decline as I aged," says Stacey. "I often had periods of years where I was 'well' and able to function like other healthy people my age. Every few years, I would have a health crisis that required attention—hospitalization, surgery, antibiotics—but then I was often able to get myself stable again. In my late thirties, though, cystic fibrosis started to catch up to me. It no longer became as easy to manage being a mom, being a full-time social worker, and being a CF patient."

In 2010, Stacey had been trying to manage a mycobacterium avium complex (MAC) infection that took hold in her lungs and still has not vacated. "I have been on IV antibiotics for months at a time," says Stacey, "I have endured bouts with blood clots, and I have tried compassionate-use treatments."

Stacey eventually came to a decision regarding her career. "I helped plan a large staff conference in a different state, all while trying to fight this nasty new lung infection. I was juggling work, business travel, CF, and my young kids. I was driving home from the airport after this intense conference and my body felt spent. Just breathing hurt. I cried in the car on the way home, knowing I wouldn't even have the time to recover when I returned home due to all of my obligations trying to be a working mother. It was during that drive home that I realized I couldn't do it anymore. I had to leave my career behind to survive." In 2012, Stacey retired from her career in medical social work.

Stacey has been on Kalydeco since 2014 but says it's difficult to tell if the CFTR modulator is making a difference because her MAC still affects her. "I switched over to Trikafta in December of 2019, but after nine months, the GI side effects became difficult to manage so I switched back to Kalydeco."

Stacey had a new mission with the start of the pandemic. "When

COVID made its appearance, I learned that not everyone in society valued my life enough to make changes to protect me," she says, "even enough to wear a simple mask to protect it. It was so upsetting to hear people say or see people post on social media that only the elderly and those with pre-existing conditions were going to die from COVID. The implication that was not so subtle from that statement is that those of us who were more vulnerable should just go away, and if we end up dying—well, we weren't contributing members of society anyway. Those thoughts were out in the open. I was angry, and by December of 2020, I fell into a deep depression. I was so sad to discover this lack of concern for the vulnerable. The introduction of a vaccine felt like a blessing. It was a way to move forward and feel safe again. I wanted and needed to unload the anxiety of the past year. I wanted to feel worthy again. I didn't want to be a month, a week, or even a day too late in grabbing that lifeline."

Ohio's vaccine rollout began in January with those eighty and older. Stacey says she was fortunate to get the vaccine at the end of January, receiving an extra "no waste" dose at the end of a night at a local pharmacy (Spectrum 1 News in Ohio televised her receiving her second dose). But while Stacey said that being vaccinated felt like "a year's worth of anxiety being washed away," she felt the need to help others to get the vaccine.

Thinking of the Japanese exchange student who was dealing with a language barrier and health issues, Stacey studied the registration process at several locations in northeast Ohio and started booking the elderly and medically fragile for appointments. "I took on the burden of fighting for the few precious appointments that became available," she says, "so that those who couldn't do it on their own had an advocate. I felt like I could be someone in their corner, showing them that I thought their life was worthy of being protected."

In mid-February 2021, Stacey learned from her mother, who saw a story on the local news, about a woman named Marla Zwinggi, who was doing the same in her Ohio town. Stacey reached out with a Facebook message, and the two connected right away. "I think we were meant to meet and were meant to be there for vulnerable people in northeast Ohio at that moment in time. We were both stay-at-home moms," says Stacey, "but our commitment to quickly try to get people vaccinated, knowing that their lives could depend upon our swift action, was profound."

Stacey and Marla joined forces and became the "Vaccine Queens," a named dubbed by Marla's husband. "I'm not sure we would have had the same impact without the catchy name," says Stacey.

Stacey and Marla worked hard on their new endeavor while still doing their best to keep things organized at home. "Both me and Marla had kids at home doing virtual school while we booked appointments," says Stacey. "I had teenagers and Marla had three young girls. Some days were filled with chaos, trying to manage the lives of our kids and our mission that we felt compelled to work toward. I was working on an eleven-year-old laptop and Marla worked at the kitchen table right next to her girls. One of the best things about our collaboration was that when one of us needed a break, the other took over the workload. We checked in often to make sure we felt like we were each managing at home."

The Vaccine Queens have since become a resource for thousands and the media (including the *Today Show*) have called on them multiple times to help share tips and strategies for finding vaccine appointments. "We work so well together and have been able to consistently help those who come to us in need," Stacey says of her and Marla's relationship. "I feel like she has the qualities I lack, and it has made us a great team. Marla is an absolute gem, and we are equally committed to a goal bigger than ourselves."

"In the short time we've known each other, Stacey has become one of my best friends," says Marla. "It is crazy that a deadly pandemic is what brought us together. Maybe it is fate. Through it all, Stacey is actually my hero. The fact that she battles cystic fibrosis and can still manage to volunteer her time for others twelve to fourteen hours a day for months is incredible. She is a remarkable individual who inspires me to keep going every single day! She is honest, kind-hearted, and trustworthy. That she could put thousands of others' needs before her own while battling CF makes her unlike anyone I have ever met before. My life is richer just by knowing her."

"The quarantine and distancing actually left me feeling okay physically during this time," says Stacey, "but I had fallen into a depression. After hearing so much from society that my life wasn't as worthy, by late 2020, I started believing it. My kids were growing up and I no longer had much to offer society. Then I started making appointments for those struggling and met Marla. Somehow, out of nothing, we built something meaningful. I am honored to hear Marla's thoughts and I echo them about her. She came into my life when I was struggling, and my life became richer after meeting her. It was so nice to meet someone else willing to do this hard work, just because it was the right thing to do."

By early April, Stacey and Marla had booked nearly 2,500 COVID-19 vaccine appointments for the elderly and medically fragile. "We run a Facebook page where we post tips and links to help thousands of others navigate the confusing and fragmented vaccination system in

Ohio," says Stacey. "We even worked on getting those confined to their homes, one of the most vulnerable groups among us, in-home vaccinations. We are doing this completely voluntarily, and I have been driven by my own experience with cystic fibrosis."

Stacey says that after her family, becoming a Vaccine Queen and making a difference for others has been her greatest accomplishment. "I believe in science, and I want people vaccinated so we can return to life as usual. I also know what it feels like when you are desperate for a lifesaving medication. I wanted to make that a reality for some of the most vulnerable among us. I feel like I was called to [do] this at this critical moment in time. I also feel honored to have been able to help so many in my community."

But while the grass roots anointment of the Vaccine Queens has been a blessing in terms of getting the word out about what they do and how they can help, what drives them are the actual folks in need. "One woman had just been diagnosed with breast cancer and needed to get the vaccine within a week, prior to starting chemo, or she would no longer be able to get vaccinated," says Stacey. "Supply was limited in Ohio at the time. I had her call me at midnight, when I knew they added new appointments at a local pharmacy. I was quick enough to grab her an appointment and I registered her over the phone. She was so relieved that she was in tears. Now she could focus on her cancer fight. I felt honored to be able to help."

In another case, an eighty-eight-year-old woman who searched for four weeks for a place to get vaccinated to no avail, was told by her daughter to call the Vaccine Queens. "We felt like Ghostbusters," says Stacey, who remembers they received an email from the elderly woman but when the Vaccine Queens sent her an email back regarding the vaccine, initially the message bounced back. Stacey and Marla only had her name but were somehow able to find her after a long search. They tracked a local business owner named Dave who was able to knock on the elderly woman's door and let her know that the Vaccine Queens were able to get her an appointment and she was able to get the vaccine the next day. The story was so incredible that it was covered by Fox 8 in Cleveland, Ohio.

Stacey says that she has remained active despite the pandemic. "I do an aerobics class three to four times per week that combines aerobic exercise and strength training. I also do a barre class once or twice a week that is entirely strength based. When COVID shut down the gyms, I started doing these classes online and I have grown comfortable with exercising at home."

Stacey also adheres to a consistent treatment routine. "I have The Vest, Flutter (a handheld device to help with clearance of mucus by exhaling), and Aerobika (a nebulizer), "however, I prefer a percussor [a handheld device which provides respiratory therapy similarly to postural drainage] to all of them. My exercise routine is also crucial to my treatment routine. I will also do hypertonic saline or Pulmozyme, mostly when experiencing an exacerbation."

"The hardest part was when we were told by [her doctor] that she would not make it past thirteen, and then past seventeen as she got older," says Daniel. "It just broke our hearts, but look at her now. Stacey is so strong, beautiful, and intelligent, and we are so blessed and so proud she is our Vaccine Queen!"

"I am so proud of the woman she has become," says Patricia. "We, then she, were very medically compliant, never denying the deadliness of CF. Stacey fought every day for her life, while she tried to live as normally as possible. I respect the great strength Stacey has shown. She is a fighter. She tried clinical trials, communicated with the CF community, and continued her treatment at Rainbow Babies and Children's Hospital and the Cleveland Clinic. What she has accomplished while maintaining her health is rather amazing. I know Stacey will never give up her fight! I love her."

Though being a Vaccine Queen currently occupies plenty of time, Stacey enjoys reading, exercising, and going to the theater, though she admits she hasn't been able to attend the theater in eighteen months. "I feel like if everyone cared about their communities, they should all be doing everything necessary to help get us out of this pandemic. I've tried to do the right thing to help others. It's frustrating when my outlets are being taken away because we can't all get on the same page." She also has a dream of traveling to Europe for the first time. "Once COVID-19 is completely under control."

In the meantime, Stacey and Marla's project continues to help others manage the pandemic anxiety and, ultimately, save lives.

"'Do all the good you can,'" says Stacey, quoting eighteenth-century English cleric John Wesley, "'by all the means you can. In all the ways you can. In all the places you can. At all the times you can. To all the people you can. As long as ever you can.'"

CHRIS MACLEOD

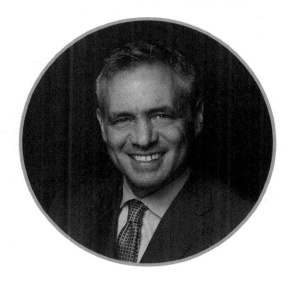

Age: 52
Resides: Toronto, Ontario, Canada
Age at Diagnosis: 2

FIGHTING FOR OTHERS: THE CF WARRIOR LAWYER

Born and raised in Saskatoon, and now residing in Toronto, lawyer and CF-patient advocate Chris MacLeod was diagnosed at the age of two when the life expectancy in Canada was around seven years.

"Chris was in [the] hospital and diagnosed with a heart condition," says his father, Rod MacLeod, "a ventricular septal defect and pulmonary stenosis when he was about two weeks old. Because of that condition, which was, in fact, managed with medication, we were advised that whenever he had a cold, he should be placed on antibiotics. That, probably, was protective, and masked the CF for a time. We were also encouraged by the doctor who looked after him then to have him live a normal life. Although the heart problem was stable, he did not thrive, despite a great appetite, and had other gastrointestinal symptoms as well, so we were concerned that there were problems apart from the heart problems. That led to further pediatric assessment."

Chris's mom, Joan Lidington, says she and Rod were going to give Chris the best life, regardless of the numbers of years he had. "When Chris was diagnosed . . . I was shocked as he had already gone through a heart diagnosis as a baby," she says. "However, there was also a sense of relief in learning the cause of symptoms he had been experiencing for some time (mainly not thriving in spite of a voracious appetite). The prognosis was not good, as children at that time were not expected to reach adulthood. I remembered the advice of the cardiologist when Chris was diagnosed with a heart defect—to allow him to have a normal life and not focus on the heart defect. His dad and I were determined that whatever time Chris had he would not be identified by his diagnosis but would have the best quality of life possible. This was not difficult as Chris always had high energy and embraced life. His enthusiasm for life and optimism were apparent as a young child."

"My family never dwelled on CF," says Chris, who has a brother, Paul, and a sister, Rachel, neither of whom has CF. "It was never discussed or dwelled on, other than to remind me to take my meds. The only questions asked were, 'What are you going to do with your life?' 'How will you deliver for your community? For your country?' No one in my family let their situation or their environment negatively impact them. I assumed that was the only option."

Rod says that he and his wife being medical professionals was both a blessing and a curse after Chris's diagnosis. "The diagnosis of CF was a scary one given the survival prospects at that time," says Rod. "As parents we were probably at a bit of an advantage since both Joan and I had medical training, so we were able to benefit from that awareness and understanding of the disease. It can be a bit of a mixed blessing as one is very aware of the challenges of the disease but, at the same time, it does help somewhat to understand it when making decisions. We were able to make some choices such as humidifying the house rather than using the mist tent—that was a common approach at the time and later was recognized to be a source of infection.

"[Chris] was always a very active child and so encouraging that activity made sense as part of the usual chest-physio approach. Both his mom and I wanted him to have a normal life with the activities and life that [any] child would have, while at the same time doing the things needed to manage the CF."

Chris did not talk about CF much growing up. He didn't discuss it with his friends unless he was asked about it. "I generally ignored it, often to my detriment," he says. Chris has had hospitalizations over the years, the worst admissions being in 1998 and in 2012 when severe infections brought him to the brink. In 2012, his lung function fell below 30 percent, resulting in his need to be on four liters of oxygen a minute.

Chris went to college at the University of Regina in the province of Saskatchewan, Canada, for a BA in political science and religious studies; law school at the University of Saskatchewan in Saskatoon, Saskatchewan, Canada; and later, McGill University in Montreal for graduate school at the Institute of Islamic Studies. Soon after, he obtained a law degree and established a boutique commercial litigation firm, now with thirty employees, in Toronto.

Chris's health was touch and go for a while. Chris says the Canadian government blocked Vertex Pharmaceuticals from delivering Kalydeco to him. "I was being released from the hospital because there was nothing more a hospital stay would do for me. I ultimately fought and secured access to Kalydeco, which was a game changer." Chris received the drug through compassionate access, and his lung function doubled, allowing him to go back to work. He has only had two hospitalizations since then. The experience was the impetus for the Cystic Fibrosis Treatment Society, which Chris founded to advocate for numerous patients when they have challenges with government, pharma, insurance companies, health charities, or hospitals.

Chris commenced the first-class action on behalf of CF patients against the government and its agencies. He also commenced the first constitutional challenge against the Canadian government. Chris says that he has fought for CF families hundreds of times to make sure they are treated fairly.

"I enjoy advocacy, in the courtroom and the board room," says Chris. "I started the CF Treatment Society because there was no organization that advocated for individuals with CF who needed assistance getting lifesaving meds. I had incredible help from so many individuals getting access to Kalydeco, so I wanted to help others." Chris also assisted in getting access to Trikafta, which he calls a "miracle medication," in Canada in September 2021; however, he admits that there are still limitations with the new approval.

"I was beyond thrilled with Trikafta finally getting public reimbursement," says Chris. Unfortunately, Chris is still unable to receive the "miracle" drug because patients with cystic fibrosis in Canada must have at least one copy of the DF508 gene to gain access to Trikafta, unlike in the United States. "I have a G551D and some other mutation" says Chris. "Sadly, I can't get on [Trikafta] in Canada, yet.

"While Kalydeco works for the G551D, I was blessed to be the first in Canada on that modulator and it saved my life," he says. "If you are on Kalydeco and have a DF508 then they move you to Trikafta because it is markedly better.

"There are 178 mutations, including the G551D, that Trikafta works well on. The FDA approved Trikafta for use on all 178 based on in vitro testing. Canada has not yet approved it for use in the 178 mutations. There are 150 of us that fall into this category in Canada. So, while I was the first on the first generation of gene modulators, I'll be in the final group fighting for access to the new modulator!

"I'm now referring to this final group as Club 150. The push is on, and I'll be advocating hard for myself and others. I believe we have a genetic-discrimination constitutional challenge."

While Chris waits for his opportunity to be approved for Trikafta, he has a relatively "normal" treatment plan for someone with CF. He takes inhaled antibiotics (Cayston) three times per day, Pulmozyme once per day, and intravenous antibiotics when necessary. He takes pancreatic enzymes with meals, does physiotherapy twice a day, and stays active by exercising at least twenty minutes per day, including jumping jacks, push-ups, planks, squats, and lifting weights. "I also try to walk fifteen thousand steps each day," he says.

Chris has just published a book called *Beating the Odds: 11 Lessons to Overcome a Health Crisis and Lead a More Resilient Life*, which he considers a manual for surviving any sort of health issue. "You control your response to whatever happens to you," he says. "Make your response bold and daring. Be the CEO of your own health."

"How he has kept strong and showed great perseverance as he has faced challenges in his life has been an inspiration to me," says Joan. "I am proud of him and his many achievements. He has used his experience and his skills to make life better for others. This is evident in his tireless efforts in advocacy for people with CF and the writing of his book to encourage others facing health crises. He is a remarkable person and an inspiration to his family and friends."

"I am very proud of him and admire him as a good person," says Rod. "He has met a lot of challenges and done so with courage and determination. And he has been generous and a strong advocate, not only for himself and others with CF in seeking access to vital medication but also in standing for others in various difficult situations, such as human rights and his pro bono services for immigrants and new Canadians."

"I've never doubted my ability to fight CF. Or anything, really," says Chris. "Everyone dies of something. I asked the question, *What would I do if I knew I could not fail?* I decided to do that, and CF became an afterthought."

12

THE 65TH WARRIOR

EVA LIPMAN

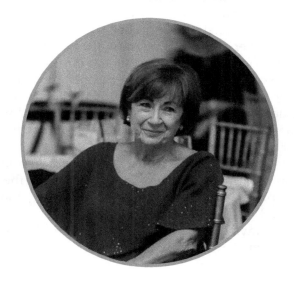

Age: 74
Resided: Atlanta, Georgia
Connection to CF: Mom to two CF warriors

A LOVING LEGACY: FIFTY YEARS OF BEING A CF MOM AND ADVOCATE

Eva Lipman, who passed away on November 18, 2020, was born Eva Elka Goldberg on September 1, 1946, in a displaced persons camp in Eshwege, Germany, shortly after the Holocaust and World War II ended. Both her parents Rose and Carl Goldberg survived despite losing several family members in the process (of the twenty thousand people who lived in Ludmir, Poland, fewer than one hundred survived).

Just prior to her third birthday, Eva and her parents came to the United States aboard the *USAT General C. C. Ballou*, which sailed from the port of Bremerhaven, Germany, on September 26, 1949, and, nine days later, arrived at New York Harbor. They were eventually sponsored by the Hebrew Immigrant Aid Society and placed in Jacksonville, Florida, where the family would learn a new language and start a new life in pursuit of the American dream.

As she grew up, Eva worked several jobs and became a second mother figure to her two younger sisters, Anita and Susie, who were both born in Jacksonville. She went on to attend the University of Florida where she became the first person in her family to attend and graduate a four-year university. While attending the University of Florida, Eva pledged the sorority, Delta Phi Epsilon (D Phi E). As a sister of the sorority, she collected donations on campus for D Phi E's national philanthropy—the Cystic Fibrosis Foundation. Family was always close to Eva's heart. Anita says that even when Eva left for college, she kept tabs on her younger siblings, even taking Anita to football games and giving her a taste of college life.

Eva graduated and became a teacher, moved to Atlanta right after her graduation, and met—and soon after, married—the love of her life, Charles Lipman, on June 8, 1969. A year later, the newlywed couple welcomed a daughter, Wendy Carol Lipman. Instead of enjoying their first days of parenthood, Charles and Eva soon noticed that their newborn daughter was not gaining weight. Wendy was diagnosed with cystic fibrosis—the same disease Eva raised money for several years earlier in college—and, sixteen days later, she was gone. She never left the hospital, was never assigned a Hebrew name (a common Jewish practice), and only one photograph was ever taken of her. Eva and Charles—neither of whom knew they were carriers of the cystic fibrosis gene, of course—were devastated.

Three years later, the couple tried again, hoping the 75-percent chance that their next child would not have cystic fibrosis would be in their favor. On September 4, 1973, right after their son, Andy, was born, he was taken into surgery because of meconium ileus. The intestinal blockage was a major symptom of cystic fibrosis and therefore Eva and Charles both knew the news they were about to receive. Later, through a positive sweat test, the diagnosis was confirmed.

At the time, Andy's life expectancy was only sixteen years. Still, Eva and Charles made a decision, as Andy grew up, to advise their family not to tell him how his sister died, in order to prevent him from being scared of the disease he and his sister shared. "Eva and I took the position that Andy was going to have a normal life—*not as normal as possible*, but *perfectly* normal," says Charles. "For that reason, we saw no reason to talk to him about cystic fibrosis, as it was not in sync with our goal that he have a fun and productive childhood. We always believed that Andy would be an exception to the numbers— they *are* just numbers—and that if we all had a positive attitude, things would go well."

Eva sacrificed her teaching career when Andy was born, due to having to take care of his medical needs. "Nothing was going to stop my mom from making sure I would live the life that her daughter was not afforded," says Andy. "Every day, Mom made sure I swallowed my enzymes so that I could absorb fats, slipped a nebulizer mask on my face to inhale my meds, and administered my postural drainage by cupping her hands and hitting my sides, back, and chest to loosen the mucus from my lungs. I regret that I told my teachers one day that Mom hit me every morning. Perhaps I could have phrased that differently. Mom had a good laugh out of it."

Though Eva was no longer working as a teacher, per se, she put her skills as a child advocate to good use. "She was the PTO president at my school, the substitute librarian, the chaperone for school trips, and the team mom for both my tennis and baseball teams," says Andy. "Mom also had the unenviable task of answering the 'Mount Everest' of questions I once asked her: *Am I going to die?* I don't remember exactly what she told me, but I know she summarized it as, 'Don't believe everything you read.' Regardless of her response, it would likely be too much for a child to absorb."

Andy eventually learned of his bleak prognosis when he read an encyclopedia article in grammar school. At one CF clinic appointment, Andy saw a poster of a weightlifter on the wall, and Eva, knowing he had already dealt with a difficult appointment in which he was coughing more than normal and hearing concern from his doctor, told Andy the person on the wall had cystic fibrosis and he could be just like him.

"Sure, she fibbed, but her white lie helped me maintain my sanity," says Andy. "I went on to become a workout junkie, and as a CF adult, my body was beginning to resemble that of the man from the poster to give hope to other young CF warriors." Andy also remembers his mom denying his doctor's plea to send him to CF camp to "learn what it is like to have CF." "She said she did not want me to compare myself to others with the disease just because I had it, but rather to live with a 'sky is the limit' mentality."

Andy says his mom made sure that he never felt left out. "I remember, around the age of eleven, going with several friends along with one of my friends' moms to Callaway Gardens about eighty miles from our home in Atlanta," says Andy. "Mom made the trip covertly and stayed in a villa nearby. She had me come over once a day so she could do my postural drainage (this was before The Vest). She made sure to shoo me out when I was done so I didn't look like a mama's boy, which I so obviously was. Mom chaperoned a school trip to Disney World to do the same. She noticed that I needed more separation, so she even taught my fourth-grade teacher, Ms. Powell, how to do my postural drainage for a trip to DC. Mom also taught my aunt Susie and, years later, my wife, Andrea, how to do my postural drainage. She was creating quite a team for me.

"Mom wasn't perfect. What mother is?" says Andy. "She was a bit overprotective as she was afraid to share any videos or fundraising documents that explained the disease because most of them were less concerned with how the patient viewed these materials and more worried how they could achieve better fundraising numbers from donors and sponsors. She also wrote my gym teacher countless excuses for me not to participate in running laps, so I did not have to watch as my peers lapped me because I didn't have the energy to run with them."

Andy says his parents did not reveal how Wendy died until his twenty-fifth birthday when he finally got the courage to ask. "I was calling Mom to read her a passage from my manuscript," says Andy, "which would later go on to be my first book, *Alive at 25: How I'm Beating Cystic Fibrosis*. I started talking about my sister in the passage and I asked Mom if it was okay to mention her. We rarely discussed her growing up. I suspected that was because it was a traumatic event for my parents. Turns out there was another reason. On that phone call, I got the nerve to finally ask the question I'd had decades to ponder but never had the nerve to ask: 'Mom, tell me how Wendy died. Was it CF?'

"I could hear the faint rustling of tissues in the background and could sense that Mom was crying. 'Yes, Andy,' she said, 'It was CF.'

"Mom would go on to tell me that she visited Wendy every year on her birthday and brought her a stuffed animal and flowers," says Andy. "She would also tell me that keeping Wendy's cause of death secret had less to do with Mom and Dad's fear of living in the past and more to do with how I would take the news.

"My parents asked my entire family not to tell me about how my sister died because they worried that I could not handle knowing the disease I would fight my entire life was the same one that killed my older sister. This was another way for them to protect me from knowing too much about the monster of a disease I inherited. The thing is that when Mom finally revealed the biggest secret kept from me during my lifetime, I wasn't upset with her or my father for not telling me when I was a child. I don't know how I would have handled it, but I know how I handled it as a twenty-five-year-old and that was using Wendy's loss as an incentive to raise money to benefit those with the disease, which is something else I learned from Mom."

In the late seventies, Eva cochaired the Santa Claus House at Perimeter Mall in Atlanta, which benefited the Cystic Fibrosis Foundation. Her job was to drive around Atlanta and ask anyone and everyone whether they would be willing to donate toys, crafts, and clothing. She claimed that all the driving actually helped her get to know her way around Atlanta better, though she'd already lived there a decade.

Eva was told by a friend that recording artist Isaac Hayes ran down West Paces Ferry quite often, so Eva had an idea and got to work. Two weeks before the event she drove down West Paces Ferry looking for Mr. Hayes and found a gentleman in a red shirt, red shorts, and a red bandana jogging, escorted by two big men she presumed to be his bodyguards. Eva pulled the car over beside the men and shouted, "Mr. Hayes!" He came over to the car window and she told him about Andy and the cause and asked if he could donate something.

"He was so nice and took down the information about the event, date, and set-up time and wrote down my name," said Eva. "He never really said whether he would help but I thanked him and told him how much that would mean to me and to everyone involved. I was nervous when I drove off but so proud that I made the decision to stop and at least try."

"The Friday morning before the event, two big men in trench coats entered and asked for my mom," says Andy. "She walked over and one of them said, 'Mrs. Lipman, Mr. Hayes would like you to have these items for your Santa Claus House and hopes you raise lots of money for cystic fibrosis.'" They gave her a few signed record albums and a framed photograph Mr. Hayes took (Mr. Hayes' hobby was photography) of the Cape of Good Hope in Africa, also signed by him. Eva kept it until she passed, and it still is framed in the house in which she lived.

Eva said she learned a lot from her chance meeting with Mr. Hayes. "It goes to show that taking a chance can bring unexpected rewards, and you never know how kind human beings can be," she said. "Had I decided not to stop and take the chance, I would have never gotten to meet the great man himself and would never have known if I could succeed or fail. My only thought at the time was to test myself and see if I could accomplish this and the worst that could happen is just getting a 'No.' Never give up on yourself, because you will be amazed at what you can achieve if you put your mind to it."

The Santa Claus House exceeded expectations that year and her example motivated Andy to start an event with his friends and family, which would later become a foundation called Wish for Wendy and which, in twenty years, has helped raise $4.5 million to benefit cystic fibrosis charities.

In the coming years, Eva and Charles became grandparents to Andy and Andrea's children, a granddaughter named Avery (now sixteen) and a grandson named Ethan (now fourteen). Eva also received volunteer awards for her hard work for the Cystic Fibrosis Foundation, which culminated in her and Charles being recipients of the 2019 Lifetime Achievement Award, honoring their half century of devotion to the goal of curing the disease. Eva also believed in giving back to a variety of charities and teaching her family the same.

Andy's sister Emily, whom Eva and Charles adopted in 1985, explains, "When it comes to giving back and being charitable, it is just what we do. Mom raised us to be that way. She took me as a young girl to a women's shelter and just being there and seeing life in a different way, we all need that. Sometimes, we get into our own little world or bubble and don't realize people around us are hurting. I enjoyed volunteering there with her, and to this day I still donate to that shelter."

As Andy grew up, Eva and Charles taught him to take responsibility for his treatments and meds and, as he became more independent, relegated themselves to the role of CF support system. Prior to Andy marrying Andrea in September 2002, Eva and Charles passed that torch on to their future daughter-in-law.

"I learned so much from Eva," says Andrea. "Not only how to do Andy's therapy but how to give back to everyone around you. She was the most generous person I have ever met. Not only with her resources but her time as well. She got so much joy giving back to others. She was not just my mother-in-law, but more importantly she was my friend."

On November 18, 2020, Eva's journey ended abruptly after a courageous battle with a rare but very aggressive form of stage IV lymphoma, which she was diagnosed just a couple of months earlier. "Her doctor confided that when she saw the initial diagnosis, she did not think my mom would last a week," says Andy. "Mom instead lived ten weeks because my mom was a warrior and that is just what warriors do."

Andy says in the months after her passing, he realized how much his mom meant to him, not only as a mother but as a CF caretaker. "I imagine that anyone who loses their mother would consider it a significant loss," he says, "but for someone with a chronic disease like cystic fibrosis, it is simply unique. CF moms are absolute champions for their children. My mom was certainly no different."

"[Eva] was a special person when I met her and even after she left us," says Charles. "She was beautiful, thoughtful, joyful, and caring. We were so lucky to have her in our lives. [She] was very knowledgeable but not sophisticated—one could say she was naïve. But that only added to her beauty and charm."

"She is and was the best human in all aspects," says Emily. "She always cared and thought about everyone before herself, especially her children."

In the months following Eva's passing, the family raised $150,000 between the Wish for Wendy Foundation and Cystic Fibrosis Foundation. They raised another $130,000 between the two charities the following year. In 2022, Emily was named LLS (Leukemia & Lymphoma Society) Woman of the Year by leading a team of family and friends called Team ForEva to raise just over $1,000,000 in Eva's memory to benefit the LLS to help inspire research that could one day lead to a cure for blood cancers like the one Eva so courageously fought.

"Mom was a superstar in the CF community," Andy says. "So many people knew her and loved her, which was only confirmed by the flooding of letters and donations from all over the country that we received after Mom's passing."

Andy's solace was that his mother would not have to bury a second child due to cystic fibrosis. "I was happy that she witnessed the birth of Trikafta, the medicine that would help me and tens of thousands of others to breathe easier with cystic fibrosis," says Andy. "My mom played a big role in the approval of that drug. Her nearly five decades of advocacy and fundraising have led to so many celebrations for the cystic fibrosis community. Still, I know that she would tell me that there is a small percentage of the CF population that is not helped by a CFTR modulator and one hundred percent of us are still without a cure. In her Lifetime Achievement Award speech, Mom said, 'We're not going to stop until that cure is found.' My family and I will make good on those words.

"Mom was my biggest fan, and I was hers," says Andy. "Her actions and her story inspired me. Mom not only taught me how to become a warrior, she showed me too."

ACKNOWLEDGMENTS

Thank you to the warriors who took time out of their lives to share their impactful story with me. My hope is that each of you feels the same sense of pride and accomplishment as I felt while bringing your remarkable stories to life. I marvel at your courage and dedication.

This book was written in memory of our sixty-fifth warrior and my incredible mother, Eva Lipman, who we lost to cancer in November 2020. My mom spent half a century making a difference for those in the cystic fibrosis community while setting a positive example to those who have the unenviable task of playing the role of parents to children, who, for many years, were limited by a dubious life expectancy—a life expectancy that has more than tripled since her only son was born. I know my mom would have been proud of every person in this book, particularly those moms and dads who played the role of both caretaker and parent—two jobs that she certainly excelled at.

We would love to hear your CF Warrior Story! Connect with us on Instagram @cfwarriorproject, on Twitter @CFWarriorProj, and use the tag #cfwarrior. For more information, please visit us at CFWarriorProject.org.

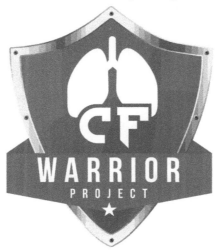

PHOTO CREDITS

Photo of Dr. Batsheva Kerem courtesy of Bruno Sharvit.

Photo of Dr. Eitan Kerem courtesy of Ilan Besor.

Photo of Amber Dawkins courtesy of Whitney Revelle Photography.

Photo of Ann T. Kates and Doris Tulcin courtesy of Ann T. Kates.

Photo of Anna Payne courtesy of Maureen Lingle.

Photo of Avery Flatford courtesy of Danny Parker.

Photo of Beth Vanstone courtesy of Madi Vanstone.

Photo of Amanda Varnes courtesy of Dina Varnes.

Photo of Alex Pangman courtesy of Lisa MacIntosh.

Photo of Dr. Bonnie Ramsey and Dr. Ann Dahlberg courtesy of Laura Taylor.

Photo of Breanna Schroeder courtesy of David F. Pu'u.

Photo of Brianna Collichio courtesy of Olivia Sherman.

Photo of Caroline Heffernan courtesy of Samantha Byrne.

Photo of Cassidy Evans courtesy of Memories by Mandy Photography.

Photo of Chelsea Spruance Stahl courtesy of Dan Mele Photography.

Photo of Larry Wayne "Chipper" Jones Jr. courtesy of B. B. Abbott.

Photo of Chris MacLeod courtesy of Giancarlo Pawelec | Pawelec Photo Inc.

Photo of Dr. Craig D. Reid courtesy of Silvia Reid.

Photo of Debra Mattson courtesy of www.weddingsmedia.com.

Photo of Dr. Francis S. Collins courtesy of the National Institutes of Health.

Photo of Dylan Mortimer courtesy of Jenae Weinbrenner.

Photo of Ella Balasa courtesy of Milken Institute.

Photo of Erinn Hoyt courtesy of Lee Gill Photography.

Photo of Ethan Payne courtesy of Cameron Packee Studios.

Photo of the Lipman Family courtesy of Styled and Snapped.

Photo of Eva Lipman courtesy of Charles Lipman.

Photo of Jacob Witten courtesy of Lisa Witten.

Photo of Parsons Family courtesy of Jaime Parsons.

Photo of Joshua Sonett courtesy of Cole Sonett.

Photo of Justin Baldoni and Claire Wineland courtesy of www.ishootamerica.com/Todd Westphal.

Photo of Katie O'Grady courtesy of Temi Bajulaiye.

Photo of Laura Bonnell Family courtesy of Mic Garofolo/Mic Clik Photography.

Photo of Lauren Luteran courtesy of Lilyana Ziemba.

Photo of Lewis Black courtesy of Joey L.

Photo of Liam Wilson courtesy of Deana Wilson.

Photo of Matt Barrett courtesy of Jess Barrett.

Photo of John Wineland, Claire Wineland, and Melissa Yeager courtesy of Avery Ward Photography.

Photo of Nicole Kohr courtesy of Open Aperture Photography.

Photo of Ross Craig courtesy of C. J. Shane.

Photo of Stacy Carmona, Micah Carmona, and Danny Carmona courtesy of Stacy Carmona.

Photo of Terry Wright courtesy of Michele Wright.

Photo of Travis Suit, LeeAnn Suit, Nikki Stellges, and Piper Suit courtesy of David Scarola.

Photo of Dr. Victor Roggli courtesy of Linda Roggli.

ABOUT THE AUTHOR

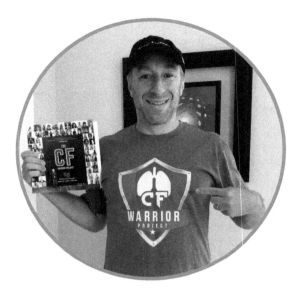

Andy C. Lipman was born and diagnosed with cystic fibrosis in 1973 and is the author of five books, all primarily focused on the disease. Additionally, Lipman is a motivational speaker who goes around the world and speaks on the importance of demonstrating a positive attitude, having a sense of humor, and staying physically fit to be successful in the battle against depression, anxiety, and CF. He is currently on the Georgia Chapter Board of the Cystic Fibrosis Foundation and a member of the National Corporate Engagement Committee Leadership Board for the Cystic Fibrosis Foundation.

In 2000, he, along with his friends and family, started Wish for Wendy, a co-ed charity softball tournament in Alpharetta, Georgia, in memory of his older sister who passed away from cystic fibrosis in 1970, three years prior to his birth. Wendy only lived sixteen days and therefore the two siblings never met. The event has raised more than $4.5 million to benefit the Cystic Fibrosis Foundation.

Lipman is a strong proponent for being compliant both with a regular exercise routine and a consistent daily medical regimen. The latter he learned from his parents, Charles and Eva Lipman, who rarely, if ever, missed a day of administrating his postural drainage therapy or forcing him to take his enzymes growing up. His daily routine includes working out with weights for thirty to forty minutes, running a 5K, doing two hours of CF treatments, and taking forty to fifty pills.

Lipman credits physical fitness, medical breakthroughs like CFTR modulator Trikafta, and a strong support system for helping him to live to the age of forty-nine, more than triple the number he and those born during that time period were expected to live.

While Lipman takes pleasure with his role in the world of cystic fibrosis, he is proudest of three things: his sixteen-year-old daughter, Avery, his fourteen-year-old son, Ethan, and his wife of twenty years, Andrea (he prefers not to mention her age due to the fact that he loves being married). He is also grateful for his parents, Charles and Eva, his sister Emily, and his many aunts, uncles, cousins, in-laws, and friends, who have all been so supportive of his many goals.

He spends his free time rooting for his Georgia Bulldogs and Atlanta Braves (who both won their first titles in decades while Andy was writing this book), coaching his children in whatever little league sport they desire to play, and counting his lucky stars that he married the woman of his dreams. Lipman credits Andrea for coming up with the idea that he should write a book about those people who have defied the odds and successfully strived despite this disease. He is excited that volume two will now show the amazing work of both those with the disease and those without it who do a lot of work to make a difference in the cystic fibrosis community.

Lipman's motto is, "Live your dreams and love your life." He believes that every single warrior in this book far and away has demonstrated those words.

THE
—— WISH FOR WENDY ——
FOUNDATION

Andy C. Lipman, along with his family and friends, created the Wish for Wendy Softball Challenge in October 2000 in memory of his older sister, Wendy Carol Lipman, who passed away from cystic fibrosis in 1971 after living only sixteen days.

Due to success of the tournament, Lipman and his family founded the Wish for Wendy Foundation in August of 2006, a nonprofit organization dedicated to increasing awareness about living with cystic fibrosis and supporting efforts to find a cure. Like the Wish for Wendy Softball Challenge, the foundation is in memory of Lipman's older sister, Wendy. In twenty-plus years, the Wish for Wendy Foundation and the softball tournament have raised more than $4.5 million to benefit cystic fibrosis charities.

Our wish for Wendy is that one day people with cystic fibrosis will no longer have to struggle with this disease.

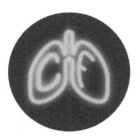

WISH FOR WENDY
FOUNDATION

CPSIA information can be obtained
at www.ICGtesting.com
Printed in the USA
BVHW061937240223
659177BV00006B/192

9 781665 304030